ECHTERNACH, John L.
(editor)

PAIN

CLINICS IN PHYSICAL THERAPY VOLUME 12

Vol. 11   Physical Therapy of the Shoulder
           Robert Donatelli, M.A., P.T., guest editor

Forthcoming Volumes in the Series

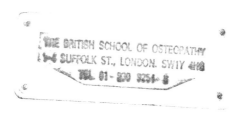
PAIN

Edited by

John L. Echternach, Ed.D., P.T.

Chairman and Professor
School of Community Health Professions
  and Physical Therapy
Director, Program in Physical Therapy
College of Health Sciences
Old Dominion University
Norfolk, Virginia

CHURCHILL LIVINGSTONE

NEW YORK, EDINBURGH, LONDON, MELBOURNE

1987

Library of Congress Cataloging-in-Publication Data

Pain.

   (Clinics in physical therapy; v. 12)
   Includes bibliographies and index.
   1. Pain—Treatment.   2. Physical therapy.
I. Echternach, John L.   II. Series.   [DNLM: 1. Pain.
W1 CL831CN v.12 / WL 704 P1442]
RB127.P3318   1987   616′.0472   86-28385
ISBN 0-443-08375-4

© **Churchill Livingstone Inc. 1987**

Distributed in the United Kingdom by Churchill Livingstone,
Robert Stevenson House, 1-3 Baxter's Place, Leith Walk, Edinburgh EH1 3AF, and by associated companies, branches, and
representatives throughout the world.

Accurate indications, adverse reactions, and dosage schedules
for drugs are provided in this book, but it is possible that they
may change. The reader is urged to review the package information data of the manufacturers of the medications mentioned.

Acquisitions Editor: *Kim Loretucci*
Copy Editor: *Miki Magome*
Production Supervisor: *Jocelyn Eckstein*

Printed in the United States of America

First published in 1987

Contributors

John L. Echternach, Ed.D., P.T.
Chairman and Professor, School of Community Health Professions and Physical Therapy; Director, Program in Physical Therapy, College of Health Sciences, Old Dominion University, Norfolk, Virginia

Jerry N. Fogel, M.S., P.T.
Director, Human Performance Service, Washington Pain and Rehabilitation Center, Washington, DC; Vice-President, Orthopaedic Section, American Physical Therapy Association, Winter Park, Florida

Yoon S. Hahn, M.D.
Assistant Professor of Surgery/Neurosurgery, Northwestern University Medical School; Assistant Head, Division of Pediatric Neurosurgery, Children's Memorial Hospital, Chicago, Illinois

Julie A. Hannan, P.T.
Physical Therapy Supervisor, Children's Memorial Hospital, Chicago, Illinois

Gary C. Hunt, M.A., P.T.
Health and Fitness Consultant, Division of Federal Employee Occupational Health, US Public Health Service/DHHS, Region VI, Dallas, Texas

John V. Lavigne, Ph.D.
Associate Professor of Clinical Psychiatry and Pediatrics, Northwestern University Medical School; Chief Psychologist, Department of Child Psychiatry, Children's Memorial Hospital, Chicago, Illinois

Sandra J. Levi, M.S.
Associate Professor, Program in Physical Therapy, College of Health Sciences, Old Dominion University, Norfolk, Virginia

George C. Maihafer, M.S.
Assistant Professor, Program in Physical Therapy, College of Health Sciences, Old Dominion University, Norfolk, Virginia

Jeffrey S. Mannheimer, M.A., P.T.
Clinical Assistant Professor, Department of Orthopedic Surgery and Rehabilitation Program in Physical Therapy, Hahnemann University, Philadelphia, Pennsylvania; President, Delaware Valley Physical Therapy Associates, Lawrenceville, New Jersey

Joseph McCulloch, Ph.D., P.T.
Associate Professor and Head, Department of Physical Therapy, School of Allied Health Professions, Louisiana State University Medical Center, Shreveport, Louisiana

Michael F. Nolan, Ph.D., R.P.T.
Associate Professor of Anatomy and Neurology, Department of Anatomy, University of South Florida College of Medicine, Tampa, Florida

Andrew Novick, P.T.
Deputy Chief, Physical Therapy Service, Biomechanics Lab Affairs, Department of Rehabilitation Medicine, Clinical Center, National Institutes of Health, Bethesda, Maryland

Michael J. Schulein, Ph.D.
Assistant Director, Acute Unit, North Dakota State Hospital, Jamestown, North Dakota

L. Alan Stone, M.A., P.T.
Administrator, Rehabilitation Services, St. John's Regional Health Center, Springfield, Missouri

Ian Wickramasekera, Ph.D.
Professor of Psychiatry and Behavioral Sciences and Director of the Behavioral Medicine Clinic and Stress Disorders Research Laboratory, Eastern Virginia Medical School, Norfolk, Virginia

Preface

An examination of the recent literature on pain shows an enormous amount of activity resulting in a plethora of published material. The purpose of this book is to gather in one source the information essential to the physical therapist dealing with pain problems. It has been my experience that members of the profession have collected bits and pieces of data on pain, but that, given the state of our current literature, it is extremely difficult to find information readily on specific types of pain patients.

The first chapter provides the background to the neurosciences, presenting the complexity and the relevance of our current knowledge of pain, anatomically and physiologically. Chapter 2 presents different methods of pain measurement in the clinical environment. Most physical therapists are familiar with these methods but few have examined the literature in which they were originally proposed, and others have learned about the methods secondhand from fellow physical therapists who practice them. The chapters on the neuromuscular and musculoskeletal systems, the low back, and the foot deal with the practical aspects of pain, which are familiar to physical therapists who confront pain patients on a daily basis.

The chapter examining traditional physical therapy approaches to pain reminds us that much of our efforts have been directed at reducing or relieving pain. We often see special pain problems that do not correspond with our understanding of traditional pain symptoms and management. In the chapters on TENS and on biofeedback and behavior modification, the authors explore these new approaches to pain problems that have not responded to typical management. Finally, the chapter on the young pain patient was one I felt was particularly needed. Although many physical therapists manage children with pain problems daily, the literature is noticeably lacking in this area.

In sum, I hope readers will find this book brings them ever closer to the answers to pain management and that it encourages them to explore further their areas of interest in pain, both within these pages and in the referenced material.

I would like to thank Kim Loretucci and the staff of Churchill Livingstone for their patience with the chapter authors and especially for their help and kindness toward the editor of this book.

John L. Echternach, Ed.D., P.T.

Contents

1 Anatomic and Physiologic Organization of Neural Structures Involved in Pain Transmission, Modulation and Perception

Michael F. Nolan

The perceptions commonly associated with the word *pain* are almost universally known to mankind. With rare exceptions every individual has had experiences that have been characterized as painful. Yet, despite the fact that pain has been studied by philosophers and scientists for thousands of years, we still know remarkably little of its nature. The causes of pain are many and varied, and are reflected in the increasing number of strategies, techniques, elixirs, programs, and methodologies which have been proposed to effect its reduction or elimination. The collective group of experiences known as pain are so numerous and individual that an accurate and encompassing definition of pain is difficult to formulate. What exists instead are words and ideas which describe individual experiences of pain and a few optimistic, though somewhat unsatisfactory, attempts at definition. These difficulties are not unexpected, however, in view of our limited understanding of the phenomenon of pain.

The fact that pain is a personal experience composed of both physical and psychological elements contributes directly to the peculiar problems encountered in its study. From a purely descriptive point of view, pain in its mild forms may be nothing more than a nuisance or a distraction. In its more severe manifestations it commands undivided and relentless attention and demands immediate and effective resolution. In these latter forms, it may be overpowering and uncompromising in its dictates.

There are other aspects of pain which are now well recognized and which guide our efforts toward further understanding. Pain of an acute nature appears to be beneficial to mankind in the sense that it serves to call attention to a real or perceived threat to health or safety. Much is known about acute pain, and in many cases, its causes can be precisely determined and effective therapeutic intervention can be utilized. Chronic pain, by contrast, is not as well understood and often develops as a consequence of unsuccessfully managed acute pain. In this regard, chronic pain may mandate a continued search for the causative factors. This too may be beneficial to the individual if it results in the eventual identification of its cause and successful treatment. However, in many instances chronic pain may be associated with genuine physiologic disorders that have evaded diagnosis, or with disease conditions such as some types of cancers which, although well recognized and easily diagnosed, are not successfully treated by currently available methods. Many pain researchers and therapists now recognize that though acute pain is frequently a symptom of underlying disease, chronic pain is a disease of its own. It is toward an understanding of the nature of chronic pain that efforts of basic science and clinical researchers need to be focused.

Unfortunately, most of what is reliably known has resulted from studies of acute pain. Furthermore, much of this work has utilized animal models. These studies have examined to the limits of technology and ethics, neuroanatomic, neurophysiologic, and behavioral components of pain. While some might argue that these studies assess merely physiologic responses to the application of noxious stimuli and not the perception of pain itself, it is undeniable that some very effective treatment techniques for man have been developed as a result of carefully designed and executed studies on animal subjects. Thus, although differences do exist in the structure, organization, and, presumably, function of different parts of the nervous system in humans and animals, striking similarities also have been found. Considering the clinical benefits that have already been derived from previous studies of the biologic basis of pain, it would appear that future inquiry in this area has the potential to significantly enhance our knowledge of pain and to directly contribute to the development of more effective treatment techniques. The following review of what is known about the neuroanatomic and neurophysiologic substrates of pain informs the reader of what has been attempted and achieved in this area in the past, and what currently serves as the basis for research efforts and clinical treatments aimed at the reduction or elimination of needless, debilitating pain.

PAIN THEORIES

For more than a century, theories concerning the mechanisms of pain transmission and perception have been proposed and subjected to experimental test. The results of these investigations have invalidated certain ideas and generated other hypotheses to take their place. Many theories have been proposed over the years, each of which has its own following of proponents and critics. Most theories of pain contain certain elements that have been supported by subsequent study as well as others which have not survived scientific scrutiny. Three particular theories are worth highlighting, not only because parts of them have survived, but because they have also stimulated critical thinking and research into the precise mechanisms of pain perception and reactions.

Intensive Theory

Perhaps the earliest view of pain resulted from common, everyday empirical observation. These observations led to the informal formulation of an intensive theory of pain. According to this theory no specific receptors, pathways, or neuronal pools were necessary for pain perception. Rather, pain resulted from excessive activity in neuronal systems normally involved in the processing of a nonpainful stimuli. The basis of this theory was the notion that any stimulus, if intense enough, could cause pain. Summation of the impulses originating from the excessive stimulus could occur either in the skin or more centrally along the pathway to the cerebrum. A more formal presentation of this pattern theory was offered by Goldscheider.[1] Subsequent reports have supported the idea of summation of impulses in both the periphery and central nervous system.[2-5]

Specificity Theory

Near the end of the 19th century the specificity theory emerged out of the doctrine of specific nerve energies proposed by Müller.[6] According to Müller, each of the five major sensations (taste, smell, hearing, vision, and touch) was conveyed via its own system of nerves to specific areas of the brain. This idea was used by von Frey who subdivided cutaneous sensation into four components: touch, heat, cold, and pain.[7] von Frey concluded that free nerve endings were the receptors for pain while the other histologically identifiable receptors, such as the Krause end bulb, Ruffini end organ, and Meissner corpuscle, were functionally and anatomically related to the other skin senses. Further extensions of this work have resulted in the search for pain fibers in peripheral nerves and pain pathways and centers within the central nervous system.

Gate Control Theory

The final theory called the gate control theory[8] takes into account many of the more recent anatomic and physiologic observations. The gate theory is closely aligned with and may be considered to be a more up to date version of the pattern theory. A key feature of this theory is the idea that a physiologic gating mechanism (located in the spinal dorsal horn and in the caudal trigeminal complex) exists, which either allows or prohibits impulses entering the central nervous system by way of peripheral nerves from being transmitted to higher centers concerned with determining the quality of the perception. The proposed gate consists of small internuncial neurons located within the substantia gelatinosa and a transmission cell (T cell) for relay of the information to more rostral levels. (Fig. 1-1) Whether or not the T cell is activated is determined by a balance between the input of large diameter (A beta) and small diameter (A delta and C) afferent fibers acting directly and through the internucial neuron. The gating mechanism can also be influenced by descending influences from a

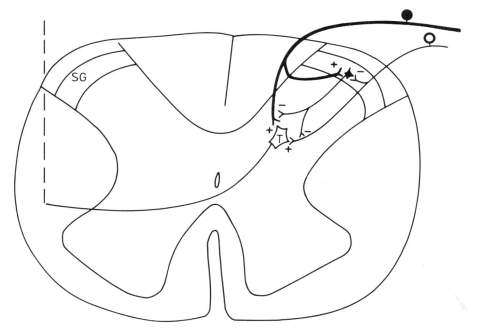

Fig. 1-1. Schematic representation of spinal structures involved in the gate control theory of pain transmission. Afferent input via both large and small diameter fibers is theorized to influence the transmission cell (T) directly and through small internuncial neurons located within the substantia gelatinosa (SG).

central control system. The theory postulates that small fiber afferent activity would stimulate the T cell resulting ultimately in the perception of pain. A collateral branch of the small afferent fiber is thought to inhibit the internuncial neuron in the substantia gelatinosa, which would reduce its presynaptic inhibitory effect on the T cell. The effect of this disinhibition would be to further enhance T cell firing by small fiber input. Large diameter afferents influence the gating mechanism somewhat differently. While large diameter fiber input activates the T cell, it also stimulates the substantia gelatinosa cell. Since the influence of the substantia gelatinosa cell is thought to be inhibitory, increased activity in this cell would counteract the direct facilitory effect of the large diameter fiber, thus closing the gate and disallowing conduction in the T cell. The gate theory was particularly attractive when first proposed; and anatomic studies have, in general, supported the gate theory by demonstrating the proposed neuronal components. However, physiologic support has been less persuasive. Furthermore, the nuclear structures and pathways that constitute the central control mechanisms were not fully understood at the time, and their influence on pain perception was left largely to speculation. History and the literature now show that descending influences are of significant importance in the transmission of pain impulses to higher centers. Nonetheless the gate theory represents a major advance in the understanding of pain mechanisms, and like all theories, has its proponents and opponents.[9-15]

Interpretation of Pain

In considering the neural basis of pain, it is important to keep in mind that the experience of pain represents an individual's interpretation of the intensity of a particular stimulus, as well as an assessment of whether or not it constitutes a significant threat to well being. These judgments are made at the level of the forebrain. Therefore, strictly speaking, cutaneous and visceral receptors, peripheral nerve fibers, and central nervous system pathways constitute a transmission system which functions in the modulation and conduction of impulses to higher levels. In this regard, pain per se is neither transduced nor conducted. A more appropriate and accurate description would emphasize the idea that receptors and pathways are concerned with relaying impulses originating from the application of noxious stimuli. This distinction is important, since it is well known that a particular stimulus may or may not be perceived as painful depending on a number of highly variable factors. These factors can be physical, psychological, or emotional in nature, and singly or in combination may significantly influence perception of a stimulus. Those stimuli which in man usually result in the perception of pain are thus appropriately referred to as noxious stimuli. The distinction between noxious and non-noxious stimuli is generally that the former either result in some degree of tissue damage, or at least, present a real potential for tissue damage, while the latter do not. For many types of stimuli this is a matter of intensity or degree, and this fact represents one of the difficulties faced by pain researchers.

PERIPHERAL SUBSTRATES

Peripheral nerves are made up of individual nerve fibers classified according to conduction velocity. Large diameter axons tend to be more thickly myelinated and conduct impulses rapidly, whereas the smaller fibers possess relatively thin myelin sheaths and conduct impulses more slowly. Those fibers that are merely enveloped by the Schwann cell are the slowest conducting of the spectrum of peripheral nerve fibers, and are referred to as the *nonmyelinated group* (Table 1-1).

The transmission of noxious stimuli in peripheral nerves is known to be associated with slowly conducting afferent nerve fibers.[16-19] Thinly myelinated (A-delta) and unmyelinated (C) afferents have been specifically identified as being important in the conduction of noxious stimuli.[20-24] It would be incorrect, however, to assume that these two afferent fiber types represent the only sources of input to ascending spinal and trigeminal projection cells. According to the gate control theory, for example, large diameter (A-beta) afferent fibers also influence the output of the second order projection cell. In addition, it is now well known that brain stem nuclei can effect discharge in *pain pathway* neurons. Thus, while A-delta and C fibers may be involved with the centripetal transmission of impulses originating from the application of noxious stimuli, other neuronal populations are known to modulate the perceptual responses to a given stimulus.

Technologic advances in neurophysiology have permitted a greater understanding of afferent mechanisms involved in pain transmission. These methods have brought about a refinement of the simple notion that small diameter fibers are involved in a major way, while larger fibers are minimally involved. Using careful dissection and single unit recording techniques, it has been possible to selectively stimulate and examine individual nerve fibers in peripheral cutaneous and muscle nerves. Selective stimulation of A-delta fibers produces a sharp, pricking sensation, whereas C-fiber activation is associated with a dull, diffuse, more deeply perceived burning type sensation.[16,18,25-29] In experiments in which A-delta and C fibers were blocked, activation of the more heavily myelinated A-beta fibers produced not pain, but rather a sensation of light pressure or tickling.[16,26,30] Furthermore, cutaneous stimulation which resulted in the sensation of light touch or vibration has been shown to travel in the more rapidly conducting fibers in peripheral nerves.[31-33]

However, this reasonably dichotomous view of pain transmission in pe-

Table 1-1. Afferent Fiber Types in Peripheral Nerves

Class	Type	Group	Diameter (μm)	Conduction Velocity (m/sec)
A	Alpha (I)	IA	12–20	70–120
		IB		
	Beta (II)		6–12	30–70
	Delta (III)		1–6	6–30
C	(IV)		0.4–1.2	0.5–2.0

ripheral nerves has been challenged by the results of several recent studies. Burgess and Perl found thinly myelinated fibers (A-delta) that were activated by non-noxious cutaneous stimuli.[34] Similar results have been reported by other investigators.[20,30,35,36] Impulses from the application of nonpainful stimuli were also found to be transmitted in unmyelinated C-type fibers.[21,22,37–40] Conversely, Willer and his coworkers reported that in man, stimulation of lower limb cutaneous nerves at intensities sufficient to activate only large diameter afferents resulted in the sensation of pricking pain.[41] Collectively, these observations weaken the specificity theory and complicate attempts to understand pain mechanisms.

Other avenues of inquiry, particularly in the area of receptors and receptor mechanisms, have provided valuable information and represent a major step forward in pain research. With the discovery that thinly myelinated and non-myelinated fibers could be activated by noxious and non-noxious stimuli, interest in identifying specific pain receptors was rekindled. If, as the data suggest, there were thin fibers that were activated by non-noxious stimuli, and others that transmitted impulses from noxious stimuli, and still others that responded to both types of stimuli, then perhaps there are several subcategories of A-delta and C fibers, each associated with a particular type of receptor. Early studies by Burgess and Perl[34] and Bessou and Perl[22] indicated that approximately 15 percent of A-delta fibers and almost 50 percent of C fibers were activated by noxious stimuli. The remaining A-delta and C fibers conducted impulses in response to non-noxious stimulation.

Receptors in the skin are responsive to a variety of stimuli (e.g., light touch, vibration, mechanical, and thermal). However, attempts to associate a specific receptor with a particular type of sensation have been largely unsuccessful. Technical problems are greater when studying fibers which respond to different types of noxious stimuli, as well as fibers that are activated by both noxious and non-noxious stimuli. A more successful approach involves examining activity in individual afferent units composed of both a peripheral nerve fiber and its associated receptors.

Afferent units from the skin can be classified in several different ways. If one considers threshold at which a unit is activated as a distinguishing criterion, individual sensory units may be classified as high or low threshold units. However, some units demonstrate a graded response to a particular stimulus and are thus difficult to clearly identify using this method. Nociceptive units are usually considered to be those with high thresholds to stimulation. An alternative approach considers the type of stimulus which activates a particular sensory unit.[42] Using this method, receptive units have been classified as mechanoreceptive and thermoreceptive. Those neurons which are activated by both mechanical and thermal stimuli are referred to as *polymodal receptive units*.

Current explanations concerning the peripheral mechanisms of pain transmission reflect an attempt to integrate these two approaches. Certain elements of both pattern and specificity theories have been supported by recent experiments and incorporated into contemporary thinking. Mechanical stimuli applied to the skin can cause pain reactions in humans and result in nocifensive responses in animals.[20,22,24] In the cat and monkey, intense mechanical stimuli has been shown to activate thinly myelinated A-delta fibers with high threshold receptors.[20,34,42] In most instances, responses were observed only when the stimulus was strong enough to produce tissue damage. Mechanoreceptive units consisting of A-delta fibers with low threshold receptors have also been identified.[36] These units discharge with high level activity in response to noxious stimulation, but unlike the high threshold mechanoreceptive units, they are also responsive to innocuous levels of stimulation. Both types of thinly myelinated units appear to play a role in pain transmission.

Mechanoreceptors are also associated with nonmyelinated (C type) primary afferent fibers. A small number of these units have high thresholds to cutaneous stimuli and may be involved along with high threshold A-delta mechanoreceptors in pain perception.[22] More commonly, C-fiber mechanoreceptive afferents demonstrate a low threshold to cutaneous stimuli, and at these low stimulation intensities are not thought to participate in pain transmission.[21,42]

Thermoreceptive units sensitive to both noxious and non-noxious temperatures are common in experimental animals and humans. Most units respond in a graded fashion to increasing or decreasing temperatures, and only a few have been found with high threshold receptors that discharge exclusively at noxious thermal levels.[38,43] Within the category of thermoreceptive units two distinct populations have been identified: cold and heat sensitive units.[44,45] A particularly interesting group of cold thermoreceptive afferents has been shown to discharge in response to sustained increases in temperature that would otherwise activate noxious heat receptors.[46] Transmission of cold stimuli occurs via thermoreceptive units associated with thinly myelinated A-delta fibers. Heat thermoreceptive units conduct impulses at both A-delta and C-fiber conduction velocities.[47–50] Like cold thermoreceptors, heat responsive units discharge in a graded way, increasing their firing with incremental increases in skin temperatures.[50–52]

Cutaneous sensory units that are responsive to both mechanical and thermal stimuli at noxious levels have been identified in the cat and monkey.[43,53] A number of these polymodal nociceptive units are associated with thinly myelinated A-delta fibers. These units appear to function in the transmission of first or pricking pain commonly associated with noxious heat stimulation.[36,42,49,54] A functionally more important group of polymodal nociceptive afferent units transmit along unmyelinated C fibers.[22,42,43] Their importance stems in part from the fact that approximately 80 to 90 percent of C-fiber nociceptors are of the polymodal type.[23,36] C-fiber polymodal nociceptive units have frequently been identified in studies in human subjects.[19,27,55] In studies in which the myelinated fiber populations have been blocked, leaving intact C-fiber nociceptive units, only a burning or second pain sensation has been perceived. However, polymodal nociceptors are not activated exclusively by painful stimuli. Van Hees and Gybels have shown that nonpainful sensations are also reported following cutaneous activation of C-fiber polymodal units.[56] In fact, recent data suggest that C-fiber polymodal nociceptors are involved in pain threshold and tolerance determination.[57] Finally, it is well known that mild heat injury of the skin results in a sensitization to further cutaneous stimulation.[58-61] Sensitized receptor units are more easily activated by a given stimulus than would otherwise be the case in uninjured skin. Recent studies have shown that heat sensitized units are of the C-fiber polymodal nociceptor type.[62-65]

Receptors in visceral structures are known to exist throughout the body.[66,67] Most visceral receptors are sensitive to a variety of mechanical or chemical stimuli. In the main, impulses transmitted along visceral afferent fibers are relayed to nuclei within the brain stem and spinal cord which function in the reflex control of those visceral structures.[68,69] Information relayed in visceral afferents is generally continuous in nature and frequently does not reach levels of conscious awareness. Impulses that do reach neural levels concerned with perception are usually interpreted in typical ways such as fullness of the bladder or bowel. However, frank pain from visceral structures such as that associated with biliary obstruction, passing kidney stones, severe muscle cramps, pulmonary occlusion, gastrointestinal inflammation, and myocardial infarction is well recognized.[70-73] Several authors have indicated that mechanoreceptors in visceral organs that transmit impulses in response to noxious stimuli are associated with C-type peripheral afferent fibers.[66,67]

The picture of peripheral pain mechanisms which has thus far emerged appears rather complicated. Thinly myelinated and unmyelinated fibers transmit impulses from both noxious and innocuous stimuli. Afferent units associated with high threshold receptors are activated by stimuli that are clearly noxious and tend not to respond to low level stimuli. Low threshold sensory units appear to respond to both nonpainful and painful stimuli and seem to be able to react to tissue threatening, as well as tissue damaging, stimuli. Physiologic overlap of these units suggests functional overlap in peripheral mechanisms, and further suggests that the ability to distinguish painful from nonpainful stimuli must occur at more centrally located points within the nervous system.

AFFERENT ORGANIZATION

Neuronal cell bodies concerned with the transmission of impulses to the central nervous system are located in dorsal root ganglia and selected cranial nerve ganglia. At spinal levels, afferent cells contribute axons which reach the cord by traveling through segmentally organized dorsal roots. As the root approaches the pial surface of the cord it divides into a number of smaller rootlets which enter the cord at the region of the dorsolateral sulcus. Microscopic examination of dorsal roots reveals a wide variety of fibers ranging from thickly myelinated A-alpha fibers to unmyelinated C fibers. The fact that afferent fibers enter the cord via the dorsal root suggested that surgical interruption of specific dorsal roots might be helpful in treating patients with severe or intractable pain conditions.[74-76] However, the results of this procedure have been inconsistent, with some patients obtaining relief and some obtaining only a temporary reduction in pain, while others had a recurrence of their pain, occasionally with much greater intensity.[76-78] Coggeshall et al have recently suggested that unmyelinated afferent fibers in the ventral roots might account for pain which persists or is increased following dorsal rhizotomy.[79]

The notion that the ventral roots contain unmyelinated afferent fibers is not new. Several reports published before 1935 suggest that sensory fibers course through the ventral roots.[80-82] Recent studies have confirmed the existence of ventral root afferent fibers using a variety of techniques.[83-89] Hosobuchi[90] and Coggeshall et al[79] have suggested that up to 27 percent of the fibers in human ventral roots are unmyelinated, and that the majority of these are probably sensory and transmit pain. More specifically, Coggeshall et al found that of the unmyelinated fibers in the ventral root half were sensory and half were preganglionic autonomic neurons.[85] Studies of the receptive fields of ventral root afferent fibers indicate that approximately one third are associated with high threshold receptors in the body wall (possibly nociceptors), with the remaining two thirds being distributed to visceral structures.[84]

Despite the fact that some afferent fibers enter the cord via the ventral root, the majority of myelinated and unmyelinated peripheral nerve fibers carrying noxious information utilize the dorsal root. Within the dorsal root, large and small diameter fibers are intermixed within individual nerve fascicles. However, as the fibers approach the dorsal root entry zone, a segregation occurs such that the large diameter, more heavily myelinated fibers tend to assume a dorsomedial position, while the thinly myelinated and unmyelinated fibers are shifted ventrolaterally in the rootlet.[91-94] Within the spinal cord, the majority of these incoming fibers terminate ipsilaterally. However, axon terminals in the contralateral gray matter have been reported.[93,95-98]

Large diameter fibers enter the cord medial to Lissauer's tract and bifurcate into ascending and descending branches before they terminate. According to Carpenter et al[99] and Glees and Soler,[100] approximately 20 percent of the ascending fibers terminate in the nuclei of the dorsal columns. The remaining large diameter peripheral afferents course ventrally along the medial edge of the dorsal horn toward the central canal. Near the base of the dorsal funiculus they curve laterally, enter the gray matter, and extend dorsally to terminate in various laminae of the dorsal horn.[93,101,102] Although most of these fibers are associated with low threshold sensory units, there are reports of nociceptive responses following their activation.[103,104]

The lateral division of the dorsal root, which contains thinly myelinated A delta and unmyelinated C fibers, is thought to play a major role in the transmission of noxious stimuli. These afferent fibers enter the spinal cord and occupy the medial portion of Lissauer's tract.[105,106] Upon entering Lissauer's tract the axons bifurcate into ascending and descending branches, each of which may travel for one to two segments before terminating the dorsal horn.[107,108]

The position of peripheral afferent fibers in Lissauer's tract has been examined experimentally by several investigators. Following dorsal root transection, degenerative responses were observed ipsilaterally in the medial part of

Lissauer's tract, while the more laterally located fibers were unaffected.[107,108] These observations are in contrast to the more recent findings of Chung and co-workers who, following dorsal rhizotomy, found degenerating fibers throughout Lissauer's tract.[109,110] Earle has indicated that in the cat, fibers in the lateral part of the tract constitute approximately 75 percent of the total population in this bundle and arise from intrinsic neurons of the cord. The origin of these intrinsic fibers was thought to be the adjacent substantia gelatinosa.[111] More recent evidence in the monkey suggests that up to 80 percent of the fibers in Lissauer's tract arise from ipsilateral peripheral nerves, leaving only 20 percent to be of propriospinal origin.[112] Reported differences in the population of primary afferents and intrinsic fibers in Lissauer's tract may be attributable to variation between species, or to relative afferent input in the segments examined. For example, peripheral afferent fibers entering at the C8 segment are quantitatively more numerous than those entering at the T7 level. Results presented as percentages might easily be biased by this fact. According to Szentagothai, intrinsic fibers running in the lateral part of Lissauer's tract may extend through as many as five or six neural segments.[106] From a functional point of view, fibers in the medial part of Lissauer's tract have been reported to transmit excitatory impulses, while intrinsic axons occupying the lateral part of this tract appear to convey inhibitory influences from nearby segments.[113] Surgical exploitation of this observation has been considered to be of value in the management of selected pain patients and has, in fact, been attempted with some success.[114]

SPINAL ORGANIZATION

Primary afferent neurons involved in the transmission of nociceptive impulses make synaptic contact with neurons in the spinal gray matter and the nucleus caudalis of the spinal trigeminal complex. Most of what is known about the mode of termination of these afferents and their physiologic interaction with second order neurons is derived from studies in the spinal cord. More recently, however, pain mechanisms involving cranial nerves have been studied. Because structures in the cord have been studied extensively for many years, this review focuses on the spinal substrate of pain transmission and perception. The reader is referred to the excellent work of Gobel[115–118] and of Kerr[119–121] for information concerning trigeminal pain mechanisms.

Recent studies concerning the anatomic and physiologic organization of spinal structures related to pain have been facilitated by the pioneering work of Rexed.[122] Rexed divided the spinal gray matter into 10 regions or laminae based on the anatomic orientation of cells within each lamina (Fig. 1-2). The division of the dorsal, intermediate, and ventral horns into fairly distinct areas allowed investigators to describe with greater accuracy various regions and cell populations under study. Rexed's studies have been particularly helpful to researchers studying spinal cord function, and several investigators have examined the physiologic characteristics of neurons in specific laminae.

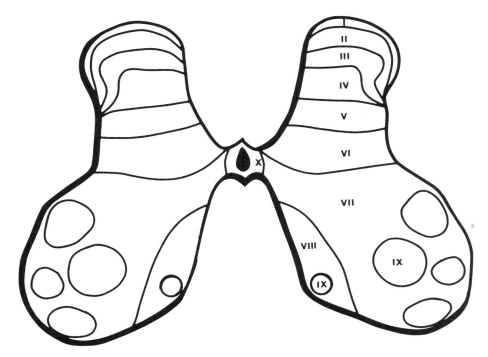

Fig. 1-2.   Schematic representation of the laminar organization of the gray matter of the spinal cord as described by Rexed.

The identification on morphologic and physiologic bases of functionally distinct populations of cells in the spinal cord has contributed significantly to the field of pain research. Many studies have shown that cells in different laminae play individual and sometimes unique roles in the processing and transmission of noxious stimuli. The following discussion of pain mechanisms in the spinal cord is approached from an anatomic perspective based on the laminar organization of the spinal gray matter.

Laminae I, II, and III

Synaptic terminals of peripheral nociceptive afferent fibers are distributed largely to the superficial layers of the dorsal horn. Specifically, these endings are distributed to lamina I, the substantia gelatinosa (lamina II), and lamina III.[123] (Fig. 1-3)

The characteristic feature of lamina I is the large marginal cell of Waldeyer. These cells are few in number but possess extensive dendritic arborizations that extend for several segments within lamina I and into the outer portion of lamina II.[105] Other smaller cells are also seen in lamina I, however, their exact role in the transmission of noxious stimuli is unclear. Primary afferent

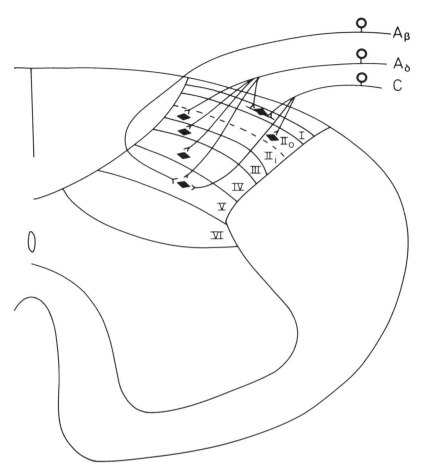

Fig. 1-3. Schematic representation of the terminal distribution within the spinal dorsal horn of different classes of primary afferent fibers involved in the transmission of noxious stimuli. Synaptic contacts are illustrated only to show the location of cells activated by specific afferent fibers. However, since most spinal neurons have extensive dendritic arborizations which reach into adjacent laminae, the exact site of synaptic interaction may be some distance from the parent cell body.

fibers traveling in the lateral division of the dorsal root terminate on the small, distal dendrites of the marginal neurons.[93,97] Light and Perl have identified these afferent fibers as being associated with high threshold mechanoreceptors transmitting along thinly myelinated A-delta fibers.[123] Following dorsal root section, terminals in contact with small, presumably distal dendrites show degenerative changes. However, axosomatic synapses and synaptic endings on the proximal dendrites of the marginal cells are largely unaffected.[124] According to Narotzky and Kerr synaptic terminals on the distal dendritic tree originate from small diameter primary afferents, while synaptic endings on cell bodies and proximal dendrites arise from internuncial cells in the substantia gelatinosa.[124] This differential synaptic arrangement might be the anatomic substrate for selective excitatory and inhibitory influences on lamina I cells as proposed by Kerr.[125] In addition to high threshold A-delta mechanoreceptors, input from A-delta thermoreceptors and polymodal C-fiber nociceptors to marginal cells in lamina I has also been reported.[126] Confirmation of high threshold A-delta and C-fiber input to the marginal layer of the dorsal horn in both cat and monkey has been provided by several investigators.[126-129]

Lamina II of the dorsal horn (substantia gelatinosa) is characterized by an abundance of very small neurons and a conspicuous lack of myelinated fibers. Ultrastructurally, the region is marked by densely packed complexes of synaptic endings collectively referred to as *glomeruli*.[115,119,130,131] The axons of substantia gelatinosa cells have short trajectories with synaptic terminations on other substantia gelatinosa cells at adjacent segments above and below their level of origin.[106] Many of the axons occupy the lateral part of Lissauer's tract and the lateral aspect of the fasciculus proprius. Several authors have noted that some substantia gelatinosa axons course through the dorsal white commissure to end in lamina II of the contralateral side.[106,132]

Recently, the substantia gelatinosa has been subdivided into an inner and outer zone based upon cellular differences as well as differences in the pattern of synaptic endings.[93,131] Synaptic terminals found in the outer zone are reported to be associated with C fibers from high threshold thermal nociceptors.[93,123] The inner zone, and to some extent lamina III, is thought to receive information from low threshold A-delta mechanoreceptors.[93,97,124] It is most likely that C fibers as well as A-delta polymodal nociceptive units also synapse in the substantia gelatinosa.

There is little question that the substantia gelatinosa is an important component of the pain transmission and modulation mechanism. However, the complex arrangement of cells, fibers, and synaptic endings in this lamina complicates efforts to study this region of the gray matter. Activation of cells in lamina II results in both inhibition and excitation of postsynaptic neurons, which further complicates attempts to clarify confusing behavioral questions.[133-137] However, recent discoveries related to putative neurotransmitters and neuromodulator substances found in the substantia gelatinosa may shed new light on this interesting nuclear area of the spinal cord.

Laminae IV, V, and VI

Laminae IV, V, and VI comprise the nucleus proprius of the dorsal horn. Unlike the substantia gelatinosa, these laminae contain numerous large neurons, many of which give rise to axons contributing to the long ascending spinal pathways. Lamina IV neurons possess dentritic processes which extend into lamina III and the substantia gelatinosa.[138] Light and Perl have shown that lamina IV cells receive synaptic contacts from low threshold A-delta fibers.[93,123] Other sources of synaptic input include plexuses of longitudinally running fibers within the lamina itself. Kerr identified these fibers as the dorsal intercornual tract and suggested that they were internuncial in origin and served to interconnect adjacent segments of the dorsal horn.[139] He further proposed that activation of these longitudinally coursing ascending and descending fibers might account for the failure of anterolateral tractotomy to completely abolish pain. Although cells in lamina IV may be activated by noxious stimuli, they are more easily and effectively discharged by innocuous tactile stimulation.[140,141]

Nerve cells in lamina V receive input from a wide variety of primary afferent fibers. Large diameter A-beta fibers as well as thinly myelinated A delta and C fibers have been shown to contact neurons in this lamina.[142–144] Physiologic studies have demonstrated that lamina V neurons have large peripheral receptive fields and receive converging input from noxious as well as non-noxious stimuli.[101,137,145,146] In addition, convergence from visceral and somatic receptive units onto lamina V neurons has also been demonstrated.[147–151] This particular observation has been used to support one explanation for the phenomenon of referred pain. From a functional perspective, wide dynamic range cells appear to behave in a manner similar to the T cell proposed by Melzack and Wall.[8] Other researchers have commented that convergence of visceral and cutaneous information onto lamina V neurons may constitute part of a mechanism whereby input from one area of the body might influence or modulate the effects of input from another area.[152,153]

Lamina V also contains neurons which respond exclusively to noxious stimulation.[154,155] Afferent fibers terminating in lamina V have been shown to be thinly myelinated A-delta fibers associated with high threshold mechanoreceptors and polymodal nociceptor C fibers. The feasibility of this interaction is not surprising given the extensive dendritic spread of lamina V cells and observation that A-delta fibers traverse the substantia gelatinosa and enter the dorsal laminae of the nucleus proprius.[97] It is interesting to note that many cells in lamina V have response characteristics similar to cells in lamina I known to be involved in the transmission of noxious stimuli. Together these two groups of neurons constitute an important link between peripheral afferent cells and more centrally located structures involved in pain transmission.

ASCENDING SYSTEMS

Within the spinal cord, ascending pathways are known to exist which transmit nociceptive impulses to higher levels. The majority of these ascending tracts are located in the anterolateral funiculus, and their role in pain perception has been recognized since the beginning of the 20th century.[156–158] Early studies suggested that pain behaviors in animals and pain responses in humans could be blocked by transection of the anterolateral quadrants.[159–163] Physiologic and behavioral studies revealed that impulses originating from the application of noxious stimuli crossed the midline in the spinal cord and ascended in the contralateral lateral funiculus.[164,165] Most investigators described the lateral spinothalamic tract as being necessary for the perception of painful stimuli, and this pathway has traditionally been referred to as the *pain pathway*.

Initially, the substantia gelatinosa was thought to be the origin of the spinothalamic tract. This notion was based on anatomic observations that incoming dorsal root fibers were lost immediately upon entering the spinal cord. Other investigators concluded that since these fibers apparently terminated in the substantia gelatinosa, and the subjacent dorsal horn, that these areas must be the location of the second order neuron in the pain pathway.[105,111] Degeneration techniques which exploit the chromatolytic responses to axotomy were the first to be used to further study this subject. Morin et al identified a number of reacting cells following anterolateral chordotomy in an attempt to identify the cells of origin of the spinothalamic tract.[166] Nolan et al used this method in neonatal kittens and demonstrated cells in all laminae, except lamina II, that projected axons to the contralateral thalamus.[167] More recent studies using antidromic stimulation and sensitive histochemical labelling techniques have also demonstrated spinothalamic tract cells throughout the spinal gray matter.[168–174] It is now well established that spinothalamic tract neurons are widely distributed in the dorsal, intermediate, and ventral gray regions of the spinal cord. A particularly interesting result of these studies was the observation that the exact distribution of spinothalamic tract cells varied between species. In cats, most spinothalamic neurons were found in the intermediate gray and medial part of the ventral horn, whereas in primates a greater proportion of these cells are located in laminae V and I of the dorsal horn.[171,172,175–178] Two recent studies have identified spinothalamic neurons within the substantia gelatinosa.[179–180] The significance of these differences is not entirely clear at present.

Evidence that spinothalamic neurons are involved in the transmission of noxious stimuli has been developed from several lines of research. Stimulation of thinly myelinated A delta and C fibers or cutaneous stimulation using frankly noxious stimuli activates spinothalamic tract cells.[101,147,181–183] Conversely, electrical stimulation in regions of the thalamus receiving and relaying pain messages results in the antidromic activation of cervical and lumbar spinal neurons in a variety of species.[168,170,175,176] Further examination of these spinal neurons has shown that they can be activated by both nociceptive and wide dynamic range afferent units.

Regarding the spinal course of spinothalamic tract axons, the major projection is via the contralateral lateral funiculus. However, small numbers of axons have been identified which ascend and terminate ipsilateral to their side of origin.[139,184] It has been suggested that in patients with unilateral pain conditions, the failure to achieve complete and lasting relief following contralateral anterolateral tractotomy may be related to the existence of an uncrossed spinothalamic projection. Furthermore, a small number of spinothalamic fibers have been identified in the ventral funiculus of the spinal cord.[185] Unlike the axons of the lateral spinothalamic tract, these fibers are widely scattered throughout the white matter medial to the medial most rootlets of the ventral root. Kerr has pointed out that ventral spinothalamic tract axons are easily distinguished from lateral spinothalamic tract fibers at spinal levels and in the lower parts of the medulla where ventral spinothalamic fibers constitute a conspicuous bundle located superficially along the lateral edge of the medullary pyramid.[185] At the level of the olive, these fibers are displaced laterally where they become intermingled with fibers of the lateral spinothalamic tract. Little is known about the laminar origin of ventral spinothalamic fibers, however, their termination has been shown to be similar to that of the lateral spinothalamic tract.[185] The anatomic similarities between these two ascending spinal pathways is such that a role in pain transmission for the ventral spinothalamic tract cannot be ruled out at this time. Kerr has remarked that the elevation in pain threshold and the sometimes disappointing results of anterolateral chordotomy might be attributable to transmission along ventral spinothalamic tract axons.[185] Additional anatomic and physiologic studies will be required before the exact function of the ventral spinothalamic tract is known.

While the spinothalamic tracts are recognized as being of primary importance in the transmission of noxious stimuli, other ascending pathways are also known to be involved. The spinoreticular tracts in particular have been the subject of many investigations. Interest in the organization of ascending pathways to the brain stem reticular formation and their role in pain mechanisms was rekindled as a result of several interesting observations in recent years. In 1969, Reynolds demonstrated in the rat that electrical stimulation of certain regions of the mesencephalon resulted in analgesia sufficient to allow intraabdominal surgery without the need for additional analgesic drugs.[186] In addition, many neurons in the brain stem reticular formation were found that were activated by noxious stimuli.[187-191] Electrical stimulation of some of these brain stem nuclei was shown to elicit escape behavior in experimental animals.[192] Examination of the physiologic response characteristics of these brain stem neurons revealed that two general categories of cells were involved in the ascending transmission of noxious stimuli: wide dynamic range cells and nociceptor-specific units.[187,193-195] Neurons with these characteristics are physiologically similar to spinal neurons known to receive A-delta and C-fiber afferent input, and indicate that nociceptive spinal and brain stem neurons might be functionally coupled.

More recent studies of spinoreticular tract cells have further supported the idea that these neurons might be important in pain mechanisms. The spinal origin of nociceptive spinoreticular neurons has been examined using both anatomic and physiologic methods. Cells projecting to the brain stem reticular formation have been found in laminae I, IV, V, and VI of the dorsal horn as well as in laminae of the intermediate and ventral gray.[196-201] Projecting fibers in the ventral and lateral funiculi have been demonstrated to be both ipsilateral and contralateral with terminations in a variety of widely scattered brain stem nuclei.[202-206] Since the spinothalamic and spinoreticular tracts have essentially identical laminar origins, and because of similarities in their physiologic properties, several investigators have suggested that spinoreticular fibers represent collateral branches of spinothalamic tract axons.[207,208] However, recent studies have identified spinal neurons with projections limited to nuclei of the brain stem reticular formation. Indeed, in the cat, relatively few spinal neurons project directly to the thalamus. In this species, the great majority of spinal cells transmitting nociceptive impulses terminate in nuclei of the brain stem reticular formation.[208-210] Interestingly, thalamic neurons receiving spinothalamic projections have also been shown to receive synaptic input from several nuclei in the brain stem reticular formation.[211-215] Thus, the reticular formation of the brain stem appears to represent a relay point for noxious impulses destined for more rostral levels of the neuraxis.

THALAMIC ORGANIZATION

Ascending pathways from the spinal cord and brain stem which transmit nociceptive information terminate in the thalamus. The synaptic endings of these pathways are distributed largely to three different regions of the thalamic nuclear complex: the ventrobasal group, the posterior nuclear group, and the medial and intralaminar nuclei. (Fig. 1-4)

Ventrobasal Group

The ventrobasal nuclei consist of nucleus ventralis posterolateralis (VPL) and ventralis posteromedialis (VPM). The traditional description of the pain pathway suggests that pain impulses from spinal levels are transmitted along the lateral spinothalamic tract to terminate in nucleus VPL. The information is then relayed in somatotopic fashion to the ipsilateral postcentral gyrus of the parietal lobe. Pain from the head utilizes an analogous pathway consisting of ascending projections in the ventral secondary tract of V with a thalamic relay in nucleus VPM.

Recent observations, however, require a modification of this oversimplified view. Although the spinothalamic tracts do contribute some fibers to the ventrobasal complex, the main source of afferent input to this nucleus is the dorsal column nuclei and the cervicothalamic tracts.[216-219] Interestingly, the majority of neurons in the ventrobasal group respond to the application of innocuous tactile and thermal stimuli.[220-224] The influence of direct spinothalamic input to the ventrobasal complex may be on those few units which have been shown to be responsive to noxious stimuli.[225-227] In human subjects, localized pain was associated with electrical stimulation in discrete regions of the ventrobasal complex.[228,229]

However, several facts mitigate against this being the only thalamic nucleus involved in the transmission and perception of pain. First, spinothalamic projections to the ventrobasal complex constitute only a small percentage of the input to that nucleus. Second, the major input to the VPM and VPL nuclei is associated with innocuous stimuli transmitted via the dorsal column-medial lemniscus system. Third, a significant spinothalamic projection has been demonstrated to thalamic nuclei other than the ventrobasal group. Finally, most of

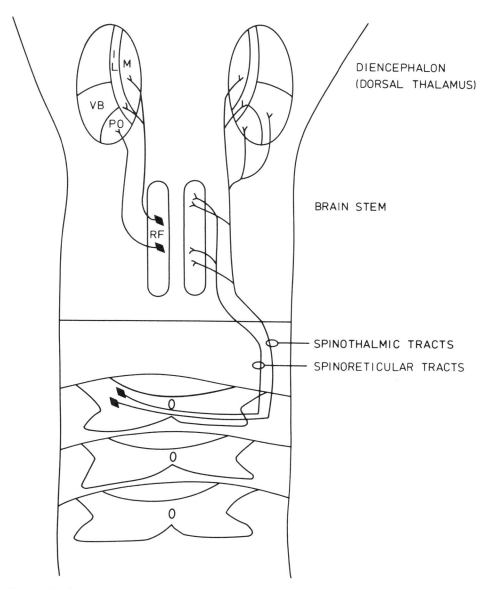

Fig. 1-4. Schematic representation of spinal projections to the brain stem reticular formation (RF) and to nuclear groups within the dorsal thalamus. Spinal projections to the dorsal thalamus terminate in the ventrobasal complex (VB), posterior nuclear group (PO) and medially in the medial (M) and intralaminar (IL) nuclear groups. Brain stem reticular formation projections to several thalamic nuclei are also illustrated.

the anterolateral tract fibers which transmit nociceptive impulses end in nuclei of the brain stem reticular formation, which in turn, relay rostrally to the medial and intralaminar nuclei of the thalamus. Thus, the role of spinothalamic projections to the ventrobasal complex appears to be limited.

Current data suggest that nociceptive information entering the ventrobasal nuclei of the thalamus is important in the sensory-discriminative aspects of pain. Specifically, the functional organization of the ventrobasal nuclei and their somatotopic projections to the primary sensory cortex seem best suited to providing information about the location of a particular stimulus. While this particular nuclear area is chiefly concerned with the processing of innocuous cutaneous information, a small number of units do respond to noxious stimulation.

Posterior Nuclear Group

A more interesting nuclear area of the thalamus in this regard is the posterior nuclear group. This nuclear region extends from the caudal pole of the ventrobasal complex to the region immediately medial to the medial geniculate nucleus. The posterior nuclear group and the ventrobasal complex have several features in common. Both nuclei receive input from the medial lemniscus, spinothalamic, and cervicothalamic tracts, and both project axons to primary and secondary somatosensory cortices.[230–232] However, significant differences have also been demonstrated. Neurons responsive to nociceptive stimuli in the posterior nuclear group tend to have bilateral receptive fields, rather than contralateral fields typical of ventrobasal neurons.[233] In addition, the posterior nuclear group contains many more neurons that are responsive to noxious stimuli, and they do appear to be somatotopically organized as are neurons of the ventrobasal complex.[234–237]

From a physiologic standpoint, the posterior nuclear group would seem to function more effectively as a thalamic relay in the pain pathway. The fact that the posterior nuclear group receives a fairly large input from nociceptive spinothalamic fibers and relays these impulses to sensory cortex provides strong support for its proposed role in pain perception. Collectively, ascending projections in the anterolateral tracts, which terminate in the posterior nuclear group, and the ventrobasal complex have been phylogenetically referred to as the neospinothalamic system.

The results of numerous laboratory and clinical investigations indicate that transmission along neospinothalamic pathways is associated with pain in a sensory-discriminative way. That is, activation of this system provides information about the location of the stimulus and its physical character (e.g., sharp, hot, intense, and brief). However, these descriptors represent only certain aspects of the pain experience. Other areas of the brain are also activated by noxious stimuli, and each contribute to the overall perception and behavioral reactions to noxious stimuli.

Medial and Intralaminar Thalamic Nuclei

Most significant in this regard is the projection to the medial and intralaminar thalamic nuclei. Direct spinal projections to the medial and intralaminar nuclei have been clearly shown by a number of investigators.[238–241] Cells giving rise to spinothalamic axons destined for the medial and intralaminar nuclei have been identified in widely scattered regions of the dorsal, intermediate and ventral horns, including laminae I and V.[242–245] Projections to the intralaminar nuclei tend to be more bilateral than projections to the ventrobasal group. Applebaum and his coworkers have further characterized these cells as high threshold and wide dynamic range units.[246] The term *paleospinothalamic system* is commonly used to distinguish projections to the medial and intralaminar nuclei from the more laterally located and anatomically distinct projections to the posterior group and ventrobasal complex.

In addition to direct spinothalamic input, the medial and intralaminar nuclei also receive a significant synaptic input from nuclei of the brain stem reticular formation.[247–248] As indicated previously, the brain stem reticular formation receives an extensive spinal projection via the anterolateral tracts, and much of this input is nociceptive. Studies of the physiologic properties of intralaminar and medial thalamic nuclei show that these cells also are activated by noxious stimulation.[249–252] Thus, it appears that the medial and intralaminar nuclei of the thalamus can be activated by a direct pathway (spinothalamic) and a phylogenetically older, multisynaptic route (spinoreticulothalamic).

CORTICAL INVOLVEMENT

The role of the cerebral cortex in pain perception is not well understood. Thalamocortical projections to the SI and SII areas from the ventrobasal complex and the posterior nuclear group are well documented.[253–259] However, the vast majority of these projections are activated by innocuous stimuli. Cortical projections from the medial and intralaminar nuclei are much more diffuse and not limited to one particular cortical area.[260]

With regard to pain projections to the cerebral cortex, most attention is focused on the SI and SII somatosensory areas, however, reports are often conflicting. In human subjects, electrical stimulation of the somatosensory cortex usually evokes paresthesia and is rarely associated with perceptions of pain.[261,262] A similar study in the monkey failed to produce evidence of avoidance behaviors or other pain reactions.[263] In contrast, surgical removal of somatosensory cortex for intractable pain has met with mixed success.[264,265] In cats, destructive cortical lesions in this area lead to an increase in the escape response threshold, rather than total loss of reactions to noxious stimulation.[266]

Physiologic recording techniques have been used to further assess the role of the cerebral cortex in pain perception. A small number of cells have been found in the somatosensory cortex that respond to noxious stimulation.[267–270]

Recently Kenshalo and Isensee identified two distinct types of neurons in the SI area in the monkey which respond to noxious stimulation.[271] One population was characterized as having a high threshold to noxious stimulation and a small contralaterally located receptive field. The responses were greatest to intense mechanical stimulation. Response characteristics of these neurons are similar in some ways to nociceptive neurons in the ventrobasal complex. The second type of cortical nociceptive neuron possessed a large, occasionally whole body receptive field and was activated by innocuous as well as noxious mechanical and thermal stimuli. These particular cells responded very much like wide-dynamic range spinothalamic tract neurons and nociceptive neurons in the medial thalamic nuclei. The authors speculated that the high threshold, cortical neurons, which may be driven by thalamic neurons in the ventrobasal complex, appear well suited to function in the sensory-discriminative aspect of pain perception. Their small receptive fields would be helpful in the localization of painful stimuli. The wide-range, large field cells apparently are better suited to provide information about the intensity of a given stimulus and may also be involved in cortical arousal.[271] Thus, thalamic projections from the ventrobasal complex, and part of the medial group of thalamic nuclei to specific nociceptive neurons in the primary somatosensory cortex, may indeed be important in the sensory discriminative components of pain. Cortical projections from the posterior group of the thalamus, which also terminate in the SI and SII regions, may also contribute to this functional system.

In addition to the SI and SII areas, other regions of the cortex are influenced by thalamic nociceptive neurons. Cells in the medial and intralaminar group in particular have diffuse cortical projections to regions including the frontal and limbic lobes. These areas are known to be involved in somatic motor function and the control of emotional behavior. It is conceivable that nociceptive input to these areas may be important in producing affective responses to a particular stimulus, and the initiation, if appropriate, of avoidance and escape behavior. The existence of significant medial thalamic projections to the hypothalamus could easily account for autonomic reactions commonly seen in association with acute and chronic pain syndromes. It seems reasonable to suppose therefore that the medial and intralaminar thalamic nuclei, together with many subcortical and cortical areas (other than SI and SII), play an important role in the motivational-affective reactions to painful stimuli.

DESCENDING SYSTEMS

Perhaps the most significant development in the study of pain mechanisms has been the recent discovery of an intrinsic neuronal system capable of altering both responses to and perception of noxious stimuli. The existence of such a system seems likely, since it was shown that electrical stimulation in selected areas of the brain produces behavioral analgesia.[186,272,273] Concurrent with the demonstration of stimulation produced analgesia (SPA), other investigators were successful in identifying opiate receptors in the mammalian brain.[274,275]

Within a short time ligands for these receptors were isolated. Naturally occurring opiate-like pentapeptides were identified in several areas of the brain and were named *enkephalins*.[276] Other larger peptides with morphine like activity (endorphins) were subsequently discovered, and their effects on pain transmission and perception have been extensively studied.[277] A comparison of these independent observations reveals extraordinary similarities. Regions of the brain rich in opiate receptors, enkephalins, and endorphins are also areas most effective in SPA.[272,278–280]

Recent studies have now clearly identified the anatomic pathways which mediate opiate and stimulation produced analgesia. Neurons in the mesencephalic periaqueductal gray (PAG) project axons caudally to the nucleus raphe magnus, the nucleus reticularis magnocellularis, and other nuclei of the pons and medulla.[281–284] These nuclei in turn send axons to spinal levels by way of the dorsal part of the lateral funiculus.[285–287] Cells in the nucleus raphe magnus release serotonin at their synaptic terminals, while nucleus reticularis magnocellularis neurons utilize other transmitter substances, possibly catecholamines.[288–290] The exact mechanisms by which descending pathways influence pain transmission are not completely understood. However, activation of these pathways in the presence of noxious stimulation results in a decrease in firing of cells giving rise to the spinothalamic and spinoreticular tracts.[291–293] Nucleus raphe magnus inhibition of nociceptive dorsal horn cells may be mediated via an enkephalin-containing interneuron link.[294–296] Thus, it appears that nuclear areas of the brain stem reticular formation can influence pain perception by reducing activity in ascending nociceptive pathways. Since many of these ascending pathways terminate in or send collateral branches to the brain stem reticular formation, a negative feedback system can be established whereby nociceptive impulses transmitted rostrally in the anterolateral tracts stimulate brain stem nuclei, which in turn reduce activity in the originally stimulated anterolateral tract neurons. Brain stem neurons involved in the descending control of pain transmission influence and can be influenced by more rostral levels of the neuraxis, including the cerebral cortex, and these mechanisms might be important in explaining various aspects of behavioral analgesia associated with sports and military battle injuries. At the present time, much work is directed toward solutions to very interesting questions concerning the biochemical and neuropharmacologic basis of pain experience. For a more complete explanation of these subjects, the reader is referred to the excellent reviews of Fields and Basbaum.[297–300]

SUMMARY

It is clear that multiple tract systems and nuclear regions of the spinal cord and brain are involved in the transmission and processing of nociceptive impulses. Each structure functions in its unique way, and working in concert with other parts of the nervous system, contributes to the total experience of pain. The discovery of specific nociceptive units and peripheral nerve fibers responsive exclusively to noxious stimuli lends support to specificity theorists. However, observations concerning parallel transmission systems and divergence of nociceptive impulses to several brain stem, thalamic, and cortical areas is not inconsistent with the notion of a pattern representation of pain. Indeed, recent anatomic, physiologic, and biochemical studies have demonstrated the extraordinarily complex organization of the nervous system. Further studies will greatly enhance our understanding of the phenomenon of pain. It is from these types of studies that reliable and effective treatment methodologies for a variety of pain syndromes can be developed. The ultimate beneficiary, of course, is the pain patient.

REFERENCES

1. Goldscheider A: Ueber den Schmerz in Physiologischer und Klinischer Hinsicht. Hirschwald, Berlin, 1894
2. Sinclair DC: Cutaneous sensation and the doctrine of specific nerve energies. Brain 78:584, 1955
3. Weddell G: Somesthesis and the chemical senses. Ann Rev Psychol 6:119, 1955
4. Gerard RW: The physiology of pain: abnormal neuron states in causalgia and related phenomena. Anesthesiology 12:1, 1951
5. Livingston WK: Pain Mechanisms. Macmillan, New York, 1943
6. Müller J: Handbuch der Physiologie des Menschen 2:249, 1840
7. von Frey YM: Beiträge zur Physiologie des Schmerzsinns. Koenigl. Saecks. Ges. Wiss, Math-Phys Classe 46:185, 1894
8. Melzack R, Wall PD: Pain mechanisms: a new theory. Science 150:971, 1965
9. Casey KL: Pain: a current view of neural mechanisms. Am Sci 61:194, 1973
10. Wall PD: The gate control theory of pain mechanisms: a re-examination and restatement. Brain 101:1, 1978
11. Wall PD: The role of the substantia gelatinosa as a gate control. Assn Res Nerv Ment Dis 58:205, 1980
12. Wall PD: The substantia gelatinosa: a gate control mechanism set across a sensory pathway. Trends in Neurosci 3:221, 1980
13. Kerr FWL: Pain: a central inhibitory balance theory. Mayo Clin Proc 50:685, 1975
14. Iggo A: Critical remarks on the gate control theory. p. 127. In Payne JP, Burt RAP (eds): Pain. J&A Churchill, London, 1972
15. Schmidt RF: The gate control theory of pain: an unlikely hypothesis. p. 124. In Payne JP, Burt RAP (eds): Pain. J&A Churchill, London, 1972
16. Collins WF, Nulsen FE, Randt CT: Relation of peripheral nerve fiber size and sensation in man. Arch Neurol 3:381, 1960
17. Hallin RG, Torebjörk HE: Studies on cutaneous A and C fiber afferents, skin nerve blocks and perception. p. 137. In Zotterman Y (ed): Sensory Functions of the Skin in Primates. Pergamon, Oxford, 1976
18. Heinbecker P, Bishop GH, O'Leary J: Pain and touch fibers in peripheral nerves. Arch Neurol Psychiat 29:771, 1933
19. Torebjörk HE, Hallin RG: Identification of afferent C units in intact human skin nerves. Brain Res 67:387, 1974
20. Perl ER: Myelinated afferent fibres innervating the primate skin and their response to noxious stimuli. J Physiol (Lond) 197:593, 1968

21. Bessou P, Burgess PR, Perl ER, Taylor CB: Dynamic properties of mechanore-ceptors with unmyelinated (C) fibers. J Neurophysiol 34:116, 1971
22. Bessou P, Perl ER: Response of cutaneous sensory units with unmyelinated fibers to noxious stimuli. J Neurophysiol 32:1025, 1969
23. Beitel RE, Dubner R: Response of unmyelinated (C) polymodal nociceptors to thermal stimuli applied to monkeys' face. J Neurophysiol 39:1160, 1976
24. Zotterman Y: Studies on the peripheral nervous mechanism of pain. Acta Med Scand 80:185, 1933
25. Collins WF, Nulsen FE, Shealy CN: Electrophysiological studies of peripheral and central pathways conducting pain. p. 33. In Knighton RS, Dumpke PR (eds): Pain. Little Brown, Boston, 1966
26. Torebjörk HE, Hallin RG: Perceptual changes accompanying controlled preferen-tial blocking of A and C fibre responses in intact human skin nerves. Exp Brain Res 16:321, 1973
27. Van Hees J, Gybels JM: Pain related to single afferent C fibers from human skin. Brain Res 48:397, 1972
28. Prattle RE, Weddell G: Observations on electrical stimulation of pain fibres in an exposed human sensory nerve. J Neurophysiol 11:93, 1948
29. Zotterman Y: Touch, pain and tickling: an electrophysiological investigation on cutaneous sensory nerves. J Physiol (Lond) 95:1, 1939
30. Hunt CC, McIntyre AK: An analysis of fibre diameter and receptor characteristics of myelinated cutaneous afferent fibres in cat. J Physiol (Lond) 153:99, 1960
31. Knibestöl M: Stimulus response functions of rapidly adapting mechanoreceptors in the human glabrous skin area. J Physiol (Lond) 232:427, 1973
32. Knibestöl M: Stimulus response functions of slowly adapting mechanoreceptors in the human glabrous skin area. J Physiol (Lond) 245:63, 1975
33. Knibestöl M, Vallbo AB: Single unit analysis of mechanoreceptor activity from the human glabrous skin. Acta Physiol Scand 80:178, 1970
34. Burgess PR, Perl ER: Myelinated afferent fibers responding specifically to noxious stimulation of the skin. J Physiol (Lond) 190:541, 1967
35. Brown AG, Iggo A: A quantitative study of cutaneous receptors and afferent fibers in the cat and rabbit. J Physiol (Lond) 193:707, 1967
36. Burgess PR, Perl ER: Cutaneous mechanoreceptors and nociceptors. p. 29. In Iggo A (ed): Handbook of Sensory Physiology. Vol. 2. Somatosensory System. Springer-Verlag, Berlin, 1973
37. Hensel H, Iggo A, Witt I: A quantitative study of sensitive cutaneous thermore-ceptors with C afferent fibers. J Physiol (Lond) 153:113, 1960
38. Iggo A: Cutaneous heat and cold receptors with slowly conducting C afferent fibers. Quart J Exp Physiol 44:362, 1959
39. Iggo A: Cutaneous mechanoreceptors with afferent C fibers. J Physiol (Lond) 152:337, 1960
40. Iriuchijima J, Zotterman Y: The specificity of afferent cutaneous C fibres in mam-mals. Acta Physiol Scand 49:267, 1960
41. Willer JC, Boureau F, Albe-Fessard D: Role of large diameter cutaneous afferents in transmission of nociceptive messages: electrophysiological study in man. Brain Res 152:358, 1978
42. Georgopoulos AP: Functional properties of primary afferent units probably related to pain mechanisms in primate glabrous skin. J Neurophysiol 39:71, 1976
43. Beck PW, Handwerker HO, Zimmermann M: Nervous outflow from the cat's foot during noxious radiant heat stimulation. Brain Res 67:373, 1974

44. Darian-Smith I, Johnson KO, Dykes R: "Cold" fiber population innervating palmar and digital skin of the monkey: responses to cooling pulses. J Neurophysiol 36:325, 1973

45. Dubner R, Sumino R, Wood WI: A peripheral "cold" fiber population responsive to innocuous and noxious thermal stimuli applied to the monkey's face. J Neurophysiol 38:1373, 1975

46. Dodt E, Zotterman Y: The discharge of specific cold fibers at high temperatures. Acta Physiol Scand 26:358, 1952

47. Hensel H: Cutaneous thermoreceptors. p. 79. In Iggo A (ed): Handbook of Sensory Physiology: Somatosensory System. Vol. 2. Springer, Heidelberg, 1973

48. Hensel H, Iggo A: Analysis of cutaneous warm and cold fibers in primates. Arch ges Physiol 329:1, 1971

49. Dubner R, Gobel S, Price DD: Peripheral and central trigeminal "pain" pathways. p. 137. In Bonica JJ, Albe-Fessard D (eds): Advances in Pain Research and Therapy. Vol. 1. Raven Press, New York, 1976

50. Sumino R, Dubner R, Starkman S: Responses of small myelinated warm fibers to noxious heat stimuli applied to the monkey's face. Brain Res 62:260, 1973

51. Hensel H, Huopaniemi T: Static and dynamic properties of warm fibers in the infraorbital nerve. Pflügers Arch ges Physiol 309:1, 1969

52. Dubner R, Sumino R, Starkman S: Responses of facial cutaneous thermosensitive and mechanosensitive afferent fibers in the monkey to noxious heat stimulation. p. 61. In Bonica JJ (ed): Advances in Neurology. Vol. 4. Raven Press, New York, 1974

53. Dubner R, Beitel RE: Neural correlates of escape behavior in rhesus monkey to noxious heat applied to the face. p. 155. In Bonica JJ, Albe-Fessard (eds): Advances in Pain Research and Therapy. Vol. 1. Raven Press, New York, 1976

54. Price DD, Hu JW, Dubner R, Gracely R: Peripheral suppression of first pain and central summation of second pain evoked by noxious heat pulses. Pain 3:57, 1977

55. Torebjörk HE: Afferent C units responding to mechanical thermal and chemical stimuli in human non-glabrous skin. Acta Physiol Scand 92:374, 1974

56. Van Hees J, Gybels J: C nociceptive activity in human nerve during painful and non-painful skin stimulation. J Neurol Neurosurg Psychiat 44:600, 1981

57. Gybels J, Handwerker HO, Van Hees J: A comparison between the discharges of human nociceptive nerve fibers and the subject's ratings of his sensations. J Physiol (Lond) 292:193, 1979

58. Fitzgerald M, Lynn B: The sensitization of high threshold mechanoreceptors with myelinated axons by heating. J Physiol (Lònd) 265:549, 1977

59. Campbell JN, Meyer RA, LaMotte RH: Sensitization of myelinated nociceptive afferents that innervate monkey hand. J Neurophysiol 42:1669, 1979

60. LaMotte RH, Thalhammer JG, Torebjörk HE, Robinson CJ: Peripheral neural mechanisms of cutaneous hyperalgesia following mild injury by heat. J Neurosci 2:765, 1983

61. Thalhammer JG, LaMotte RH: Spatial properties of nociceptor sensitization following heat injury of the skin. Brain Res 231:257, 1982

62. Torebjörk HE, LaMotte RH, Robinson CJ: Peripheral neural correlates of magnitude of cutaneous pain and hyperalgesia: simultaneous recordings in humans of sensory judgements of pain and evoked responses in nociceptors with C-fibers. J Neurophysiol 51:325, 1984

63. Campbell JN, Meyer RA: Sensitization of unmyelinated nociceptive afferents in monkey varies with skin type. J Neurophysiol 49:98, 1983

64. Perl ER, Kumazawa T, Lynn B, Kenins P: Sensitization of high-threshold receptors with unmyelinated (C) afferent fibers. Prog Brain Res 43:263, 1976
65. Witt I, Griffin JP: Afferent cutaneous C-fibre reactivity to repeated thermal stimuli. Nature 194:776, 1962
66. Iggo A: Physiology of visceral afferent systems. Acta Neuroveget 28:121, 1966
67. Leek BF: Abdominal visceral receptors. p. 113. In Neil E (ed): Handbook of Sensory Physiology. Vol. III/I. Springer, Berlin, 1972
68. Paintal AS: Vagal sensory receptors and their reflex effects. Physiol Rev 53:159, 1973
69. Kalia M, Senapati JM, Pareda B, Panda A: Reflex increase in ventilation by muscle receptors with nonmedullated fibers (C fibers). J Appl Physiol 32:189, 1972
70. Mense S, Schmidt RF: Activation of group IV afferent units from muscle by algesic agents. Brain Res 72:305, 1974
71. White JC: Cardiac pain: anatomic pathways and physiologic mechanisms. Circulation 16:644, 1957
72. Uchida Y, Murao S: Excitation of afferent cardiac sympathetic nerve fibers during coronary occlusion. Amer J Physiol 226:1094, 1974
73. Brown AM: Excitation of afferent cardiac sympathetic nerve fibers during myocardial ischaemia. J Physiol (Lond) 190:35, 1967
74. Abbe R: Resection of the posterior roots of spinal nerves to relieve pain, pain reflexes, athetosis and spastic paralysis: Dana's operation. Med Rec 79:377, 1911
75. Bennet W: On the resection of the posterior spinal nerve roots (rhizotomy): painful amputation stump. Br J Surg 2:234, 1914
76. Loeser JD: Dorsal rhizotomy for the relief of chronic pain. J Neurosurg 36:745, 1972
77. Groves EWH: On the division of the posterior spinal nerve roots: (1) for pain, (2) for visceral crises, (3) for spasm. Lancet 2:79, 1911
78. Onofrio BM, Campa HK: Enduration of rhizotomy: review of 12 years of experience. J Neurosurg 36:751, 1972
79. Coggeshall RE, Applebaum ML, Fazen M, et al: Unmyelinated axons in human ventral roots, a possible explanation for the failure of dorsal rhizotomy to relieve pain. Brain 98:157, 1975
80. Sherrington CS: On the anatomical constitution of nerves of skeletal muscles; with remarks on recurrent fibers in the ventral spinal nerve root. J Physiol (Lond) 17:211, 1894
81. Kidd LJ: Afferent fibres in ventral spinal roots. Br Med J 2:359, 1911
82. Windle WF: Neurones of the sensory type in the ventral roots of man and other mammals. Arch Neurol Psychiat 26:791, 1931
83. Coggeshall RE: Afferent fibers in the ventral root. Neurosurg 4:443, 1979
84. Clifton GL, Coggeshall RE, Vance WH, Willis WD: Receptive fields of unmyelinated ventral root afferent fibers in the cat. J Physiol (Lond) 256:573, 1976
85. Coggeshall RE, Coulter JD, Willis WD: Unmyelinated fibers in the ventral root. Brain Res 57:229, 1973
86. Coggeshall RE, Ito H: Sensory fibres in the ventral roots L_7 and S_1 in the cat. J Physiol (Lond) 267:215, 1977
87. Kato M, Hirata Y: Sensory neurons in the spinal ventral roots of the cat. Brain Res 7:479, 1968
88. Light AR, Metz CB: The morphology of the spinal cord efferent and afferent neurons contributing to the ventral roots of the cat. J Comp Neurol 179:501, 1978
89. Maynard CW, Leonard RB, Coulter JD, Coggeshall RE: Central connections of

ventral root afferents as demonstrated by the HRP method. J Comp Neurol 172:601, 1977

90. Hosobuchi Y: The majority of unmyelinated afferent axons in human ventral roots probably conduct pain. Pain 8:167, 1980

91. Ranson SW: An experimental study of Lissauer's tract and the dorsal roots. J Comp Neurol 24:531, 1914

92. Ranson SW, Billingsly PR: The conduction of painful afferent impulses in the spinal nerves. Am J Physiol 40:571, 1916

93. Light AR, Perl ER: Re-examination of the dorsal root projection to the spinal dorsal horn including observations on the differential termination of coarse and fine fibers. J Comp Neurol 186:117, 1979

94. Snyder RL: The organization of the dorsal root entry zone in cats and monkeys. J Comp Neurol 174:47, 1970

95. Anderson FD: Distribution of dorsal root fibers in the cat spinal cord. Anat Rec 136:154, 1960

96. Rethelyi M, Trevino DL, Perl ER: Distribution of primary afferent fibers within the sacrococcygeal dorsal horn: an autoradiographic study. J Comp Neurol 185:603, 1979

97. Light AR, Perl ER: Spinal termination of functionally identified primary afferent neurons with slowly conducting myelinated fibers. J Comp Neurol 186:133, 1979

98. Culberson JL, Haines DE, Kimmel DL, Brown PB: Contralateral projection of primary afferent fibers to mammalian spinal cord. Exp Neurol 64:83, 1979

99. Carpenter MB, Stein BM, Shriver JE: Central projections of spinal dorsal roots in the monkey. II Lower thoracic, lumbosacral and coccygeal dorsal roots. Am J Anat 123:75, 1968

100. Glees P, Soler J: Fibre content of the posterior column and synaptic connections of nucleus gracilis. Z Zellforsch 36:381, 1951

101. Wagman IH, Price DD: Responses of dorsal horn cells of Macaca Mulatta to cutaneous and sural nerve A and C-fiber stimuli. J Neurophysiol 32:803, 1969

102. Price DD, Hull CD, Buchwald NA: Intercellular responses of dorsal horn cells to cutaneous and sural A and C-fiber stimuli. Exp Neurol 33:291, 1971

103. Willer JC, Boureau F, Albe-Fessard D: Human nociceptive reactions: effects of spatial summation of afferent input from relatively large diameter fibers. Brain Res 201:465, 1980

104. Willer JC, Albe-Fessard D: Further studies on the role of afferent input from relatively large diameter fibers in transmission of nociceptive messages in humans. Brain Res 278:318, 1983

105. Pearson AA: Role of gelatinous substance of spinal cord in conduction of pain. Arch Neurol Psychiat 68:515, 1952

106. Szentagothai J: Neuronal and synaptic arrangements in the substantia gelatinosa Rolandi. J Comp Neurol 122:219, 1964

107. Ranson SW: The tract of Lissauer and the substantia gelatinosa Rolandi. Am J Anat 16:97, 1914

108. Ranson SW: The course within the spinal cord of the nonmedullated fibers of the spinal dorsal roots: a study of Lissauer's tract in the cat. J Comp Neurol 23:259, 1913

109. Chung KC, Langford LA, Applebaum AE, Coggeshall RE: Primary afferent fibers in the tract of Lissauer in the rat. J Comp Neurol 184:587, 1979

110. Chung KC, Coggeshall RE: Primary afferent axons in the tract of Lissauer in the cat. J Comp Neurol 186:451, 1979

111. Earle KM: The tract of Lissauer and its possible relation to the pain pathway. J Comp Neurol 96:93, 1952
112. Coggeshall RE, Chung K, Chung JM, Langford LA: Primary afferent axons in the tract of Lissauer in the monkey. J Comp Neurol 196:431, 1981
113. Denny-Brown D, Kirk EJ, Yanagisawa N: The tract of Lissauer in relation to sensory transmission in the dorsal horn of the spinal cord of the macaque monkey. J Comp Neurol 151:175, 1973
114. Hyndman OR: Lissauer's tract section. A contribution to chordotomy for the relief of pain: a preliminary report. J Int Coll Surg 5:394, 1942
115. Gobel S: Synaptic organization of the substantia gelatinosa glomeruli in the spinal trigeminal nucleus in the adult cat. J Neurocytol 3:219, 1974
116. Gobel S: Neurons with two axons in the substantia gelatinosa layer of the spinal trigeminal nucleus of the adult cat. Brain Res 88:333, 1975
117. Gobel S: Dendroaxonic synapses in the substantia gelatinosa glomeruli of the spinal trigeminal nucleus of the cat. J Comp Neurol 167:165, 1976
118. Gobel S: Golgi studies of the neurons in layer I of the dorsal horn of the medulla (trigeminal nucleus caudalis). J Comp Neurol 180:375, 1978
119. Kerr, FWL: The ultrastructure of the spinal tract of the trigeminal nerve and the substantia gelatinosa. Exp Neurol 16:359, 1966
120. Kerr FWL: The fine structure of the subnucleus caudalis of the trigeminal nerve. Brain Res 23:129, 1970
121. Kerr FWL: The organization of primary afferents in the subnucleus caudalis of the trigeminal: a light and electron microscopic study of degeneration. Brain Res 23:147, 1970
122. Rexed B: The cytoarchitectonic organization of the spinal cord in the cat. J Comp Neurol 96:415, 1952
123. Light AR, Perl ER: Differential termination of large diameter and small diameter primary afferent fibers in the spinal dorsal gray matter as indicated by labelling with horseradish peroxidase. Neurosci Lett 6:59, 1977
124. Narotzky RA, Kerr FWL: Marginal neurons of the spinal cord: types, afferent synaptology and functional considerations. Brain Res 139:1, 1978
125. Kerr FWL: Pain: a central inhibitory balance theory. Mayo Clin Proc 50:685, 1975
126. Kumazawa T, Perl ER: Excitation of marginal and substantia gelatinosa neurons in the primate spinal cord: indications of their place in dorsal horn functional organization. J Comp Neurol 177:417, 1978
127. Kumazawa T, Perl ER: Differential excitation of dorsal horn marginal and substantia gelatinosa neurons by primary afferent units with fine (A delta and C) fibers. p. 67. In Zotterman Y (ed): Sensory Functions of the Skin in Primates. Pergamon, Oxford, 1976
128. Kumazawa T, Perl ER: Primate cutaneous receptors with unmyelinated C fibres and their projection to the substantia gelatinosa. J Physiol (Paris) 73:287, 1977
129. Christensen BN, Perl ER: Spinal neurons specifically excited by noxious or thermal stimuli: marginal zone of the dorsal horn. J. Neurophysiol 23:293, 1970
130. Ralston HJ: The organization of the substantia gelatinosa Rolandi in the cat lumbosacral spinal cord. Z Zellforsch 67:1, 1965
131. Ralston HJ: The fine structure of laminae I, II and III of the macaque spinal cord. J Comp Neurol 184:619, 1979
132. Rethelyi M, Szentogathai J: The large synaptic complexes of the substantia gelatinosa. Exp Brain Res 7:258, 1969

133. Wall PD, Merrill EG, Yaksh TL: Responses of single units in laminae II and III of cat spinal cord. Brain Res 160:245, 1979
134. Wall PD: Excitability changes in afferent fibre terminations and their relation to slow potentials. J Physiol (Lond) 142:1, 1958
135. Wall PD: The origin of a spinal cord slow potential. J Physiol (Lond) 164:508, 1962
136. Gregor M, Zimmermann M: Characteristics of spinal cord neurons responding to cutaneous myelinated and unmyelinated fibres. J Physiol (Lond) 221:555, 1972
137. Mendell L: Physiological properties of unmyelinated fiber projections to the spinal cord. Exp Neurol 16:316, 1966
138. Scheibel ME, Scheibel AM: Terminal axonal patterns in the cat spinal cord: II The dorsal horn. Brain Res 9:32, 1968
139. Kerr FWL: Neuroanatomical substrates of nociception in the spinal cord. Pain 1:325, 1975
140. Wall PD: Cord cells responding to touch, damage and temperature of skin. J Neurophysiol 23:197, 1960
141. Price DD, Mayer DJ: Physiological laminar organization of the dorsal horn of M. Mulatta. Brain Res 79:321, 1974
142. Handwerker HO, Iggo A, Zimmermann M: Segmental and suprasegmental actions on dorsal horn neurons responding to noxious and non-noxious skin stimuli. Pain 1:147, 1975
143. Le Bars D, Guilbaud B, Jurna I, Besson JM: Differential effects of morphine on responses of dorsal horn lamina V cells elicited by A and C–fibre stimulation in the spinal cat. Brain Res 115:518, 1976
144. Ralston HJ, Ralston DD: The distribution of dorsal root axons to laminae IV, V and VI of the macaque spinal cord: a quantitative electron microscope study. J Comp Neurol 212:435, 1982
145. Hillman P, Wall PD: Inhibitory and excitatory factors influencing the receptive fields of lamina V spinal cord cells. Exp Brain Res 9:284, 1969
146. Price DD, Wagman IH: The physiological roles of A and C-fiber inputs to the dorsal horn of M Mulatta. Exp Neurol 29:383, 1970
147. Pomeranz B, Wall PD, Weber WV: Cord cells responding to fine myelinated afferents from visceral muscle and skin. J Physiol (Lond) 199:511, 1968
148. Foreman RD: Viscerosomatic convergence onto spinal neurons respond to afferent fibers located in the inferior cardiac nerve. Brain Res 137:164, 1977
149. Hancock MB, Foreman RD, Willis WD: Convergence of visceral and cutaneous input onto spinothalamic tract cells in the thoracic spinal cord of the cat. Exp Neurol 47:240, 1975
150. Selzer M, Spencer WA: Convergence of visceral and cutaneous afferent pathways in the lumbar spinal cord. Brain Res 14:331, 1969
151. Selzer M, Spencer WA: Interactions between visceral and cutaneous afferents in the spinal cord: reciprocal primary afferent fibre depolarization. Brain Res 14:349, 1969
152. Fields HL, Meyer GA, Partridge LD: Convergence of visceral and somatic input onto spinal neurons. Exp Neurol 26:36, 1970
153. Hancock MB, Rigamonti DD, Bryan RN: Convergence in the lumbar spinal cord of pathways activated by splanchnic nerve and hindlimb cutaneous nerve stimulation. Exp Neurol 38:337, 1973
154. Cervero F, Iggo A, Ogawa H: Nociceptor driven dorsal horn neurons in the lumbar spinal cord of the cat. Pain 2:5, 1976
155. Price DD, Browe AC: Responses of spinal cord neurons to graded noxious and non-noxious stimuli. Brain Res 64:425, 1973

156. Spiller WG: The location within the spinal cord of the fibers for temperature and pain sensations. J Nerv Ment Dis 32:318, 1905
157. May WP: The afferent path. Brain 29:742, 1906
158. Ranson SW, von Hees CL: The conduction within the spinal cord of afferent impulses producing pain and the vasomotor reflexes. Am J Physiol 38:128, 1915
159. Walker AE: The spinothalamic tract in man. Arch Neurol Psychiat 43:284, 1940
160. Rassmusen AT, Peyton WT: The location of the lateral spinothalamic tract in the brainstem of man. Surg 10:699, 1941
161. Weaver TA, Walker AE: Topical arrangement within the spinothalamic tract of the monkey. Arch Neurol Psychiat 46:877, 1941
162. Poirier LJ, Bertrand C: Experimental and anatomical investigation of the lateral spinothalamic and spinotectal tracts. J Comp Neurol 102:745, 1955
163. Price DD, Wagman IH: Characteristics of two ascending pathways which originate in the spinal dorsal horn of M. Mulatta. Brain Res 26:406, 1971
164. White JC, Richardson EP, Sweet WH: Upper thoracic chordotomy for relief of pain: postmortem correlation of spinal incision with analgesic level in 18 cases. Ann Surg 144:407, 1956
165. Gardner E, Cuneo HM: Lateral spinothalamic tract and associated tracts in man. Arch Neurol Psychiat 53:423, 1945
166. Morin F, Schwartz HG, O'Leary JL: Experimental studies of the spinothalamic and related tracts. Acta Psychiat Neurol Scand 26:371, 1951
167. Nolan MF, Curtis RL, Anderson FD: The laminar location of cervical spinal neurons contributing to the crossed ascending pathways in the kitten. Exp Neurol 57:231, 1977
168. Dilly PN, Wall PD, Webster KE: Cells of origin of the spinothalamic tract in the cat and rat. Exp Neurol 21:550, 1968
169. Giesler GJ, Menetrey D, Guilbaud G, Besson JM: Lumbar cord neurons at the origin of the spinothalamic tract in the rat. Brain Res 118:320, 1976
170. Albe-Fessard D, Levante A, Lamour Y: Origin of spinothalamic tract in monkeys. Brain Res 65:503, 1974
171. Carstens E, Trevino DL: Laminar origins of spinothalamic projections in the cat as determined by retrograde transport of horseradish peroxidase. J Comp Neurol 182:151, 1978
172. Trevino DL, Carstens E: Confirmation of the location of spinothalamic neurons in the cat and monkey by the retrograde transport of horseradish peroxidase. Brain Res 98:177, 1975
173. Hayes NL, Rustioni A: Spinothalamic and spinomedullary neurons in macaques: a single and double retrograde tracer study. Neuroscience 5:861, 1980
174. Willis WD, Kenshalo DR, Leonard RB: The cells of origin of the primate spinothalamic tract. J Comp Neurol 188:543, 1979
175. Trevino DL, Coulter JD, Willis WD: Location of cells of origin of spinothalamic tract in lumbar enlargment of the monkey. J Neurophysiol 36:750, 1973
176. Trevino DL, Maunz RA, Bryan RN, Willis WD: Location of cells of origin of the spinothalamic tract in the lumbar enlargement of the cat. Exp Neurol 34:64, 1972
177. Trevino DL, Coulter JD, Maunz RA, Willis WD: Location and functional properties of spinothalamic cells in the monkey. p. 167. In Bonica JJ (ed): Advances in Neurology. Vol. 4. Raven Press, New York, 1974
178. Albe-Fessard D, Levante A, Lamour Y: Origin of spinothalamic and spinoreticular pathways in cats and monkeys. p. 157. In Bonica JJ (ed): Advances in Neurology. Vol. 4. Raven Press, New York, 1974
179. Giesler GJ, Cannon JT, Urca G, Liebeskind JC: Long ascending projections from

substantia gelatinosa Rolandi and subjacent dorsal horn in the rat. Science 202:984, 1978

180. Willis WD, Leonard RB, Kenshalo DR: Spinothalamic tract neurons in the substantia gelatinosa. Science 202:986, 1978

181. Beall JE, Applebaum AE, Foreman RD, Willis WD: Spinal cord potentials evoked by cutaneous afferents in the monkey. J Neurophysiol 40:199, 1977

182. Foreman RD, Applebaum AE, Beall JE, et al: Responses of primate spinothalamic tract neurons to electrical stimulation of hindlimb peripheral nerves. J Neurophysiol 38:132, 1975

183. Foreman RD, Schmidt RF, Willis WD: Effects of mechanical and chemical stimulation of fine muscle afferents upon primate spinothalamic tract cells. J Physiol (Lond) 286:215, 1979

184. Carstens E, Trevino DL: Anatomical and physiological properties of ipsilaterally projecting spinothalamic neurons in the second cervical segment of the cat's spinal cord. J Comp Neurol 182:167, 1978

185. Kerr FWL: The ventral spinothalamic tract and other ascending systems of the ventral funiculus of the spinal cord. J Comp Neurol 159:335, 1975

186. Reynolds DV: Surgery in the rat during electrical analgesia induced by focal brain stimulation. Science 164:444, 1969

187. Casey KL: Somatic stimuli, spinal pathways and size of cutaneous fibers influencing unit activity in the medial medullary reticular formation. Exp Neurol 25:35, 1969

188. Casey KL: Responses of bulboreticular units to somatic stimuli eliciting escape behavior in the cat. Int J Neurosci 2:15, 1971

189. Le Blanc HJ, Gatipon GB: Medial bulboreticular responses to peripherally applied noxious stimuli. Exp Neurol 42:264, 1974

190. Benjamin RM: Single neurons in the rat medulla responsive to nociceptive stimulation. Brain Res 24:525, 1970

191. Burton H: Somatic sensory properties of caudal bulbar reticular neurons in the cat (Felis domesticus). Brain Res 11:357, 1968

192. Casey KL: Escape elicited by bulboreticular stimulation in the cat. Int J Neurosci 2:29, 1971

193. Perl GS, Anderson KV: Effects of nociceptive and innocuous stimuli in the firing patterns of single neurons in the feline nucleus reticularis gigantocellularis. p. 259. In Bonica JJ, Albe-Fessard D (eds): Advances in Pain Research and Therapy. Vol. 1. Raven Press, New York, 1976

194. Perl GS, Anderson KV: Response patterns of cells in the feline caudal nucleus reticularis gigantocellularis after noxious trigeminal and spinal stimulation. Exp Neurol 58:271, 1978

195. Anderson SD, Basbaum AI, Fields HL: Response of medullary raphe neurons to peripheral stimulation and to systemic opiates. Brain Res 123:363, 1977

196. Menetrey D, Chaouch A, Besson JM: Location and properties of dorsal horn neurons at origin of spinoreticular tract in lumbar enlargement of the rat. J Neurophysiol 44:862, 1980

197. Kevetter GA, Haber LH, Yezierski RP, et al: Cells of origin of the spinoreticular tract in the monkey. J Comp Neurol 207:61, 1982

198. Maunz RA, Pitts NG, Peterson BW: Cat spinoreticular neurons: locations, responses and changes in responses during repetitive stimulation. Brain Res 148:365, 1978

199. Fields HL, Wagner GM, Anderson SD: Some properties of spinal neurons projecting to the medial brainstem reticular formation. Exp Neurol 47:118, 1975

200. Fields HL, Clanton CH, Anderson SD: Somatosensory properties of spinoreticular neurons in the cat. Brain Res 120:49, 1977

201. Fields HL, Anderson SD, Wagner GM: The spinoreticular tract: an alternate pathway mediating pain. Trans Amer Neurol Assn 99:211, 1974

202. Wiberg M, Blomqvist A: The spinomesencephalic tract in the cat: its cells of origin and termination pattern as demonstrated by the intraaxonal transport method. Brain Res 291:1, 1984

203. Zemlan FP, Leonard CM, Kow LM, Pfaff DW: Ascending tracts of the lateral columns of the rat spinal cord: a study using the silver impregnation and horseradish peroxidase techniques. Exp Neurol 62:298, 1978

204. Brodal A, Walberg F, Taber E: The raphe nuclei of the brainstem in the cat. III. Afferent connections. J Comp Neurol 114:261, 1960

205. Breazile JE, Kitchell RL: Ventrolateral spinal cord afferents to the brainstem in the domestic pig. J Comp Neurol 133:363, 1968

206. Brodal, A: Spinal afferents to the lateral reticular nucleus of the medulla oblongata in the cat. J Comp Neurol 91:259, 1949

207. Mehler WR, Feferman ME, Nauta WJH: Ascending axon degeneration following anterolateral chordotomy. An experimental study in the monkey. Brain 83:718, 1960

208. Anderson FD, Berry CM: Degeneration studies of long ascending fiber systems in the cat brainstem. J Comp Neurol 111:195, 1959

209. Rossi GF, Brodal A: Terminal distribution of spinoreticular fibers in the cat. Arch Neurol Psychiat 78:439, 1957

210. Fields HL, Anderson SD: Comparison of spinoreticular and spinothalamic projections in the cat. p. 279. In Bonica JJ, Albe-Fessard D (eds): Adv Pain Res Ther. Vol. 1. Raven Press, New York, 1976

211. Eccles JC, Nicoll RA, Taborikova H, Willey TJ: Medical reticular neurons projecting rostrally. J Neurophysiol 38:531, 1975

212. Bowsher D, Mallart A, Petit D, Albe-Fessard D: A bulbar rely to centromedianum. J Neurophysiol 31:288, 1968

213. Mancia M, Broggi G, Margnelli M: Brainstem reticular effects on intralaminar thalamic neurons in the cat. Brain Res 25:638, 1971

214. Pearl GS, Anderson KV: Interactions between nucleus centrum medianum and gigantocellularis nociceptive neurons. Brain Res Bull 5:203, 1980

215. Bowsher D: Diencephalic projections from the midbrain reticular formation. Brain Res 95:211, 1975

216. Lund RD, Webster KE: Thalamic afferents from the spinal cord and trigeminal nuclei: an experimental anatomical study in the rat. J Comp Neurol 130:313, 1967

217. Boivie J: Anatomical observations on the dorsal column nuclei and their thalamic projection and the cytoarchitecture of some somatosensory thalamic nuclei. J Comp Neurol 178:17, 1978

218. Whitlock DG, Perl ER: Thalamic projections of spinothalamic pathways in monkeys. Exp Neurol 3:240, 1961

219. Bowsher D: Properties of ventrobasal thalamic neurones in cat following interruption of specific afferent pathways. Arch Ital Biol 109:59, 1971

220. Poggio GF, Mountcastle VB: The functional properties of ventrobasal thalamic neurons studied in unanesthetized monkeys. J Neurophysiol 26:775, 1963

221. Kruger L, Albe-Fessard D: Distribution of response to somatic afferent stimuli in the diencephalon of the cat under chloralase anesthesia. Exp Neurol 2:442, 1960

222. Paulos DA, Benjamin RM: Responses of thalamic neurons to thermal stimulation of the tongue. J Neurophysiol 31:28, 1968

223. Burton H, Forbes DJ, Benjamin RM: Thalamic neurons responsive to temperature changes of glabrous hand and foot skin in squirrel monkey. Brain Res 24:179, 1970

224. Harris FA: Wide field neurons in somatosensory thalamus of domestic cats under barbiturate anesthesia. Exp Neurol 68:27, 1980

225. Gaze RM, Gordon G: The representation of cutaneous sense in the thalamus of the cat and monkey. Quart J Exp Physiol 39:279, 1954

226. Perl ER, Whitlock DG: Somatic stimuli exciting spinothalamic projections to thalamic neurons in cat and monkey. Exp Neurol 3:256, 1961

227. Shigenaga Y, Matano S, Okada K, Sakai A: The effects of tooth pulp stimulation in the thalamus and hypothalamus of the rat. Brain Res 63:402, 1973

228. Halliday AM, Logue V: Painful sensations evoked by electrical stimulation in the thalamus. p. 221. In Somjen GG (ed): Neurophysiology Studied in Man. Exerpta Medica, Amsterdam, 1972

229. Hassler R: Dichotomy of facial pain conduction in the diencephalon. p. 123. In Hassler R, Walker AE (eds): Trigeminal Neuralgia. WB Saunders, Philadelphia, 1970

230. Bowsher D: The termination of secondary somatosensory neurons within the thalamus of Maccaca Mulatta: an experimental degeneration study. J Comp Neurol 117:213, 1961

231. Kruger L: The thalamic projections of pain. p. 67. In Knighton RS, Dumpke PR (eds): Pain. Little Brown, Boston, 1966

232. Mehler WR: Some observations on secondary ascending afferent systems in the central nervous system. p. 11. In Knighton RS, Dumpke PR (eds): Pain. Little Brown, Boston, 1966

233. Poggio GF, Mountcastle VB: A study of the functional contributions of the lemniscal and spinothalamic systems to somatic sensibility. Bull Johns Hopk Hosp 106:226, 1960

234. Berkley KJ: Response properties of cells in ventrobasal and posterior group nuclei of the cat. J Neurophysiol 36:940, 1973

235. Curry MJ: The exteroceptive properties of neurones in the somatic part of the posterior group (PO). Brain Res 44:439, 1972

236. Nyquist JK, Greenhoot JH: Unit analysis of non-specific thalamic responses to high intensity cutaneous input in the cat. Exp Neurol 42:609, 1974

237. Dong WK, Wagman IH: Modulation of nociceptive responses in the thalamic posterior group of nuclei. p. 455. In Bonica JJ, Albe-Fessard D (eds): Advances in Pain Research and Therapy. Vol. 1. Raven Press, New York, 1976

238. Mantyh PW: The terminations of the spinothalamic tract in the cat. Neurosci Lett 38:119, 1983

239. Boivie J: An anatomical reinvestigation of the termination of the spinothalamic tract in the monkey. J Comp Neurol 186:343, 1979

240. Holloway JA, Fox RE, Iggo A: Projections of the spinothalamic tract to the thalamic nuclei of the cat. Brain Res 157:336, 1978

241. Mantyh PW: The spinothalamic tract in the primate: a re-examination using wheatgerm agglutinin conjugated to horseradish peroxidase. Neurosci 9:847, 1983.

242. Kevetter GA, Willis WD: Collaterals of spinothalamic cells in the rat. J Comp Neurol 215:453, 1983

243. Giesler GJ, Menetrey D, Basbaum IA: Differential origins of spinothalamic tract projections to medial and lateral thalamus in the rat. J Comp Neurol 184:107, 1979

244. Giesler GJ, Yezierski RP, Gerhart KD, Willis WD: Spinothalamic tract neurons

that project to medial and/or lateral thalamic nuclei; evidence for a physiologically novel population of spinal cord neurons. J Neurophysiol 46:1285, 1981

245. Craig AD, Burton H: Spinal and medullary lamina I projection to nucleus submedialis in medial thalamus: a possible pain center. J Neurophysiol 45:443, 1981

246. Applebaum AE, Leonard RB, Kenshalo DR, et al: Nuclei in which functionally identified spinothalamic tract neurons terminate. J Comp Neurol 188:575, 1979

247. Becker DP, Gluck H, Nulsen FE, Jane JA: An inquiry into the neurophysiological basis for pain. J Neurosurg 30:1, 1969

248. Mancia M, Otero-Costas J: Nature of midbrain influences upon thalamic neurons. Brain Res 49:200, 1973

249. Chang HT: Integrative action of thalamus in the process of acupuncture for analgesia. Scient Sin 16:25, 1973

250. Perl GS, Anderson KV: Response of cells in faline nucleus centrum medianum to tooth pulp stimulation. Brain Res Bull 5:41, 1980

251. Dong WK, Ryu H, Wagman IH: Nociceptive responses of neurons in medial thalamus and their relationship to spinothalamic pathways. J Neurophysiol 41:1592, 1979

252. Urabe M, Tsubokawa T, Wantabe Y: Alteration of activity of single neurons in the nucleus centrum medianum following stimulation of the peripheral nerve and application of noxious stimuli. Jap J Physiol 16:421, 1966

253. Jones EG, Powell TPS: The cortical projection of the ventroposterior nucleus of the thalamus in the cat. Brain Res 13:298, 1969

254. Jones EG, Powell TPS: Connexions of the somatosensory cortex of the rhesus monkey: III Thalamic connections. Brain 93:37, 1970

255. Burton H, Jones EG: The posterior thalamic region and its cortical projection in new and old world monkeys. J Comp Neurol 168:249, 1976

256. Friedman DP, Jones EG: Focal projection of electrophysiologically defined groupings of thalamic cells on the monkey somatic sensory cortex. Brain Res 191:249, 1980

257. Saporta S, Kruger L: The organization of projections to selected points of somatosensory cortex from the cat ventrobasal complex. Brain Res 178:275, 1979

258. Graybiel AM: The thalamo-cortical projection of the so-called posterior nuclear group: a study with anterograde degeneration methods in the cat. Brain Res 49:229, 1973

259. Macchi G, Angelesi F, Guazzi G: Thalamocortical connections of the first and second somatic sensory areas of the cat. J Comp Neurol 111:387, 1959

260. Jones EG, Leavitt RY: Retrograde axonal transport and the demonstration of nonspecific projections to the cerebral cortex and striatum from thalamic intralaminar nuclei in the rat, cat and monkey. J Comp Neurol 154:349, 1974

261. Penfield W, Boldrey E: Somatic motor and sensory representation in the cerebral cortex of man as studied by electrical stimulation. Brain 60:389, 1937

262. Libet B: Electrical stimulation of cortex in human subjects, and conscious sensory aspects. p. 743. In Iggo A (ed): Handbook of Sensory Physiology. Vol. II. Springer-Verlag, Berlin, 1973

263. Delgado JMR: Cerebral structures involved in transmission and elaboration of noxious stimulation. J Neurophysiol 18:261, 1955

264. Lende RA, Kirsch WM, Drukman R: Relief of facial pain after combined removal of postcentral and precentral cortex. J Neurosurg 34:537, 1971

265. Corkin S, Milner B, Rasmussen T: Contrasting effects of postcentral gyrus and posterior parietal excisions. Arch Neurol 23:41, 1970

266. Berkley KF, Parmer R: Somatosensory cortical involvement in response to noxious stimulation in the cat. Exp Brain Res 20:363, 1974
267. Carreras M, Andersson SA: Functional properties of neurons of the anterior ectosylvian gyrus of the cat. J Neurophysiol 26:100, 1963
268. Morse RW, Vargo RA: Functional neuronal subsets in the forepaw focus of somatosensory area II of the cat. Exp Neurol 27:125, 1970
269. Whitsel BL, Petrucelli LM, Werner G: Symmetry and connectivity in the map of the body surface in somatosensory area II of primates. J Neurophysiol 32:170, 1969
270. Lamour Y, Willer JC, Guilbaud G: Neuronal responses to noxious stimulation in the rat somatosensory cortex. Neurosci Lett 29:35, 1982
271. Kenshalo DR, Isensee O: Responses of primate SI cortical neurons to noxious stimuli. J Neurophysiol 50:1479, 1983
272. Mayer DJ, Liebeskind JC: Pain reduction by focal electrical stimulation of the brain: anatomical and behavioral analysis. Brain Res 68:73, 1974
273. Mayer DJ, Wolfle TL, Akil H, et al: Analgesia from electrical stimulation in the brainstem of the rat. Science 174:1351, 1971
274. Pert CB, Aposhian D, Snyder SH: Phylogenetic distribution of opiate receptor binding. Brain Res 75:356, 1974
275. Pert CB, Kuhar MJ, Snyder SH: Opiate receptor: autoradiographic localization in rat brain. Proc Natl Acad Sci USA 73:3729, 1976
276. Hughes J, Smith TW, Kosterlitz HW, et al: Identification of two related pentapeptides from the brain with potent opiate agonist activity. Nature 258:577, 1975
277. Loh HH, Tseng LF, Wei E, Li CH: β-endorphin is a potent analgesic agent. Proc Natl Acad Sci USA 73:2895, 1976
278. Lewis VA, Gebhart GF: Evaluation of the periaqueductal central gray (PAG) as a morphine specific locus of action and examination of morphine-induced and stimulation-produced analgesia coincident at PAG loci. Brain Res 124:283, 1977
279. Pert A, Yaksh T: Sites of morphine induced analgesia in the primate brain: relation to pain pathways. Brain Res 80:135, 1974
280. Yaksh TL, Yeung JC, Rudy TA: Systematic examination in the rat brain of sites sensitive to the direct application of morphine: observation of differential effects within the periaqueductal gray. Brain Res 114:83, 1976
281. Fields HL, Anderson SD: Evidence that raphe spinal neurons mediate opiate and midbrain stimulation produced analgesia. Pain 5:333, 1978
282. Lovick TA, West DC, Wolstencroft JH: Responses of raphespinal and other bulbar raphe neurons to stimulation of the periaqueductal gray in the cat. Neurosci Lett 8:45, 1978
283. Behbehani MM, Pomeroy SL, Mack CE: Interaction between central gray and nucleus raphe magnus: role of norepinephrine. Brain Res Bull 6:361, 1981
284. Gebhart GF, Sandkuhler J, Thalhammer JG, Zimmermann M: Inhibition of spinal nociceptive information by stimulation in midbrain of the cat is blocked by lidocaine microinjected in nucleus raphe magnus and medullary reticular formation. J Neurophysiol 50:1446, 1983
285. Basbaum AI, Clanton CH, Fields HL: Opiate and stimulation produced analgesia: functional anatomy of a medullospinal pathway. Proc Natl Acad Sci USA 73:4685, 1976
286. Basbaum AI, Morley NJE, O'Keefe J, Clanton CH: Reversal of morphine and stimulus-produced analgesia by subtotal spinal cord lesions. Pain 3:43, 1977
287. Hayes RL, Price DD, Bennett JJ, et al: Differential effects of spinal cord lesions on

narcotic and non-narcotic suppression of nociceptive reflexes: further evidence for the physiologic multiplicity of pain modulation. Brain Res 155:91, 1978

288. Akil H, Mayer DJ: Antagonisms of stimulation-produced analgesia by p-CPA, a seratonin synthesis inhibitor. Brain Res 44:692, 1972

289. Hayes RL, Newlon PG, Rosecrans JA, Mayer DJ: Reduction of stimulation-produced analgesia by lysergic and diethylamide, a depressor of serotonergic neural activity. Brain Res 122:367, 1977

290. Messing RB, Lytle LD: Serotonin containing neurons: their possible role in pain and analgesia. Pain 4:1, 1977

291. Fields HL, Basbaum AI, Clanton CH, Anderson SD: Nucleus raphe magnus inhibition of spinal cord dorsal horn neurons. Brain Res 126:441, 1977

292. Guilbaud G, Oliveras JL, Giesler G, Besson JM: Effects induced by stimulation of the centralis inferior nucleus of the raphe on dorsal horn interneurons in cats' spinal cord. Brain Res 126:355, 1977

293. Willis WD, Haber LH, Martin RF: Inhibition of spinothalamic tract cells and interneurons by brainstem stimulation in the monkey. J Neurophysiol 40:968, 1977

294. Hokfelt T, Elde R, Johansson O, et al: The distribution of enkephalin immunoreactive cells bodies in the rat central nervous system. Neurosci Lett 5:25, 1977

295. Simantov R, Kuhar M, Uhl G, Snyder SH: Opioid peptide enkephalin: immunohistochemical mapping in the rat central nervous system. Proc Natl Acad Sci USA 74:2167, 1977

296. Atweh SF, Kuhar MJ: Autoradiographic localization of opiate receptors in rat brain: I. spinal cord and lower medulla. Brain Res 124:53, 1977

297. Fields HL, Basbaum AI: Brainstem control of spinal pain transmission neurons. Ann Rev Physiol 40:217, 1978

298. Fields HL, Basbaum AI: Anatomy and physiology of a descending pain control system. p. 427. In Bonica JJ, Liebeskind JC, Albe-Fessard D (eds): Advances in Pain Research and Therapy. Vol. 3. Raven Press, New York, 1979

299. Basbaum AI, Fields HL: Endogenous pain control mechanisms: review and hypothesis. Ann Neurol 4:451, 1978

300. Fields HL: Brainstem mechanisms of pain modulation. p. 241. In Kruger L, Liebeskind JC (eds): Advances in Pain Research and Therapy. Vol. 6. Raven Press, New York, 1984

2 | Evaluation of Pain in the Clinical Environment

John L. Echternach

Pain is a common component of nearly every condition which clinicians are called upon to treat. An examination of the clinical notes on most patients reveals that changes in pain and especially diminished or relieved pain are always important features of the clinical record. Since pain as a symptom is so common, attempts to evaluate and measure pain have held a prominent place.

There is a limerick that expresses some of the difficulties encountered when evaluating pain in the clinical environment. The limerick goes as follows:

> There was a faith healer from Deal
> Who said, although pain isn't real
> When I sit on a pin and it punctures my skin
> I dislike what I fancy and feel.[1]

This limerick illustrates, as does the illustration Werner used in her textbook (Fig. 2-1), the two major components of pain—the interpretive/emotional component and localizing/sensation component.[2] Anyone who has experienced pain can attest to these two components.

The evaluation and measurement of pain has always presented problems because it has been considered highly subjective in nature. An examination of the literature on pain (see Ch. 1) reveals that we have learned a great deal about the neural structures involved in the sensation of pain as well as the function of these structures.

It is equally clear though that, in dealing with patients, we are still dealing

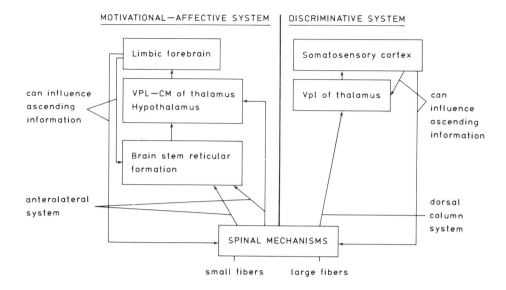

MOTIVATIONAL—AFFECTIVE SYSTEM | DISCRIMINATIVE SYSTEM

VPL=ventral posterolateral nucleus

CM=centrum medianum nucleus

Fig. 2-1. The two major components of pain. (Werner JK: Neuroscience: A Clinical Perspective. Reprinted with permission from WB Saunders, Philadelphia, 1980.)

with a topic that is highly subjective and which continues to defy measurement with the same objectivity we can bring to measurement of many other clinical phenomenon.

The evaluation or appraisal of treatment effectiveness is a critical component of therapeutic intervention used in the treatment of injury, disease, or malfunctioning of patients, and alleviation or modification of pain. Therefore, a variety of methods for evaluating and measuring pain have been proposed and a great deal of research has been conducted in evaluating the pain response.

In this chapter, we examine the most commonly used methods of pain evaluation and very briefly discuss some of the laboratory research on pain measurement.

BASIC CONCEPTS

It is important from the outset of this discussion to understand the differences between pain response in a laboratory setting for experimental purposes and in a clinical setting where the patient's pain reactions are an expression of the symptoms of the disease or condition affecting the patient. The laboratory situation can help us understand the pain phenomenon better but it does not replicate what happens in the clinical environment. For this reason, it then can be said that all attempts at measuring pain in the clinical environment are methods to try to improve the objectivity of the highly subjected and private response of the patient. When discussing measurements of any kind in the laboratory or in the clinical environment, it is important to keep in mind two important concepts related to measurement.

The first concept is *validity*. I think it is fair to question whether the patients' response to painful stimuli and descriptions of the pain are accurate measures of the amount of pain. In other words, are we measuring what we truly say we are measuring?

The second important consideration in measurement is *reliability*. Here we are concerned about whether the measurements can be repeated in the same way by different examiners or from one examination to the next by the same examiner. To look at the problem of reliability, we examine two issues. First, as the patient is examined from one period of time to the next, does the patient suddenly change his or her understanding of the pain phenomenon, giving different responses from one examination to the next? Second, since the examiner is also interpreting the patient's response as well as the patient interpreting his responses, does the examiner suddenly change his understanding of the patient's problem from one examination to the next, again affecting the reliability of the information being gathered?

When using the word *pain* in the clinical environment, there is a tendency to confuse the meaning. One use of pain is to see if the patient can experience a response to a noxious stimuli. This is probably the easiest of the pain questions to answer, but even here there can be a difference of opinion about what is being measured. As part of the neurologic examination, it is common to measure a patient's responses to various sensory imputs, such as light touch, hot and cold, and painful stimuli such as a pin prick and deep pressure. These responses are important when obtaining information about the extent and location of a lesion the patient has which may alter these sensory imputs.

The most important use of the word *pain* in the clinical environment is pain as a response to injury or disease and as a symptom. Pain as a symptom has been cited by some authors as the primary reason that the care of individuals by health professionals evolved. The very earliest contact between a patient and a physician was because the patient suffered a painful symptom and needed relief. Nearly all the modern interest in pain as a problem has been directed at understanding how to relieve this symptom. Many of the chapters in this book are devoted to some of the newer methods of controlling pain such as behavior modification, hypnosis, biofeedback, and trancutaneous electrical nerve stimulation (TENS). The symptom of pain is the most important aspect of assessing pain in the clinical environment.

EVALUATION OF THE PAIN PATIENT

As we deal with patients with pain problems, it has become evident that acute pain in many conditions is often manageable and that the failure of treatment of pain that has resulted in chronic pain is where the major interest in pain lies. However, in assessing pain it is important to be able to assess the pain problems of the acute as well as the chronic pain patient. Treating the primary cause of acute pain in a patient, whether it is trauma or disease often solves the pain problem. Whereas, in patients with chronic pain it may be that treatment has only been partially successful or has been successful in all aspects of the problem except in relieving the major symptom of pain. Many investigators in discussing acute versus chronic pain have made the point that acute pain is much more "physiologic" in that it is more clearly pinpointed, more easily described, and more easily understood by both clinician and patient alike. As problems with pain become more chronic they are subject to interpretation by the patient and take on more behavioral and emotional aspects. As these behavioral and emotional aspects increase, assessment of the pain problem becomes more difficult.

There are two important reasons why the clinician is involved in evaluation of a patient's pain response. First, the clinician tries to determine the underlying cause of the patient's pain, what structure or structures may be responsible for the painful stimulus, and under what conditions pain occurs. The first examination of the patient with pain is to determine the baseline level of the pain problem. This aspect of the evaluation is discussed later on in this chapter.

The second important reason for evaluating a patient's pain problem is to determine if the interventions that are made by the clinician have altered the pain in any significant way. These two reasons are very much related. If we were not going to intervene in the patient's problem with the hope of improving their pain then the baseline information about the patient's pain problem is essentially meaningless. Occasionally, you will find the clinician who says, "I am not nearly as concerned about the patient's pain as I am about the underlying problem, because if I can alter the underlying problem I will alter the pain situation." This is not always true since there are times when it appears that the patients underlying problem no longer exists but the patient continues to have significant pain symptoms.

The Interview

The first collection of information about pain from a patient is usually in the form of an interview (history taking) during which the patient responds to the examiner's questions. The examiner often will use the concept of pain variables and direct the questions to descriptions of these variables. Four variables of pain are often included. These are (1) intensity, (2) quality, (3) temporal aspects, and (4) physical characteristics. Under each of these variables, an attempt is made by the examiner to get the patient to describe the pain.

Intensity relates to the severity of the pain while quality relates to such characteristics as burning, pinching, and pulsing sensations. Temporal aspects examine such aspects of pain as constancy, periodic or intermittant, or brief attacks. Physical characteristics may try to define where the pain is experienced, is it localized, radiating, or diffused?

Further questions about pain during the interview determine if pain is made worse by any position or activity, or if some activities lessen the pain.

Some clinicians feel that the failure to manage pain problems results from an inadequate initial examination of the pain problem. A detailed history and the first examination may be the most important aspect of understanding and managing pain problems. Proper dissection of the pain story can be accomplished by questions about pain that are specific and in a logical sequence. This method facilitates clinical reasoning in important ways. When a patient is being evaluated, not only for the pain problem (or for any problem), the clinician often hypothesizes causes for the problems that the patient presents. An important part of this may be to hypothesize a cause or a mechanism for the patient's pain. This hypothetical reasoning process might lead the clinician to treat the underlying causes and not just the patient's symptoms. Giving a complete description of the patient's pain by directing and guiding the patient through an interview on pain serves the important function of establishing a baseline for comparison on subsequent examinations.

METHODS OF PAIN EVALUATION

The section deals with a series of methods for evaluating pain in the clinical environment. It emphasizes information about the methods and not necessarily the effectiveness of the various methods. The first area is a group of procedures used to help patients estimate their pain for the clinician.

Sternbach's Pain Estimate Method

Sternbach feels that the traditional diagnostic approaches to pain evaluation often penalizes the patient with psychogenic pain and, therefore, these methods must be supplemented with methods which help the patient explain why he or she is in pain and cannot live with it.[3] Sternbach emphasizes that one of the first considerations should be a simple method to obtain a description of the severity of the pain.

The method Sternbach has proposed is called the "pain estimate" wherein he asks the patient to assign a number to the intensity of the pain on a scale from 0 to 100. He feels that nearly everyone is familiar with percentages, which helps in using this scale. The specific instructions are as follows:

> We need to get a more accurate idea of how severe your pain is. On a scale of 0 to 100, in which 0 is no pain at all, and 100 is pain so severe you'd commit suicide if you had to endure it more than a minute or two, what number would you give your *average* pain? What is your average pain *these days*?[3]

Sternbach explains that the definition of the score 100 as suicide was necessary because some very dramatic patients while seeming calm and relaxed would report scores of 100. Sternbach uses this score, which he calls a magnitude production score, to compare with another method described later as an ischemic pain test, which he calls magnitude matching.

Verbal Pain Report

The next method has been called the verbal pain report or a verbal rating scale. Figure 2-2 shows several variations in this method for evaluating both intensity of pain as well as amount of pain relief achieved.[4,5]

The chief objection to this method has been that it provides only a very general rating of pain and that adjectives such as moderate and severe can give only vague approximation of the pain experience, showing the limitations of language. Others have noted that a human's verbal ability gives the only definable method for describing pain experiences.[6]

The subject remains controversial with some feeling that information derived this way can be extremely misleading and others finding it a simple and effective way to gather patient responses.[7,8]

Visual Analogue Scales

Visual analogue scales have become widely used and are a method that meets some of the objections to verbal report methods since they allow the patient more freedom to respond in expressing the pain experience between the

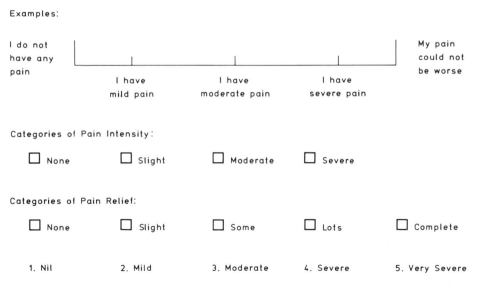

Fig. 2-2.   Verbal pain report: rating scales.

extremes of "no pain" to "my pain could not be worse" or similar descriptions. Figures 2-3 and 2-4 show several examples of visual analogue scales. The most common ones used are a line 100 mm in length with no pain being at the left and severe pain described on the right. The patient is instructed to make a mark on the line at a right angle at a point which represents the level of pain at the time of responding.[4] The distance is measured in millimeters from the left side to the patient's mark and is recorded as a pain score. The process is repeated during the time the patient is being treated for pain, which could be several times in a day or during each treatment and/or evaluation session.[4,5,9]

The visual analogue scales in Figure 2-4 show variations of this method.[10] The horizontal scales in this instance are all oriented from right to left for "no pain" to "severe pain" and also show scales which are vertical in nature. The method is very simple but requires that the patient is aware of how to use the rating scale.[4,5] As with the verbal report scales, there are patients who respond differently based on personality characteristics. Some patients respond to the expectation of those treating them. With repeated use of the scales with the same patient, it can be noted that some patients' responses will tend to cluster at one end of the scale while some patients are "all over" the scale from one use of the rating to those that follow.[9]

The use of visual analogue scales has been expanded by some authors (such as the method seen in Table 2-1 proposed by Kopala and Matassarin-Jacobs[11]) to evaluate pain effects on various aspects of daily life. Mannheimer

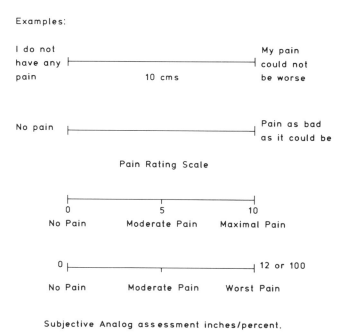

Fig. 2-3.   Visual analogue scale.

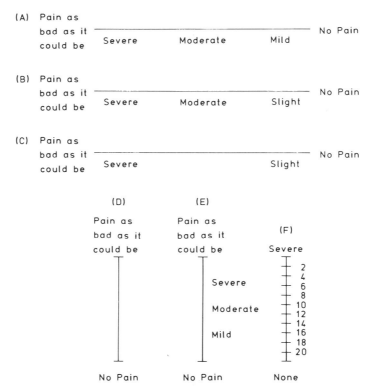

Fig. 2-4.   Visual analogue scale. (Scott J, Huskisson EC: Graphic representation of pain. Pain 2:175, 1976.)

Table 2-1. Effects of Pain on Daily Life Scale

On a scale of 1 to 10 (1, no interference by pain; 10, maximum interference by pain) have the client indicate the areas of life currently affected and the severity of that interference. Ask the client if this is the usual level and interference and if not, is it greater or less.

Areas of life affected

Sleep	Marital relations/sex
Appetite	Home activities (housework)
Elimination	Driving
Concentration	Walking
Work/school	Leisure activities
Interpersonal relationships	Emotional status

(Adapted from assessment tool by E. Matassarin-Jacobs, In Kopala B, Matassarin-Jacobs E: Sensory-perceptual-pain assessment. p. 341. In Bellack J, Bamford P (eds): Nursing Assessment: A Multidimensional Approach. Wadsworth, Belmont, CA, 1984.)

and Lampe combine the visual analogue scale with two other pain assessment methods.[9] The first is a pain questionnaire followed by pain diagrams (see Appendix 2-1). The pain questionnaire asks the patient to fill in (or allow space for the examiner to fill in) responses to a series of questions about the patient's pain. This is followed by a section which covers pain location. To help define more clearly the pain location, the patient is asked to state which of a selection of words describes the pain best. The subject is then asked to use the visual analogue scale to rate the pain in the sitting, standing, and lying positions.

The remainder of the assessment is for the examiner to record palpation/range of motion information, position observations, neurologic signs, and other details of the physical examination. This format permits the area of pain and behavior of the pain to be recorded along with an estimate of the intensity of the pain.

Body Diagrams

The approach of Mannheimer and Lampe[9] uses body diagrams which the therapist fills out indicating both the quality and intensity of the pain. Kopala and Matassarin-Jacobs use a similar approach of marking on a human diagram, the sites, intensities, and qualities of the patient's pain (Fig. 2-5).[11] Pain diagrams have also been used in which the patient fills in the diagram indicating sites of origin of the pain and to where the pain radiates. Melzack in the McGill-Melzack pain assessment questionnaire uses this approach (Fig. 2-6).[12] In Part 1, the patient is instructed to indicate where (on the diagram) the pain is located and by placing an E or an I to indicate external or internal pain. This information is combined with other types of information the patient provides, which are discussed later. One observation about patient generated pain diagrams has been that the amount of time and care the patient takes may indicate something about the psychological overtones of pain for the patient. Also, a recent study compared patient generated pain diagrams with therapist generated pain diagrams and found that they did not match, which raised the question of accuracy of reporting pain using this method.[13]

McGill-Melzack Pain Assessment Questionnaire

A method used to evaluate pain in a clinical environment can involve the language associated with describing the pain. The McGill-Melzack pain questionnaire uses this approach and Part 2 of the questionnaire asks the patient to describe what the pain feels like.[12] The instructions can be seen in Figure 2-6 wherein the patient is asked to circle those words that best describe the pain at the present time. Part 3 asks the patient to describe how the pain changes with time and gives the patient a selection of words having to do with periodicity such as continuous, steady, rythmic, and transient. Part 4 asks the patient to describe whether the pain is mild or, on a scale up to five, excruciating.

The client should be asked to identify:

1. Location - use "Person" diagram
   mark all sites

2. Intensity (mild, moderate,
   severe; 1 - (least) - 10 (most)

3. Quality (aching, burning, pricking,
   stabbing, throbbing, sharp, dull,
   shooting)

4. Chronology (acute, chronic,
   recurrent, intermittent, onset,
   duration of episode)

5. Precipitating factors (injury,
   onset in relation to any event
   or period of time)

6. Associated symptoms (pain may cause
   nausea, crying, constipation, etc)

7. Effects upon activities of daily
   living

8. Measures used to relieve pain
   (invasive and non-invasive)

9. Analgesic history (medication
   taken, amount, frequency,
   effectiveness, side effects)

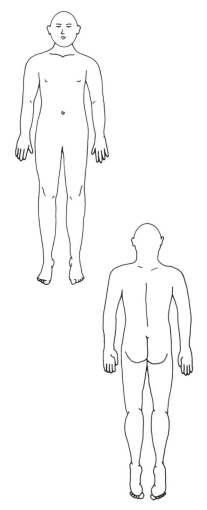

Fig. 2-5. Pain diagram for marking current or significant past reports of pain. (Reprinted with permission of the present publisher, Jones and Bartlett Publishers, Inc. from Kopala B, Matassarin-Jacobs E: Sensory-perceptual pain assessment. p. 338. In Bellack J, Bamford P (eds): Nursing Assessment: A Multidimensional Approach. Wadsworth Health Sciences, Belmont, CA, copyright 1984.)

Tursky Word Scales

Other investigators have used what they consider to be dimensions of pain, such as asking for sensory intensity as one dimension, expressions of pleasantness or unpleasantness as a second dimension, and painfulness as the third dimension.[5] This is very similar to a technique of Tursky in which he talks about the relative scales used for three dimensions of pain (Table 2-2).[14] The

Table 2-2. Relative Scale Values for Three Dimensions of Pain

Intensity		Reaction		Sensation	
Excruciating	227	Agonizing	153	Piercing	113
Intolerable	167	Intolerable	145	Stabbing	109
Very intense	154	Unbearable	128	Shooting	106
Extremely strong	135	Awful	98	Burning	80
Severe	132	Miserable	97	Grinding	79
Very strong	129	Distressing	50	Throbbing	75
Intense	123	Unpleasant	43	Cramping	67
Strong	101	Distracting	36	Aching	58
Uncomfortable	58	Uncomfortable	35	Stinging	50
Moderate	50	Tolerable	23	Squeezing	46
Mild	23	Bearable	23	Numbing	40
Weak	15			Itching	25
Very weak	10			Tingling	17
Just noticeable	8				
Extremely weak	8				

(Modified from Tursky B: The development of a pain perception profile: A psychological approach. p. 171. In Weisenberg M, Tursky B (eds): Pain: New Perspectives in Therapy and Research. Plenum Press, New York, 1976)

three dimensions of pain that Tursky used were intensity, reaction, and sensation. Tursky's technique was based on the idea of cross modality matching. He used hand grip, line length, or similar objective measures to establish magnitude standards that could then be cross matched with another variable such as experimental pain. He then used these magnitude standards with patients so they could rate their clinical pain. One of the advantages of this method is that it quantifies verbal descriptions and helps to clarify the dimensional qualities of pain. For example, when subjects were asked to score both intensity and unpleasantness of pain separately, they would only scale intensity; but when they were provided with verbal descriptions for judging unpleasantness, they were able to judge both dimensions independently (Table 2-3).[5]

Table 2-3. Verbal Pain Descriptors[a]

Sensory Intensity	Unpleasantness	Painfulness
Nothing	Neutral	Not painful
Faint	Annoying	Faintly painful
Weak	Slightly annoying	Mildly painful
Very weak	Very annoying	Somewhat painful
Mild	Unpleasant	Slightly painful
Very mild	Slightly unpleasant	Moderately painful
Moderate	Very unpleasant	Rather painful
Strong	Distressing	Quite painful
Barely strong	Slightly distressing	Decidedly painful
Intense	Very distressing	Pretty painful
Slightly intense	Intolerable	Very painful
Very intense	Slightly intolerable	Unusually painful
Extremely intense	Very intolerable	Extremely painful

[a] Verbal descriptors of sensory intensity, unpleasantness, and painfulness quantified by cross-modality procedures. Twelve descriptors for each dimension are shown in order of ascending magnitude. These words have been used to assess pain produced experimentally and pain from acute and chronic clinical syndromes.

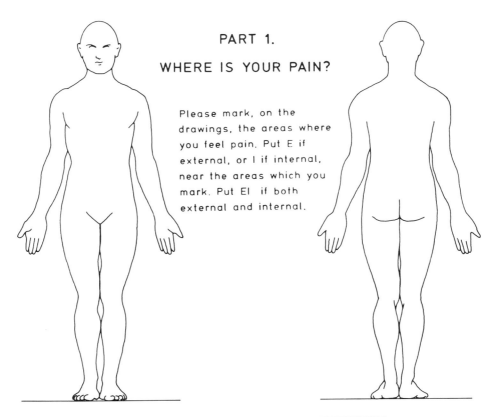

PART 1.

WHERE IS YOUR PAIN?

Please mark, on the
drawings, the areas where
you feel pain. Put E if
external, or I if internal,
near the areas which you
mark. Put EI if both
external and internal.

Patient's name_____Age_____

Hospital No._____

Clinical category (e.g. Cardiac, Neurological, etc.):_____

Diagnosis:_____

_____

_____

Analgesic (if already administered):

1. Type_____

2. Dosage_____

3. Time given in relation to this test_____

Patient's intelligence: Circle number that represents best estimate.

1 (low)   2   3   4   5 (high)

••••••••••••••••••••••••••

This questionnaire has been designed to tell us more about your pain.
Four major questions we ask are:

1. Where is your pain?

2. What does it feel like?

3. How does it change with time?

4. How strong is it?

It is important that you tell us how your pain feels now. Please
follow the instructions at the beginning of each part.

Fig. 2-6. The McGill-Melzack pain assessment questionnaire, Parts 1 to 4. (Melzack
R: The McGill pain questionnaire: major properties and scoring methods. Pain 1:277,
1975.)

Part 2. What Does Your Pain Feel Like?

Some of the words below describe your present pain. Circle ONLY those words that best describe it. Leave out any category that is not suitable. Use only a single word in each appropriate category--the one that applies best.

1	2	3	4	5
Flickering	Jumping	Pricking	Sharp	Pinching
Quivering	Flashing	Boring	Cutting	Pressing
Pulsing	Shooting	Drilling	Lacerating	Gnawing
Throbbing		Stabbing		Cramping
Beating		Lancinating		Crushing

6	7	8	9	10
Tugging	Hot	Tingling	Dull	Tender
Pulling	Burning	Itchy	Sore	Taut
Wrenching	Scalding	Smarting	Hurting	Rasping
	Searing	Stinging	Aching	Splitting
			Heavy	

11	12	13	14	15
Tiring	Sickening	Fearful	Punishing	Wretched
Exhausting	Suffocating	Frightful	Gruelling	Blinding
		Terrifying	Cruel	
			Vicious	
			Killing	

16	17	18	19	20
Annoying	Spreading	Tight	Cool	Nagging
Troublesome	Radiating	Numb	Cold	Nauseating
Miserable	Penetrating	Drawing	Freezing	Agonizing
Intense	Piercing	Squeezing		Dreadful
Unbearable		Tearing		Torturing

Part 3. How Does Your Pain Change With Time?

1. Which word or words would you use to describe the pattern of your pain?

1	2	3
Continuous	Rhythmic	Brief
Steady	Periodic	Momentary
Constant	Intermittent	Transient

2. What kind of things relieve your pain?

_____
_____
_____
_____

3. What kind of things increase your pain?

_____
_____
_____
_____

Part 4. How Strong Is Your Pain?

People agree that the following 5 words represent pain of increasing intensity. They are:

1	2	3	4	5
Mild	Discomforting	Distressing	Horrible	Excruciating

To answer each question below, write the number of the most appropriate word in the space beside the question.

1. Which word describes your pain right now? _____
2. Which word describes it at its worst? _____
3. Which word describes it when it is the least? _____
4. Which word describes the worst toothache you ever had? _____
5. Which word describes the worst headache you ever had? _____
6. Which word describes the worst stomach-ache you ever had? _____

51

Tursky combined the ideas of relative scale values of pain and cross modality matching to develop a four-part pain perception profile. The first part measures sensation threshold; the second uses a magnitude estimation procedure to judge induced pain; the third involves the psychophysical scaling of the verbal pain descriptors which are then used to measure pain on the three dimensions of intensity, reaction, and sensation as noted in Table 2-2; and the fourth allows the use of the psychophysically scaled descriptors in a diary format for repeated assessment of pain over a period of time. I have not seen this method used very often in the clinical environment and the procedure may have proven to be too complex for many clinicians to use. It does, however, seem to provide a research method for gathering pain information. It appears that some investigators have used the word scales provided by Tursky and others because they are shorter than the McGill pain questionnaire and do not seem to be as repetitious when used as a relative scale value for the three dimensions of pain. It has been suggested that these ratio values can be used without the matching hand grip or line length magnitude estimate. Perhaps further research is needed to answer all the validity and reliability questions about the extent of pain matching to these scales.

Experimental Pain Induction Methods

Wolff, in discussing the problem of measurement of pain, has noted the lack of an accepted scientific definition of pain.[15] He states that this lack has made the use of the measurement of pain in clinical environments and the use of experimentally induced pain difficult but feels that both approaches have made important contributions to understanding clinical pain. Experimental pain induction methods have used five different broad categories of stimulation. Discussed briefly, these are thermal, mechanical, chemical, electrical, and miscellaneous.

Electrical stimulation, thermal stimulation, and a method categorized as miscellaneous (the use of a tourniquet) for ischemic pain induction based on experimental methodology have been used in the clinical environment for the purposes of pain matching. Sternbach combines the magnitude production or pain estimate method discussed earlier with magnitude matching to develop the tourniquet/pain ratio.[3] He cites the method developed by Smith et al to develop ischemic pain measures.[16]

Sternbach's method briefly is as follows. The blood is drained from the nondominant arm by means of a tight rubber bandage which is removed after a blood pressure cuff is inflated well above systolic pressure. The patient is then instructed to squeeze a hand exerciser slowly 20 times and a stopwatch is started. The patient reports when the pain equals his or her usual clinical pain in intensity, even though it may be a different kind of pain. The cuff is left on until the patient reports that the pain is the maximum that can be tolerated. The clinical pain level and the maximum pain tolerance are both recorded. Tourniquet/pain ratio score is computed by dividing the time to reach the clinical pain level by the time to reach the maximum tolerance and multiplying the result by 100. This gives a score comparable to the pain estimate, such as 45 or 60. Sternbach then compares this score with the patient's pain estimate. Sternbach feels that the tourniquet pain ratio is a more meaningful score because the relationship in the tourniquet-pain ratio is based on the patient's clinical pain level in relation to the maximum that can be tolerated. Sternbach feels that this score is related to what Wolff has described as the pain endurance factor.[17] Gracely conducted a study in which subjects were asked to match their pain from their problem to the electrical stimuli by various matching methods.[18] One of the studies he did using electrical stimulation compared a patient's response to electrical stimulation of tooth pulp to an acute cold stimulus. In a small group of patients that matched electrical stimulation of tooth pulp to chronic myofascial pain a good matching of pain was shown. The investigation concluded that chronic pain as experienced by the patient can be matched reliably to the acute pain of the electrical stimulus.

The use of thermal stimuli has been well documented in the experimental literature starting with the work of Hardy, Goodell, and Wolff in the 1950s involving the development of the device called the dolorimeter.[19] Table 2-4 shows a rating scale for categorizing strength of thermal experience. The categorization ranges from "nothing" to "very painful."[20] Withdrawal was the final category; but this was not presented to the subjects but was an observation that was made by the experimenter. Much of the work done with thermal stimulus has been in the evaluation of the analgesic effects of drugs and is not applied directly to pain matching techniques in the clinical environment. The use of thermal stimulus by Hardy et al[19] implied that pathologic pain could be matched to the pain induced by heat. Pathologic pain was given an intensity value in dols according to the matching intensity of the heat-produced pain.

A similar method has been developed by Kast using a patient-operated apparatus that applies pressure to the fingertip.[21] The amount of air pressure required to establish intensity of the experimental pain equal to the pathologic pain serves as a measurement of the pathologic pain. Kast found that when he compared his pressure method to other methods—such as the estimate of pathologic pain, behavioral signs, and the patient's report of pain relief—the

Table 2-4. Rating Scale for Categorizing Strength of Thermal Experience

Instruction to Patient:
    "We wish to determine your ability to feel warmth, heat, and faint pain. A variety of heat intensities, including zero, will be applied to your arm. Some stimuli will be so weak that you will feel nothing at all, others will be hot, while others will produce a painful sensation. If you feel that the stimulus is getting too hot, remove the projector from the skin. Here is a list of possible responses to help you maintain consistency."

Rating Scale:
Nothing—Detect something—Faintly warm—Warm—Hot—Very hot—Very faint pain—Faint pain—Painful—Very painful—Withdrawal[a]

    [a] The withdrawal category was used for analysis, but was not on the list presented to the subject.

methods correlated highly with each other.[21] The theoretic basis for sensory matching is relatively simple. An experimentally induced sensory form of pain can be compared by the patient at the point of comparative equalization of the pathologic pain. The experimental sensory modality is under the control of the examiner and changes in the patient's pathologic pain can be quantified.

Stewart[22] has pointed out two difficulties in sensory matching: (1) the patient must be in pain at the time of the comparison estimate and (2) the severity of the clinical pain may be so extreme that the introduction of either experimental pain or another sensory matching method may be both ethically and physiologically impossible. Stewart feels that this, therefore, limits the technique to individuals with relatively mild pain who have the ability to cooperate and to concentrate on the tests being done. She feels this might be difficult for patients who are extremely ill or who are heavily medicated.

The experimental pain induction methods that are most widely used use electrical stimulation.[15] It is an ideal stimulus because it is easily controlled by the experimenter; it is a unique subjective sensation: it is different from pain and does not stimulate a single selective receptor but stimulates many different types of sensory receptors.

Comprehensive and Specialized Approaches

Some authors have discussed the McGill pain questionnaire as an example of a more comprehensive approach to the analysis of pain since the pain questionnaire tries to look at several aspects of pain, not just the intensity component.[4,5] Some clinicians feel that this more comprehensive approach as exhibited by Melzack[12] and by Mannheimer and Lampe[9] as examples of comprehensive pain questionnaires may provide the most useful information to the clinician in many types of cases since the approach is to look at as many aspects or dimensions of the patient's pain as possible (See Fig. 2-6 and Appendix 2-1).

Other specialized pain indexes have been developed for specialized conditions. An example is that developed by Hendler for the screening of chronic back pain.[23] Hendler developed a method called "the ten minute screening test for chronic back pain patients" in conjunction with others at the Johns Hopkins Hospital Chronic Pain Treatment Center (see Appendix 2-2). A score of 14 points or less suggests that the patient is an objective pain patient and is reporting a normal response to pain. A score of 15 to 20 points suggests that the patient has features of a subjective and exaggerated pain. This implies that the patient had prepain adjustment problems and does have an organic lesion but that chronic pain produces a more extreme response in this kind of patient. A score of 21 to 31 points suggests that the patient is an exaggerated pain patient. Surgical intervention should be carried out with these patients with extreme caution because this type of patient has a prepain personality that may justify the complaint of chronic pain; instead this patient would benefit from a treatment center program with an emphasis on an attitude change towards the chronic pain.

Backache:

1. My back never bothers me at all.
2. My back hardly ever bothers me.
3. I sometimes have a twinge of pain in my back.
4. I often have a twinge of pain in my back.
5. Often my back hurts quite a lot.
6. I often have really bad backache.
7. I have really bad backache all of the time.

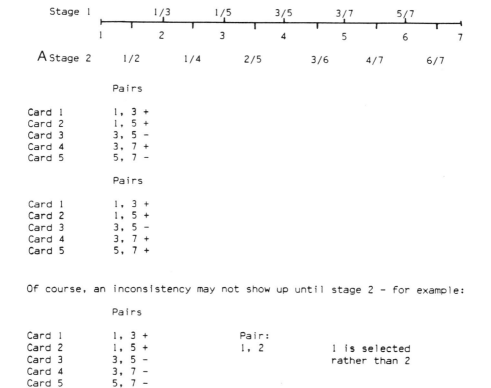

Of course, an inconsistency may not show up until stage 2 - for example:

Fig. 2-7. Ingham's scale for backaches. (A) Midpoints of scale values (B) Methods of scoring pain symptom scales. (Ingham JG: Quantitative evaluation of subjective symptoms. Proc R Soc Med 62:492, 1969.)

A score of 32 points or greater suggests to Hendler and his group that a psychiatric consultation is needed. He feels that these patients are in the severe depression, suicide, or psychotic group and present serious problems in management.

Another specialized pain index for low back pain was developed by Ingham and was an attempt by him to reduce response bias or response set so that the patient could report symptoms more clearly.[24] Ingham felt that symptoms should be able to be reported on a continuum, and he developed scales for a variety of conditions. I am reporting here only his scale for backaches since that is the one that is most likely to be of interest to the readers of this text (Fig. 2-7). Ingham's method on first inspection appears to be simple but his scoring method is extremely complicated and reading the references may be necessary to understand it completely.[22,24,25] Essentially, the statements are presented to the subject in pairs and the subject is required to choose the statement that is closer to the truth. Figure 2-7 shows the scale values for presenting the pairs. The purpose in presenting the pairs is to see if the patient is consistent so that a true evaluation of the patient's description of the pain can be obtained.

One final example of a pain profile is presented in Table 2-5. This was developed by Picaza, Ray, and Sheely who looked at four aspects of pain.[26] The percentage of time that pain was present, severity of the pain, the effect of pain

Table 2-5. Pain Profile of Picaza, Ray, and Shealy[a]

Percent of time pain present	0—None 1—Up to 25% 2—26–50% 3—52–75% 4—76–100%
Severity of pain	0—None 1—Mild 2—Discomforting 3—Distressing 4—Horrible or Excruciating
Effect of pain on physical activity	0—None 1—Up to 25% incapacitated 2—26–50% incapacitated 3—51–75% incapacitated 4—76–100% incapacitated
Use of drugs	0—None 1—Aspirin and mild analgesics 2—Tranquilizers and sedatives in moderation 3—Moderately addicting drugs (alcohol, codeine, Darvon, Talwin) 4—Strongly addicting drugs (narcotics and large doses of those in No. 3)
Effects of pain upon mood	0–4 (Panic; total incapacity)

[a] The pain profile is graded in each of five categories with 0 (normal) to 4 (maximum disability).

(Shealy CN, Shealy M: Behavioral techniques in the control of pain: a case for health maintenance vs. disease treatment. p. 21. In Weisenberg M, Tursky B (eds): Pain: New Perspectives in Therapy and Research. Plenum Press, New York, 1976.)

on physical activity, and the use of drugs were graded on a scale of 0 to 4. Then the effects of pain upon patient mood was also evaluated by the examiners on a scale of 0 to 4. A pain profile was developed so that they could add up scores for patients and then as the patients progressed through a treatment program for pain control, they could see if the scores in the pain profile changed and in what area the changes were taking place. They looked at both the total scores and the scores in the different categories as methods for evaluating patients' responses to treatment.

SUMMARY

This chapter presents clinicians with information that can possibly be used in the clinical environment for the assessment of pain. The methods have been presented with enough description that the clinician might be able to use the method in a clinical environment. To avoid creating bias for or against a particular method, a great deal of evaluative information is not presented. An understanding of the great variety of methods available for the measurement of pain in the clinical environment should prove useful to clinicians for selecting the method that is most appropriate for the type of patient or client group that they are dealing with. No one method of collecting pain information or evaluating pain information can be universally applied to patients since the types of patients and the needs of clinicians varies so greatly. Clinicians should verify or expand upon the knowledge presented in this chapter by using the methods presented, becoming familiar with the literature on clinical assessment of pain, and making judgments about what works best for them in assessing pain problems in their clinical practice. Patients will benefit from the increased understanding by clinicians of the complexities of the problems associated with pain and the challenges and pitfalls in the attempt to measure this complex phenomenon.

REFERENCES

1. Reed L: The Complete Limerick Book, p. 87. Jarrolds Publishing, London 1925
2. Werner JK: Neuroscience: A Clinical Perspective. WB Saunders Philadelphia, 1980
3. Sternbach RA: Pain Patients, Tracts and Treatment. Academic Press, New York, 1974
4. Bond MR: Pain, Its Nature, Analysis and Treatment. Churchill Livingstone, Edinburgh, 1979
5. Gracely RH: Pain measurement in man, p. 111. In Ng LKY, Bonica JJ (eds): Pain: Discomfort and Humanitarian Care. Elsevier/North Holland, New York, 1980
6. Hilgard FR: Pain as a Puzzle for Psychology and Physiology. Am Psychol, 24: 103, 1969
7. Poultan EC: Quantitative subjective assessments are almost always biased, sometimes completely misleading. Br J Psychol, 68:409, 1977

8. Stevens SS: Psychophysics: Introduction to Its Perceptual Neural and Social Prospects. John Wiley and Sons, New York, 1975

9. Mannheimer JS, Lampe GN: Clinical Transcutaneous Electrical Nerve Stimulation. FA Davis, Philadelphia, 1984

10. Scott J, Huskisson EC: Graphic representation of pain. Pain, 2:175–184, 1976

11. Kopala B, Matassarin-Jacobs E: Sensory-perceptual-pain assessment. p. 341. In Bellack J, Bamford (eds): Nursing Assessment: a Multidimensional Approach. Wadsworth, Belmont, CA, 1984

12. Melzak R: The McGill pain questionnaire: major properties and scoring methods: Pain, 1:277, 1975

13. Cummings GS, Routon JL: Validity of unassisted pain drawings by patients with chronic pain (Abstract). Phys Ther, 5:668, 1985

14. Tursky B: The development of a pain perception profile: A psychophysical approach. p. 171. In Weisenberg M, Tursky B (eds): Pain: New Perspectives in Therapy and Research, Plenum Press, New York, 1976

15. Wolff BB: Measurement of human pain. p. 173. In Bonica JJ (ed): Pain, Research Publications: Association for Research in Nervous and Mental Disease. Raven Press, New York 1980

16. Smith GM, Lowenstein E, Hubbard JH, Beecher HK: Experimental pain produced by the submaximum effort tourniquet technique: further evidence of validity. J Pharma Exp Ther 163:468, 1968

17. Wolff BB: Factor analysis of human pain responses: pain endurance as a specific pain factor. J Abnormal Psychol 78:292, 1971

18. Gracely RH: Advances in Pain Research and Therapy. Bonica JJ, Liebeskind JC, Albe-Fessard D (eds), Vol. 3. Raven Press, New York, 1979

19. Hardy JD, Wolff HG, Goodell H: Pain Sensations and Reactions. Hafner Publishing, New York, 1952

20. Clark WC: Pain sensitivity and the report of pain: an introduction to sensory decision theory. p. 195. In Weisenberg M, Tursky B (eds): Pain: New Perspectives in Theory and Research. Plenum Press, New York, 1976

21. Kast EC: An understanding of pain and its measurement. Med Times, 94:1501, 1966

22. Stewart ML: Measurement of clinical pain p. 107. In Jacox AK (ed): Pain: A Source Book for Nurses and Other Health Professionals. Little Brown, Boston 1977

23. Hendler N: Psychological tests for chronic pain. p. 101. In Diagnosis and Nonsurgical Management of Chronic Pain. Raven Press, New York, 1981

24. Ingham JG: Quantitative evaluation of subjective symptoms. Proc R Soc Med 62:492, 1969

25. Ingham JG: A method of observing symptoms and attitudes. Br J Soc Clin Psychol 4:131, 1965

26. Shealy CN, Shealy M: Behavorial techniques in the control of pain: a case for health maintenance vs. disease treatment. p. 21. In Weisenberg M, Tursky B (eds): Pain: New Perspectives in Therapy and Research. Plenum Press, New York, 1976

Appendix 2-1*

PAIN ASSESSMENT FORM

Name: _____ Age: _____ Date: _____
Occupation: _____ Injured at work: _____ Presently working: _____
Date of injury: _____ or Onset of pain: _____ Gradual _____ Sudden _____
Description of accident: _____
_____
_____
_____

PAIN DESCRIPTION

What does your pain feel like? _____
Is it present constantly? _____ periodically? _____
Is it present at certain times during the day? _____ night? _____
When your pain is present, how long does it last? _____
What positions, movements, or activities increase or bring on pain? _____
_____
What positions, movements or activities decrease your pain? _____
_____
Are you able to sleep at night without pain? _____
Do you have a firm mattress? _____ Are you awakened by pain? _____
What is your primary sleeping position? _____
_____
What pain medications, if any are you taking? _____
_____ How frequently? _____
How long have you been taking this medication? _____
How much pain relief does the medication provide? _____
Does anything else affect your pain? _____
_____ Food   _____ Coughing or sneezing $\oplus$ = Increase
_____ Weather changes   _____ Exertion $\ominus$ = Decrease
_____ Finger pressure   _____ Noise
_____ Menstruation   _____ Light
_____ Heat
_____ Ice
Since the onset of pain, has it been: decreasing _____ , increasing _____ , or remaining
the same _____ .
Have you had a similar problem in the past? If so, when? _____
What treatment if any did you receive at that time? _____
_____ Was it helpful? _____
Have you already received treatment elsewhere for your present problem? _____ If so,
specify the type of treatment which you received _____
Was it beneficial? _____
Place an "X" next to the statements that apply to you.
_____ Grinding your teeth   _____ Visual disturbances
_____ Facial or head pain   _____ Gastrointestinal discomfort
_____ Vomiting _____ Frequency _____ Does this ↓ or ↑ pain _____
_____ Pain during or after eating   _____ Pain upon chewing

PAIN LOCATION

Where did your pain start? _____

Has it changed location or spread to other areas? _____

_____

Are there any areas where discomfort is most intense? _____

Where? _____

Are there any areas where you don't feel any sensation? _____

_____

Use the diagrams on the back of this page to draw the distribution and quality of your pain. Try to be as specific as possible in regard to the exact type or quality of pain.

COMPLETING THE DIAGRAMS

First decide which of the following words best describes your pain or discomfort . . .

Achy, sharp, shooting, burning, tingling (pins and needles or numbness), sensitive to touch.

Use the following pages to show areas of pain that may intensify only while standing, sitting, or lying down. We would like you to rate your pain on a scale of 10 as it exists in each position.

Pain Rating Scale

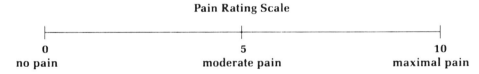

0	5	10
no pain	**moderate pain**	**maximal pain**

Thank you for your cooperation in filling out this form for us. It will further help to clarify your complaints of pain and aid us in your evaluation.

_____

* Appendix 2-1 from Mannheimer JS, Lampe GN: Clinical Transcutaneous Electrical Nerve Stimulation. p. 190–197. FA Davis, Philadelphia, 1984

PALPATION/ROM ASSESSMENTS

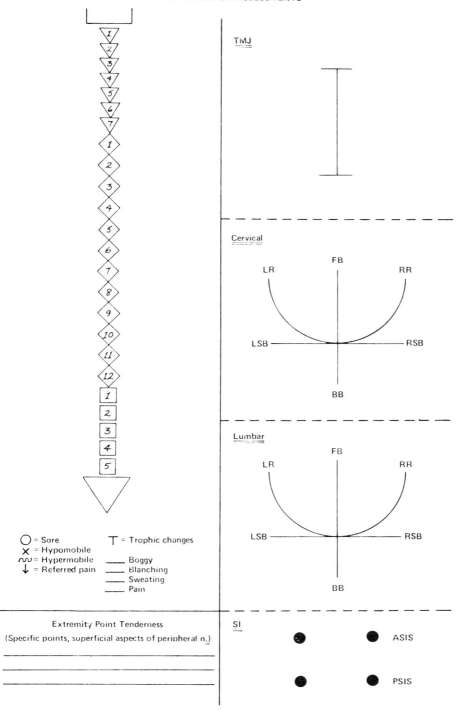

TMJ

Cervical

FB

LR   RR

LSB ——————— RSB

BB

Lumbar

FB

LR   RR

LSB ——————— RSB

BB

SI

ASIS

PSIS

○ = Sore   T = Trophic changes
✗ = Hypomobile
∿ = Hypermobile   ____ Boggy
↓ = Referred pain   ____ Blanching
                              ____ Sweating
                              ____ Pain

Extremity Point Tenderness
(Specific points, superficial aspects of peripheral n.)

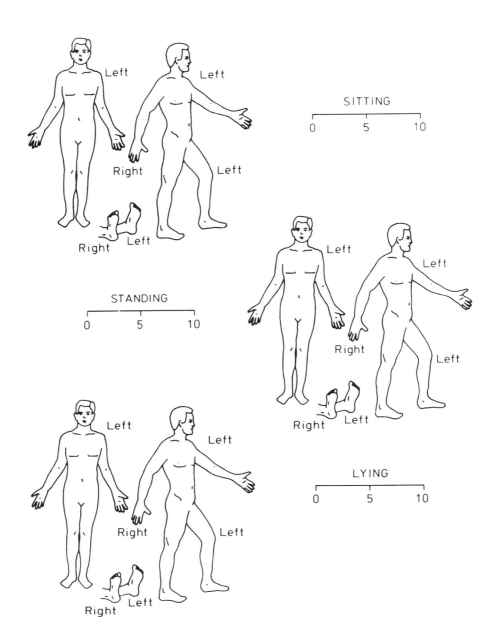

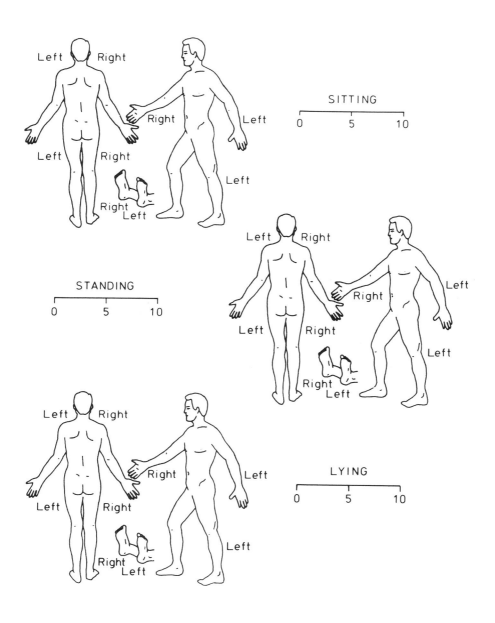

SITTING

STANDING

LYING

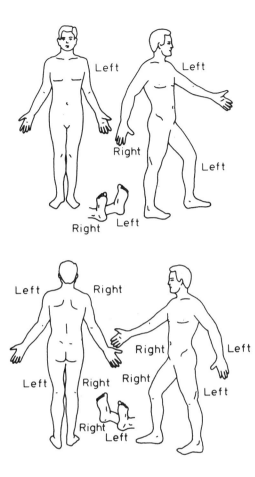

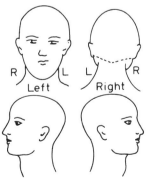

POSTURE

_____ Forward head
_____ Dowager's hump
_____ Alar scapula
_____ Round shoulders
_____ Kyphosis
_____ Scoliosis
_____ Lordosis
_____ Contractures
_____ Atrophy
_____ Leg length
_____ Edema
_____ Pronation/supination of foot

MYOTOME ASSESSMENT

Cervical _____
_____

Lumbar _____
_____

B&B signs _____

NEUROLOGIC ASSESSMENT

Sensation _____
Reflexes _____
Dural signs _____

                              DF   FB   Med Hip Rot
SLR Ⓛ _____
    Ⓡ _____
Ely _____
Ober _____
Tinel _____
Adson's _____
Other tests: _____
_____
_____
_____
_____
_____
_____
_____
Gait _____
Sitting posture _____
Walking posture _____
    Aids _____
Facial expression _____

(continued)

MOBILITY (peripheral)

TMJ _____
AC _____
SC _____
Shoulder _____
Elbow _____
Forearm _____
Wrist _____
Hand _____
Hip _____
Knee _____
Ankle _____
Foot _____
Painful arc _____
Capsular pattern _____
Pain with resistance _____
   Upon _____
   End feel _____
   Compression _____
   Distraction _____
Crepitation _____

REPEATED (SPINAL) MOTIONS

	Standing	**Lying down**
FB		
BB		
LSG		
RSG		
Compression		
Distraction		

Appendix 2-2: The Hendler 10 Minute Screening Test for Chronic Back Pain Patients[a]

1. How did the pain that you now experience occur?
   a. Sudden onset with accident or definable event. 0
   b. Slow, progressive onset without acute exacerbation. 1
   c. Slow, progressive onset with acute exacerbation without accident or event. 2
   d. Sudden onset without an accident or definable event. 3

2. Where do you experience the pain?
   a. One site, specific, well defined, consistent with anatomic distribution. 0
   b. More than one site, each well defined and consistent with anatomic distribution. 1
   c. One site, inconsistent with anatomic considerations, or not well defined. 2
   d. Vague description, more than one site, of which one is inconsistent with anatomic considerations, or not well defined or anatomically explainable. 3

[a] Compiled in conjunction with Mary Viernstein, Ph.D., Pat Gucer, B.A., M.S., and Donlin Long, M.D., Ph.D., The Chronic Pain Treatment Center, The Johns Hopkins Hospital, Baltimore, Maryland 21205 (Revised 1978). (From Hendler N: Psychological tests for chronic pain. p. 101. In Diagnosis and Nonsurgical Management of Chronic Pain. Raven Press, New York, 1981.)

3. Do you ever have trouble falling asleep at night, or are you ever awakened from sleep? If the answer is no, score 3 points and go to 4.

3a. What keeps you from falling asleep?
   a. Trouble falling asleep every night because of pain.   0
   b. Trouble falling asleep because of pain more than three times a week.   1
   c. Trouble falling asleep because of pain less than three times a week.   2
   d. No trouble falling asleep because of pain.   3
   e. Trouble falling asleep which is not related to pain.   4

3b. What awakens you from sleep?
   a. Awakened by pain every night?   0
   b. Awakened from sleep by pain more than three times a week.   1
   c. Not awakened from sleep by pain more than twice a week.   2
   d. Not awakened from sleep by pain.   3
   e. Restless sleep, or early morning awakening with or without being able to return to sleep, both unrelated to pain.   4

4. Does weather have any effect on your pain?
   a. The pain in always worse in both cold *and* damp weather.   0
   b. The pain is always worse with damp weather *or* cold weather.   1
   c. The pain is occasionally worse with cold or damp weather.   2
   d. The weather has no effect on the pain.   3

5. How would you describe the type of pain that you have?
   a. Burning, or sharp, shooting pain, or pins and needles, or coldness or numbness.   0
   b. Dull, aching pain, with occasional sharp shooting pains, not helped by heat, or experiencing hyperasthesia.   1
   c. Spasm type pain, or tension type pain, or numbness over the area, which is helped by massage or heat.   2
   d. Nagging or bothersome pain.   3
   e. Excruciating, or overwhelming, or unbearable pain, which is relieved by massage or heat.   4

6. How frequently do you have your pain?
   a. The pain is constant.   0
   b. The pain is nearly constant, 50 to 80% of the time.   1

c. The pain is intermittent, 25 to 50% of the time.   2
d. The pain is only occasionally present, less than 25% of the time.   3

7. Does movement of position have any effect on the pain?
    a. The pain is unrelieved by position change or disuse, with a history of previous operations for the pain.   0
    b. The pain is worsened by use, or standing, walking, and relieved by lying down or disuse.   1
    c. There are variable effects on the pain with position change and use.   2
    d. There is no change in the pain with use or position change, without a history of previous operations for the pain.   3

8. What medications have you used in the past month?
    a. No medications at all.   0
    b. Use of non-narcotic pain relievers or non-benzodiazepam tranquilizers or use of antidepressants.   1
    c. Less than three times a week narcotic use or hypnotic use, or benzodiazepam.   2
    d. Greater than four times a week narcotic use or hypnotic use of benzodiazepam.   3

9. What hobbies do you have, and can you still participate in them?
    a. Unable to participate in any hobbies formerly enjoyed.   0
    b. Reduced number of hobbies or activities relating to a hobby.   1
    c. Still participates in hobbies but with some discomfort.   2
    d. Participates in hobbies as before.   3

10. How frequently did you have sex and orgasms before the pain and how frequently do you have sex and orgasms now?
    a. Good sexual adjustment prior to pain (three to four times per week), with no difficulty with orgasm; now sexual contact 50% or less and coitus interrupted by pain.   0
    a1. (For people over 45)
        Good sexual adjustment (two times a week) and 50% reduction in frequency since the pain.   0
    a2. (For people over 60)
        Good sexual adjustment (sexual contact one time a week) and a 50% reduction in coitus since the pain.   0
    b. Good prepain adjustment, with no difficulty with. orgasm; now loss of interest in sex and/or difficulty with orgasm or erection.   1

c. No change in sexual activity before versus after
the pain.   2
d. Unable to have any sexual contact since the
pain, and difficulty with orgasm or erection prior
to the pain.   3
e. No sexual contact prior to the pain or absence of
orgasm prior to the pain.   4

11. Are you still (working) (doing your household
chores)?
a. Works everyday at the same prepain job, or
same level of household duties.   0
b. Works everyday but the job is not the same as
prepain job, with reduced responsibility or physi-
cal activity.   1
c. Works sporadically or reduced household
chores.   2
d. Not at work, or everyone does household
chores.   3

12. What is your income now compared to the time before your injury or the acquisition of the pain, and
what are the sources of your income?
a. Any one of the following answers scores   0
1. Experiencing financial difficulty with family
income 50% or less prepain income.
2. Was retired and still is retired.
3. Patient is still working and is not experiencing
financial difficulty.
b. Experiencing financial difficulty with family income 50 to 75% of the prepain income.   1
c. Patient unable to work, and receives some compensation so that the family income is at least
75% of the prepain income.   2
d. Patient unable to work, receives no compensation but the spouse works, and the family income
is still 75% of the prepain income.   3
e. The patient does not work, his family income
from disability or other compensation sources is
80% or higher than the gross pay before the pain,
and the spouse does not work.   4

13. Are you suing anyone, or is anyone suing you, or do
you have an attorney helping you with compensation
or disability payments?
a. No suit pending, and does not have an attorney.   0
b. Litigation is pending, but is not related to the
pain.   1
c. The patient is being sued as the result of an acci-
dent.   2

      d. Litigation is pending or workmen's compensa-
tion case with a lawyer involved.   3

14. If you had three wishes for anything in the world,
what would you wish for?
    a. "Get rid of the pain" is the only wish for all three
answers.   0
    b. "Get rid of the pain" is one of the three wishes.   1
    c. Does not mention getting rid of the pain, but has
specific wishes, usually of a personal nature,
such as acquiring more money and having a better relationship with spouse or children.   2
    d. Does not mention pain, general nonpersonal type
wishes (i.e., peace for the world).   3

15. Have you ever been depressed or thought of suicide?
    a. Admits to depression, or history of depression
secondary to pain, associated with crying episodes and thoughts of suicide.   0
    b. Admits to depression, guilt, and anger secondary
to pain.   1
    c. Prior history of depression before the pain or a
financial or personal loss prior to the pain; now
admits to some depression.   2
    d. Denies depression, crying spells, or "feeling
blue"   3
    e. History of a suicide attempt prior to the pain.   4

TOTAL

    A score of 14 points or less suggests that the patient is an objective pain patient, and is reporting a normal response to chronic pain. One may proceed surgically with this patient if indicated, and usually finds this kind of patient quite willing to participate in all modalities of therapy including exercise and supportive psychotherapy. Occasionally, a person with conversion reaction or posttraumatic neurosis will score less than 14 points since he or she experiences subjective distress on an unconscious level.

    A score of 15 to 20 points suggests the patient has features of an objective and exaggerating pain patient. This implies that a person with a poor premorbid (prepain) adjustment has an organic lesion that has produced the normal sequential psychological response to pain, but that the chronic pain produces a more extreme response.

    A score of 21 to 31 points suggests that the patient is an exaggerating pain patient. Surgical or interventional procedures may be carried out with caution, and this type of patient usually has a premorbid (prepain) personality and may utilize the complaint of chronic pain. This type of patient may benefit from a chronic pain treatment center program, with an emphasis on attitude change toward the chronic pain.

A score of 32 points or greater suggests that a psychiatric consult is needed. These patients freely admit to a great many premorbid (prepain) problems and a great deal of difficulty coping with the chronic pain they now experience. Surgical or interventional procedures should not be carried out without prior approval of a psychiatric consultant. Severe depression, suicide, and psychosis are potential problems in this group of affective pain patients.

3 | Traditional Approaches to Pain

Sandra J. Levi
George C. Maihafer

Traditionally, physical agents of heat and cold have been used by physical therapists in the treatment of painful conditions. These agents continue to be used because they appear to be successful at relieving pain. Even though their use has been popular, it was not until the last 20 years that the mechanism of pain relief has begun to be understood. A basic understanding of the way in which the application of heat and cold function in the relief of pain will allow one to selectively and appropriately apply these physical agents to bring about the maximal relief of pain.

TRADITIONAL APPROACH TO PAIN MANAGEMENT

To understand the present reliance on traditional modalities for pain management, one must first be aware of past viewpoints and therapeutic approaches taken by American health care practitioners. Pain, whether it be acute, chronic, or at any point along that spectrum, has been viewed as a symptom which should be eliminated for the benefit of the patient. Rather than emphasize pain as a tool for measuring degree of involvement, progress, or appropriateness of care, health care practitioners have often considered the relief of pain as being a primary goal in patient care. The fundamental premise in health care—to relieve suffering—has placed strong emphasis on pain control, expecting related symptoms to be corrected and controlled subsequent to this relief. The development of a wide range of drugs by the pharmaceutical industries for pain relief and their acceptance by society is an example of this belief. Physical therapy, has also emphasized pain management as one of its central roles in rehabilitation. The profession naturally turned to the energies of heat, cold, water, and electricity for answers in pain management. Taken in this context, physical therapy in the United States has been closely identified with the modality equipment it uses for pain relief. As the profession has grown and matured, specific questions regarding modality selection for pain relief have been introduced. Which modality, or even energy, works best with acute pain? Which works best with chronic pain? What are the characteristic differences between acute and chronic pain? Are the effects of our treatment for pain truly measurable? This chapter addresses these issues and hopefully, provides the clinician with a clearer understanding of the current role of traditional physical agents in the relief of pain.

THERAPEUTIC HEAT AND COLD IN THE RELIEF OF PAIN

The degree to which pain is amenable to treatment by heat and cold modalities will depend on the type of pain and its cause. Delta-fiber pain, C-fiber pain, and visceral pain should be differentiated from each other.

A-delta fibers are large diameter, myelinated fibers on which impulses travel rapidly. *Delta* fibers have an average diameter of 3 μm, and the average conduction velocity is 18 to 20 m/sec. The patient perceives this type of pain to have a rapid onset and to be "pins and needles" or stinging in nature. This type of pain is associated with acute conditions such as localized trauma. Physical agents, particularly cold applications, may have a limited role in the modulation of this type of pain.

C fibers have a small diameter and are unmyelinated. C fibers are .5 to 2 μm in diameter and their average conduction velocity is .5 to 2 m/sec. Because impulses travel slowly on these fibers, this type of pain has a slow onset. The patient perceives this type of pain to be burning in nature. Concomitant significant biologic and psychological problems are common with C-fiber pain. In addition to the increased heart rate, blood pressure, and sweating associated with the autonomic nervous system's response to acute pain, psychological symptoms such as anxiety, depression, and fear often influence the perception of pain. C-fiber pain may often be modified by heat or cold treatments.

Visceral pain is associated with the autonomic nervous system. This type of pain is perceived as an ache and is indicative of a problem in the patient's internal organs. Treatment of the underlying condition, rather than pain modulation, is generally of primary concern in patients with visceral pain, although heat application may have some value in the management of this type of pain.

An understanding of the mechanism of thermal stimulation is important in understanding how physical agents influence pain. When a thermal stimulus is applied to a local area of skin, the change in temperature is registered on temperature receptors. Thermal receptors are stimulated by a change in metabolic activity; cold decreases metabolic activity and heat increases it. Thermal detection is a result of chemical stimulation and not physical stimulation.

The ability to perceive a thermal stimulus varies with the type and concentration of receptors. There are three to four times as many cold receptors as heat receptors in skin. The concentration of these temperature receptors varies with the part of the body. The lips have 15 to 20 times more receptors per square inch than the broad surfaces of the body. In contrast, the fingers have three to five times more receptors per square inch than the broad body surfaces. The perception of heat and cold is determined by the relative amounts of temperature receptors stimulated. Therefore a .1°C temperature change can be detected if the whole body is stimulated, but a 1°C change may not be detected if applied to a very small area.

Thermal signals are carried by almost the same pathways as pain signals. The large diameter, myelinated A-delta fibers and the small diameter, unmyelinated C fibers also carry temperature signals. They travel a few segments up or down in the track of Lissauer (posterolateral fasciculus) and terminate mainly in lamina I, II, and III of the dorsal horns. They then cross and travel in the anterolateral spinal thalamic tract of the spinal cord to the reticular area of the brain stem, the hypothalmus, and a few other associated nuclei. The anterior hypothalmus deals with heat stress whereas the posterior hypothalmus controls cold regulation.

As mentioned previously, C-fiber pain has associated biologic and psychological components. Musculoskeletal pain of this type may be reduced by the effect of heat or cold on some of these components. Aspects to be considered in the application of physical agents include the pathology causing the pain, secondary muscle spasm, ischemia resulting from tension conditions, and the sensory input being perceived by the patient.

The effect of heat and cold on the pathology underlying a painful condition should be considered when applying a physical agent. The application of heat to a part can be used to stimulate and enhance normal tissue function. It is assumed that the restoration of normal tissue function will influence the pain associated with a pathologic condition. Local tissue temperature above 45°C and below 13°C are associated with tissue necrosis.[1] Therefore, the aim of treatment is to provide a limited tissue temperature change that is great enough to alter tissue function, but is small enough to prevent tissue damage. One aspect of the traditional approach to the treatment of pain involves the influence of heat and cold directly on the tissue pathology.

Muscle spasm is commonly associated with painful areas. A pain–muscle spasm–more pain–more muscle spasm cycle is created. Physical agents can be used to reduce the pain associated with muscle spasm. As a result the escalation of pain due to muscle spasms can often be controlled.

In tension conditions, pain and ischemia may be related. Heat is known to increase local circulation, and cold has increased circulation as a latent effect. A physical agent may be used to control pain by altering local blood flow.

Heat and cold modalities may also influence pain perception by providing a counterirritant to the painful stimuli. According to the gate theory of Melzack and Wall,[2] a person's perception of pain is modulated by the amount of competing sensory stimulation. It follows that if the afferent system is flooded with sensory input from a heat or cold physical agent, the perception of pain would be reduced.

The challenge to the physical therapist is to determine what type of physical agent at which treatment dosage will provide the maximal pain relief.

CLINICAL COMPARISONS OF ACUTE AND CHRONIC PAIN

The defining of acute versus chronic pain and their respective clinical manifestations, has been a dilemma for physical therapists in their practices. When does an acute pain patient cross over into the chronic pain category? Some clinicians may use time as the deciding factor. Acute pain may exist from 48 to 72 hours, at which point, the patient is considered in the subacute stage; the subacute stage may extend for 2 to 3 weeks, until chronic pain manifestations take place. The time schedule may be different for some clinicians, but it has provided physical therapists with practical boundaries, based on a predetermined criterion, by which they may classify their patients' response. Unfortunately, this rather simplistic method has too much generalization to apply to many patients reporting pain. A time schedule doesn't take into account possibilities of reinjury, exacerbations, factors specific to age or pathology, or even individual's general tolerances and responses to pain.

More recent attempts by Bonica[3] and Sternbach[4] to differentiate acute versus chronic pain by physiologic responses and patient behavior appear to be more useful to the physical therapist. As is discussed later in this chapter, Bonica's research has devised three categories of chronic pain based on the physical sites or psychological gain to the patient. Sternbach reports that acute and chronic pain can be accurately categorized according to their characteristics, with longevity being one of the criteria. Acute pain has a sudden onset and short duration. The patient frequently exhibits heightened sympathetic nervous system responses such as increased blood pressure and temperature and sweating. The patient is usually able to localize the pain at or near the lesion. The pathology usually is easily diagnosed, treated, and resolved, since the pain is performing its normal biologic function as a protective mechanism or danger sign.

In contrast, chronic pain's onset is weeks or months after the injury, with a duration which may extend into years. The pain is frequently referred away from the lesion, serving no biologic purpose or meaning. The chronic pain patient may become depressed, lethargic, or hypochondriacal, with long standing abuse of medications noted. The chronic pain patient may have incorporated the pain into his normal life style, making accurate assessment of treatment effects difficult to determine. Reliance on a single, traditional modality approach for the chronic pain patient is generally unsuccessful, since active patient participation, attitudinal changes, and lifestyle adjustments are essential for pain relief.

Certain modalities are used with greater success in the relief of acute pain or as adjunct therapy in a comprehensive approach to chronic pain treatment. Most authors agree[1,5] that all of the traditional modalities may play a role in the subacute stage of pain, in varying degrees based on clinical evaluation of symptoms. Feibel and Fast report that the deep heating of joint structures result in tissue temperature rises typical of joint inflammatory diseases.[6] They propose, therefore, that careful consideration should be taken before diathermy is applied to relieve chronic pain in joints (e.g., rheumatoid arthritis). Table 3-1 is a representative chart of various pain relief modalities, with suggested applications. Care should be taken whenever applying standardized approaches to individual patients. A thorough understanding of the underlying pathology and its response to heating is necessary before modality application commences.

Table 3-1. Pain Relief Modalities

Modality	Depth of Penetration	Treatment Applications for Pain
Infrared lamp	3 mm	Ideal for acute injuries due to sedatitive affects. Consensual heating properties allow reflex heating when circulatory impairment is present.
Paraffin	3 mm	Most effective for distal segments in acute or chronic pain conditions. Its ability to block external stimuli, soften tissues and promote significant temperature increases superficially are the greatest assets.
Hot packs	3 mm	Especially effective when selective heating of the subcutaneous tissue is desired as in the treatment of pain due to muscle spasms.
Cold packs	3 mm	Especially effective for chronic pain and when heating modalities are contraindicated.
Shortwave diathermy	1–3 cm	Ideal for subacute stages when deep heating is required. Equipment tends to be costly with greatest number of precautions/contraindications. Should not be used over joints in chronic stages.
Microwave diathermy	1–5 cm in presence of <1 cm fat layer	Very effective modality for deep heating in subacute and chronic soft tissue injury. Like SWD, similar precautions must be taken.
Ultrasound	3–5 cm	Very effective modality for deep heating of structures. It can safely be used in the presence of large layers of subcutaneous fat and in the presence of most metal implants.

CLINICAL EVALUATION OF PAIN

Bonica classifies chronic pain patients, and their perception into three categories: (1) persistent peripheral noxious stimulants, (2) neuraxis pain, and (3) learned pain behavior.[3] The first group includes patients with pain symptoms related to peripheral structures that may encompass systemic disorders or be local in origin (i.e., cancer, arthritis). Group two includes peripheral or central nervous system dysfunction resulting in direct neurologic affects on pain. Group three encompasses those patients who receive secondary gain from their symptoms of pain.[1] In clinical practice these categories may become mixed, with signs and symptoms often fitting all three classifications.[7]

To the clinical practitioner, recent developments in the evaluation techniques used by orthopedic physical therapists (see Ch. 5) may assist in assessment of chronic or acute pain patients. The information gathered during the history and subjective-objective examination may provide a more reliable rationale for conventional modality selection. Kaltenborn stresses the importance of obtaining a detailed clinical picture of the patient's immediate painful symptoms.[8] During the initial examination, the clinician identifies the localization of pain through the use of a body chart. The original onset and characteristics of the pain are also clearly defined through specific clarification by the patient. Questions dealing with influence on the pain (what causes or affects the pain?) and pain associations (what symptoms accompany the pain?) provide additional information which becomes critical when assessing a modality's effect on pain. Additional questions which will affect the choice of modality selection are those dealing with relief (what improves the patient's condition?) related or similar symptoms, and the effect of pain on normal bodily functions. Questions involving level of activity, social and medical history, and occupation will provide critical information to the clinician in planning the treatment regimen. A careful interview of the patient will identify the boundaries of the painful behavior and perhaps help eliminate the use of ineffective modalities.

Selection of a treatment modality should not be made by the trial and error approach, rather physical agents should be selected by cross matching the specific characteristics of a painful condition with predictable results of the application of a particular physical agent on that condition. To achieve the successful responses desired in the application of modalities for pain relief, a careful re-examination and interview is essential. The authors recommend the re-evaluation be made at the completion of the modality's application, approximately 30 minutes later and 24 to 48 hours following to determine where treatment modifications are needed. Ongoing evaluation during the course of treatment gives the therapist the essential information required to assess long term benefits. The lack of follow-up evaluation often results in confusion, frustration, or indecision on the appropriate plan of action in treatment for pain relief.

A detailed understanding of the physical effects, both local and systemic, of conventional modalities, is necessary for the successful treatment of pain behavior. Likewise, the physical manifestations and characteristics of pain must be readily understood during the initial patient evaluation. Previous chapters have dealt with the neurophysiologic response to pain and the current methods of measurement. How the patient responds to painful stimuli and, in turn, reports these symptoms, will affect the choice of modality selection.

Campbell and Laheurta have classified three distinct categories of nociceptor nerve fibers that pain produces.[9] The first responds only to strong mechanical stimuli; the second responds to both noxious mechanical and noxious heat stimuli; and the third category of polymodel nociceptors representing 90 percent of all afferent C fibers responds to mechanical, chemical, heat, and cold stimuli. Their study of pain-producing thresholds found that frequencies of 1.5/sec of electrical stimulation were always perceived by their subjects as painful. In conclusion, however, they determined that no single experimental test with accurate measurements could be correlated with the clinical assessment of pain.

GENERAL CONTRAINDICATIONS

The first rule of health care ethics is to cause the patient no harm. Heat and cold modalities are contraindicated for some patients. Heat generally should not be used (1) during the first 48 hours following trauma, (2) in acute conditions that are exacerbated by heat, or (3) in the very young because of their immature thermoregulatory systems.

Neither heat nor cold should be used over an area of impaired sensation or an area of circulatory impairment, in the presence of a severe cardiac or respiratory condition, and for people who cannot be relied on to report signs of adverse responses to treatment. Contraindications to specific physical agents will be addressed when the agent is reviewed.

INFRARED ENERGIES

Very little research to date has directly measured, in quantitative terms, the effect of infrared irradiation on the nociceptive response system. The few studies reported in the literature during the past 50 years have measured local temperature changes, blood flow differences, or have provided descriptive endorsements for the palliative measures achieved through application of infrared irradiation.[5] In recent years, infrared lamps have rarely been selected by physical therapists as the modality of preference in the treatment of painful conditions. Today, this modality is more often utilized in the management of other patient problems such as drying wounds and temperature regulation of treatment environment.

When application of infrared energy is determined to be appropriate, most clinics now utilize hot packs or paraffin. Massage and whirlpool also are commonly used in pain management.[10] Reasons for the decline in use of infrared lamps include (1) the limitation of penetration of the heat source as tissue temperature rises have been reported at only a depth of 3 mm, (2) the lack of control of external stimuli (air currents) to the painful area, and (3) the patient's psychological need for a more direct or dramatic treatment response to his report of pain.

Infrared energy is theorized to be an effective modality in pain management when pain etiology is suspected to be of local and superficial origin. Receptors found in the superficial skin may be stimulated above pain threshold levels when trauma or dysfunction results in cell damage with subsequent release of proteolytic enzymes. The enzymes, in turn split bradykinin from the globulins found in interstitial fluid. Bradykinin, once released, is a powerful vasoconstrictor, increasing capillary permeability, while stimulating pain receptors.[11] In theory, infrared energy increases superficial metabolic and phagocytic activity with an accompanying increase in leucocytic migration. A more direct rationale for infrared energy's role in pain control may lie in its relationship to superficial blood flow. Muscle spasm increases the local metabolic rate, while decreasing blood flow results in an accumulated oxygen debt (i.e., ischemia). It has been noted that, superficially, infrared energy increases blood flow, thereby relieving any superficial ischemia present. In addition, it is postulated that relief and relaxation of deeper structures (muscles) may be achieved through the reflex arc mechanism.[7] Studies have been performed which dispute the infrared energy's affect on deep ischemia; demonstrating an actual decline in deep blood flow during the first 10 minutes of superficial heating and tissue temperature rise.[1] Because of its past clinical importance and its unique characteristics of the infrared energies, a review of the clinical management of pain through the use of infrared lamps is still worthy of further consideration.

Infrared Lamps

The transfer of heat energy from an infrared source to an object is an example of radiation. Infrared therapy is the oldest form of heat application for pain. The Greeks and Romans constructed solaria to use the sun's rays for therapeutic treatment.[7] Infrared irradiation is found to exhibit wave lengths from 7,600 to 150,000 angstrom units. This zone of the electromagnetic spectrum is subdivided into a near infrared (7,600 nm–15,000 nm) and far infrared (15,000–150,000 nm) (Fig. 3-1). The effect of far infrared rays on subjects is a selective heating and tissue temperature rise of the surface epidermis. Because of the poor vascular supply to the epidermis, poor dissipation of the heat results; this causes a counterirritant reaction with eventual local tissue damage.[12] For this reason, infrared lamps used in clinics are found to utilize the near infrared spectrum. Infrared energy absorption, in addition to being governed by the wavelength of irradiation, is also affected by the intensity and distance of light source from the treated body part. The inverse square law states that the level of intensity of infrared irradiation varies inversely with the square of the distance from the source. In practical application, an infrared lamp placed 30 inches from the patient will increase its intensity fourfold if moved to 15 inches from the treated area. Lambert's Cosine Law stipulates

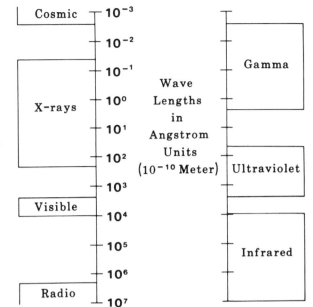

Fig. 3-1. Zone of electro-magnetic spectrum.

that the energy intensity is proportional to the cosine of the angle between the light source beam and perpendicular to the treated part (Fig. 3-2).[5] These two laws, when controlled by the discerning clinician, highlight the versatility and treatment opportunities for application of infrared energy for pain management. Patients who are unable to tolerate rapid or high tissue temperature rises over a 20 minute treatment due to lowered ability for thermal dissipation, or general discomfort, may tolerate a more gradual, carefully controlled application of infrared at a greater distance or angle for a longer period of time.

One form of treatment for pain management which is somewhat unique for infrared energies, is the use of irradiation for consensual heating. Again, literature and research have not thoroughly investigated this phenomenon. Clinical use of infrared lamps for consensual heating is not a treatment frequently reported in the literature nor a procedure often observed in the clinic. The direct heating of a large body segment resulting in a significant local rise in superficial tissue temperature, often causes an indirect elevated temperature of tissues not found in the field of treatment application. In a practical example, application of infrared rays to the cervico-thoracic region may result in achieving the same effects, albeit to a lesser degree, in the lumbosacral or lower extremity region. Downey noted that afferent nerve impules from the skin receptors pass to the central nervous system via C fibers and/or the sympathetic nervous system.[13] Distal increases of blood flow or temperature or decreased gamma fiber activity may occur due to the response of a reflex arc or higher levels of temperature control found in the hypothalamus. One study by Newton and Lehmkuhl analyzed the muscle spindle response to localized ap-

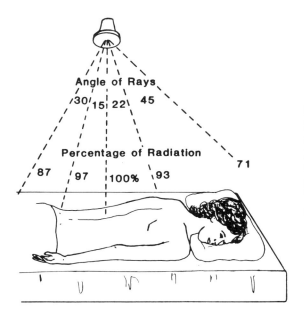

Fig. 3-2. Law of the Cosine for infrared radiation application. (Licht S: History of Therapeutic Heat and Cold. p. 11. In Lehmann JF (ed): Therapeutic Heat and Cold. 3rd Ed. © 1982 The Williams & Wilkins Co., Baltimore.)

plication of ice versus consensual heating by infrared lamps.[14] The frequency of action potential firing (recorded over the dorsal root filaments) was increased during an elevated body temperature of 40°C, and decreased during a reduced temperature of 10°C. The greatest reduction of spasticity due to muscle spindle excitability occurred when the muscle was cooled locally while the overall body temperature was maintained through consensual heating. This, therefore, calls into question the role that infrared and muscle spindle response, through reflex action, plays in pain management. If pain is caused by muscle spindle excitability and action potential firing, local cold applications appear to be indicated over the use of infrared irradiation. The latter's role in consensual heating may assist in achieving the desired effects, however, by maintaining overall body temperature.

An additional characteristic or response to infrared irradiation is the overall psychological perception, by the patient, of sedation. General sedation is a term or symptom which has not been quantitatively defined or analyzed. It is postulated that a general decrease in sympathetic activity accompanies the perception of this sedation. The use of infrared irradiation, applied locally and for consensual effects, causes the sedative quality expressed by patients. This may be the underlying justification for infrared application to decrease pain.

The strongest indication for the use of infrared in consensual heating conditions is for those individuals who, due to peripheral vascular or neurologic disorders, are unable to tolerate direct local application of infrared, without risking possible tissue damage. Upon assessment of the patient's conditions, infrared lamp therapy may be indicated, but the segment's ability to readily dissipate heat is found to be impaired. Increased vasodilation and superficial tissue relaxation of the lower extremities may be achieved by heating large areas of the back through consensual heating. Infrared irradiation should be the modality preferred for pain relief for patients who, for various reasons, are unable to tolerate direct contact application of the other infrared energy modalities.[1] This restriction may be due to hypersensitivity of the pressure mechanoreceptors which transmit responses along the same neuroaxial system as pain. The observation that the other forms of superficial heat tend to precipitate a greater local sweating response from patients, which may irritate the skin, eventually resulting in rashes or eczema, may also indicate the need to use infrared irradiation.

Infrared lamp therapy has been used clinically for preventive measures in pain management as a result of over exposure to ultraviolet rays. Various reports have documented infrared therapy as either enhancing or dispersing the potency of ultraviolet applications. Montgomery evaluated the compounding effects of infrared and ultraviolet irradiation upon normal skin.[15] Four scenarios involving the sequencing and amount of application of these two modalities were assessed. The results were inconclusive; subjects' erythemal effects were enhanced and diminished in each case of application. The author suggests that greater investigation into this question is required before treatment recommendations can be made.

In summary, infrared irradiation is a modality which offers the clinician a varied range of treatment options when superficial heating is indicated. The preference of moist heat or ice in pain management by therapists and patients alike have limited the scope of infrared lamps use in recent years. Further research into the consensual heating effects on human subjects, measurement of local application on pain thresholds, and infrared's role in relationship to ultraviolet rays would provide clinicians with more accurate information when determining treatment selection. The rule of applying cold to acute injuries and various forms of heat to chronic problems is still prevalent and practiced in the clinic. Current literature supports this premise, but further study is necessary before we can determine infrared irradiation's direct affect on the many different types of pain presented to the clinical practitioner today.

Hot Packs

Hot water and other forms of conductive heating have been used to relieve pain since man learned how to build and utilize fires. The modern form of heat packs were developed in the 1940s. Today, a hot pack consists of a series of attached pouches in which a form of silicon dioxide has been placed. The packs are manufactured in a variety of shapes and sizes as are the hot water storage units. Silicon dioxide has an affinity for water and each molecule has the capacity to absorb approximately 17 water molecules. Hot packs, therefore, approximate water in their thermal characteristics.

Hot packs are generally stored in thermostatically controlled hot water units until they are to be used. The thermostat is set so that the temperature is maintained between 65 and 90°C. The application of water temperatures greater than 45°C cause tissue damage. Special covers or dry towelling is placed around hot packs to prevent skin burn and to slow hot pack cooling. The initial temperature of a hot pack should be at least 65°C due to the rapid cooling that occurs when hot packs are removed from hot water. If a hot pack will not be used for an extended period of time, it should be placed in a plastic bag and stored in a freezer.

Hot packs provide intense superficial heating. Their use is indicated when selective heating of the skin and subcutaneous tissue is desired, such as in the treatment of muscle spasm. Hot packs are especially useful in pain management because with proper application other external environmental stimuli, such as air currents, are eliminated. The expected result is that skin should feel warm after a few minutes and that hyperemia may appear. If the 5-minute check indicates either mottling or coolness, the layers of towelling need to be increased or decreased accordingly. The maximal skin temperature rise occurs at about 8 minutes, and the usual treatment duration is 20 to 30 minutes.[16]

There are relatively few contraindications to the use of hot packs other than those commonly associated with the general use of heat. Hot packs should not be applied to an area of acute inflammation or trauma, or to a patient who is unable to perceive or report heat sensation normally. The major contraindication specific to hot packs is treatment in the area of a skin infection that may be exacerbated by water or heat.[17]

Paraffin

The law of specific energies is frequently used as justification whenever any conventional modality is applied for pain relief. Simply stated, any particular sense organ will transmit only one unique sensation, no matter what stimuli is used to obtain the response.[3] Building on this theory further, Fischer and Solomon suggest that when there is more than one form of sensory stimulation (e.g., heat and pain), the body's perception of either is substantially reduced. This has been substantiated by quantitatively measuring the diminished response to pin prick following local heat application.[18] The use of paraffin for treatment of locally perceived pain peripherally, is an excellent example of clinical applications to these principles. Paraffin, like infrared and hot packs, has enjoyed widespread use throughout medical history. During the early 1900s the first descriptions of paraffin baths and their widespread popular acceptance in British hospitals were reported in the literature.[5] The therapeutic use of paraffin today is confined, for the most part, to applications of the distal segments (hand or feet). Treatment indications reported have included patients exhibiting subacute, chronic, traumatic, and inflammatory conditions, especially arthritis. Limitation of motion due to postoperative or immobilization conditions also are frequent indications for paraffin. Application of paraffin is another method of delivering infrared energy specifically to areas that are difficult to heat with anything other than a liquid medium. In addition to exhibiting the properties discussed under infrared irradiation, paraffin greatly increases local perspiration, softens the skin, and promotes a stronger hyperemia.[17]

The three most commonly reported methods of paraffin application are immersion bath, dip followed by immersion, and the glove technique.[1,12,16,17] during the *immersion* method, the segment is lowered into the paraffin bath and held in position for 20 minutes. Care must be taken that the patient not come into direct contact with the machine's heating plates, usually found at the bottom of the tank. This method is the most effective in raising the local tissue temperature to higher levels and consequently, superficial burns may occur if careful monitoring is not observed. The *dip-immersion* method allows the patient to dip the body segment two or three times, building up a wax layer, followed by the 20 minute immersion. Although not as effective as the first technique at elevating tissue temperatures, the dip-immersion method is often more easily tolerated by patients. The *glove technique* allows the patient to dip the segment eight to twelve times, forming a wax glove which is then wrapped in plastic or wax paper and a terry cloth towel to maintain the heat.

Contraindications for paraffin treatments reported in the literature include open wounds, skin infections, acute conditions, sensory loss of the body segment being treated, heat sensitive patients, and peripheral vascular disease.[17] Some patients may experience uncomfortable itching, or even tickling sensations following paraffin applications. Since these perceptions are carried along the same nerve endings as pain, this phenomenom tends to support the law of specific energies and must be taken into account when pain management is the goal of the clinician.

The specific heat of paraffin combined with mineral oil is .45 in relationship to that of water. When cooling, there is less specific energy transmitted to surrounding tissues, thereby allowing the temperature of paraffin baths to safely exceed that of whirlpool or other infrared modalities during application. Paraffin baths are generally maintained at 53 to 54° C for hand treatments. Slightly lower temperatures are advised when used in treating feet, because of the diminished ability to transfer heat in the lower extremities. Patients with chronic pain have reported and perceived greater benefits in relief from the use of paraffin rather than whirlpool or infrared irradiation. Griffin hypothosizes that, in paraffin, the cutaneous pain receptors are cut off from external stimuli if a solid layer is build up by repeated immersion to a thickness of 5 mm or more.[1] In addition, the insulating capability of paraffin decreases the amount of heat loss through evaporation during treatment, providing longer relief time and a greater local rise in tissue temperatures. Further investigation into the various modes of paraffin application and whirlpool on chronic pain patients would greatly assist the substantiation of these theories. Certainly paraffin controls evaporative heat loss by preventing perspiration to escape during treatment and preventing air currents to flow directly over moist skin.

Thermosensitive receptors in the skin have an electrical discharge with a frequency dependent on absolute temperatures of the skin. A change in local temperature will result in a change in receptor activity. The afferent nerve impulses pass directly to the central nervous system via C fibers or the sympathetic nerves.[18] Blood flow to the skin of the hand is primarily controlled by sympathetic vasoconstrictor nerves. The increased blood flow noted during and immediately after the application of paraffin is accomplished by a corresponding inhibition of tone of the vasoconstrictor nerves. The sympathetic vasoconstrictors are felt to be directly controlled and responsive to local heating. If pain relief is directly a result of improved circulation, a direct correlation between pain relief and inhibition of the sympathetic nervous system is also apparent.

The relief of pain by removing adhesions or restrictions of periarticular structures is a commonly accepted practice. Often clinicians speak of the vital and direct role paraffin plays in improving passive, physiologic motion. Hamilton investigated the use of heat, cold, and exercise in the mobilization of the proximal interphalangeal joint of 27 hand patients, each presenting with soft tissue restrictions.[19] He found a significant gain in passive motion was obtained by the use of passive range of motion techniques, with no significant change in motion noted when either cold or paraffin modalities were applied. The use of paraffin for improvement of range may be best be described, therefore, by its role of decreasing pain, thereby allowing range to be achieved without spasm or discomfort.

As with the other modalities, further investigation into paraffin's role in pain management is indicated. Study of its local effect on pain nerve fiber endings and reflex activity within the central nervous system would provide the clinician with a greater understanding of this modality's role. The importance placed on the isolation of the painful extremity from external stimuli by using paraffin rather than other conventional modalities is also an area of investigation which could provide us with more clues to the efficacious treatment of pain.

Fluidotherapy

Fluidotherapy is a relatively new modality in physical therapy clinics. It consists of a unit in which hot air is blown through a mass of very fine solids. This semisolid material acts like a liquid, but provides dry heat. Heat transfer occurs by convection. The dosage to the extremity is determined by the temperature of the air and by the duration of the treatment.

Fluidotherapy should be considered to be a form of superficial heat, similar to hot packs and paraffin. It has been shown to be effective in causing a tissue temperature rise in the capsules of hand joints.[20] It causes a greater tissue temperature rise than the dip method of paraffin and a 39°C whirlpool. It is not known whether fluidotherapy has better pain relieving qualities than other forms of superficial heat but indications and contraindications for its use correspond to those for the use of paraffin.

SHORTWAVE DIATHERMY

Diathermy has been described as energy transferred into deeper tissue layers by a high frequency current. The heating transfer is accomplished by means of conversion, where the energy penetrating these structures is converted into heat.[12] With the development, at the turn of the century, of high frequency currents and the manufacture of commercial equipment for clinical application, the heating of deeper tissues for pain relief became a reality. Original units required spark gaps for current generation; electrodes were designed of flexible metal plates which required a lubricant for safe application. Frequent electrical burns and inconsistencies in current levels were hinderances toward effective widespread use.[1] In the 1930s the Federal Communications Commission (FCC) undertook the regulation of current and power output requirements for all diathermy units. Present day shortwave diathermy functions at a frequency of 27.12 MHz with a .6 percent allowable fluctuation in performance.[21] Secondary frequencies of 13.56 and 40.68 MHz with .05 percent fluctuation were also authorized as acceptable.

Any electric current has the property of generating both an electrical and a magnetic field. Tissues exhibiting high fat levels will resist and, hence, absorb the energy generated from the electrical field, converting it into heat. Tissues of higher electrolyte content (e.g., muscles and tendons) will oscillate when subjected to a high magnetic field and be heated in the process. Taking into consideration the dual properties exhibited by shortwave diathermy, careful and correct application of this modality will cause local tissue rises in temperature at a depth of penetration of 2 to 3 cm.[22] Failure of technique and application of the modality to patients with 1 cm or more of subcutaneous fat, will result in heat absorption in the superficial fat layers to dangerous levels with little or no effect on the underlying deeper structures. In recent years, solid state circuitry has greatly enhanced the ease of this modality's application and the beneficial effects achieved by the magnetic field's penetration.[1]

Most literature describes present diathermy units as being either condensor or induction coil types. In the condensor technique, the body segment to be treated is placed between two capacitor plates and becomes part of the circuit. Air space plates, glass enclosed capacitor plates, rubber or plastic condensor pads, and internally inserted metal electrodes are variations of capacitor plates used in this technique. The induction coil type has the complete circuitry rigidly housed within the unit. A drum or monode electrode would be examples of the equipment used in induction coil application. With the exceptions of vaginal or rectal applications, dosage levels are dependent on body tissues' composition and therefore cannot be accurately predicted. Rather, optimal dosage is determined by the patient's subjective feelings of warmth and the therapist's careful observation of any superficial reactions.

Most sources agree shortwave diathermy's greatest effect is in relieving chronic pain due to skeletal muscle or subcutaneous tissue involvement, when improving local circulation and decreasing spasm is indicated.[1,12,16] Due to its ability to penetrate deeper tissue layers, shortwave diathermy is preferred over the infrared energy modalities when deeper tissues are suspected to be the origin of pain. Like infrared irradiation, towelling is used to absorb perspiration during treatment, and is indicated for those patients who exhibit dermatologic reactions during skin hydration.

Shortwave diathermy has also been reported to be effective in the treatment of pelvic and rectal inflammatory diseases. Of the 100 patients diagnosed with pelvic inflammatory disease in Cherry's report, 72 percent were entirely relieved of symptoms after receiving treatments of 30 minute duration with vaginal local tissue temperature rises of 42 to 43°C.[23] The pelvic region has been shown to tolerate greater temperature applications due to the well developed circulation surrounding the vaginal walls. Conductive heating, as seen in infrared applications, however, is ineffective due to the insulating capacity of the pelvic fat and muscle.[16] The internal diathermy electrodes are equipped with a temperature gauge, so dosage levels of diathermy can be more accurately determined during application. Pelvic diathermy dosages should result in tissue temperatures of 40 to 42°C to be effective in these cases. Shortwave diathermy application for relief of pain in rectal or vaginal conditions is rarely performed in clinics today.[24] The lack of understanding of its effects by physicians resulting in few referrals, the emphasis on pharmaceutical therapies, and the clinicians' personal preferences against this treatment application are the probable causes.

The use of electromagnetic waves to generate heat in tissues carries with it the responsibility of understanding the many contraindications specific to this mode of treatment. Any metal within the electromagnetic field will concentrate the energy at that point. This includes external metal devices (metal in tables, chairs, watches, jewelry) and internal appliances (plates, arthroplasties, screws). Diathermy application is also strongly contraindicated in patients with cardiac pacemakers. It is also contraindicated during pregnancy and menstruation, over epiphysial plates of children, and in patients with malignancies. In addition, the general contraindication for heat modalities also apply.[1,16,17]

The effects of shortwave diathermy on tissues at the local site of treatment include elevation in temperature, greater capillary permeability, enzyme activity changes, and decrease in muscle spindle sensitivity to stretch. In the clinic, pain relief is associated with the relaxation of muscle spasm following heat application. Shortwave diathermy has also been reported to improve tendon extensibility and increase pain thresholds of peripheral nerves' area of supply.[25] Effects and reactions occurring distant to the site of application have been reported to include consensual heating of distant tissues, initial vasoconstriction of blood vessels of deeper tissues, decreased peristalsis, and general relaxation and sedation of striated muscles.[26,27]

McCray and Patton measured pain relief at trigger points of patients, comparing moist heat and shortwave diathermy's effect.[10] The measurement tool was a pressure algometer calibrated in kilograms. Nineteen subjects with 31 trigger points were examined, and the researchers determined that the trigger points were divided clinically into two types. The sensitive type reported moderate pain at 2,000 g or less; trigger points withstanding greater force were classified as the moderate type. "Moderate levels of pain" were determined in a functional ability context. Moderate pain as described to the patients would be of such intensity that the subject would be unable to read a paper or write a letter without seeking relief. The results indicated that both modalities relieved the sensitive trigger point types. In reviewing the results of the moderate trigger point pain relief, shortwave diathermy was superior to hot packs at the statistical level of .0581.

Shortwave diathermy does not enjoy as widespread a use in clinical practice as it did in the 1940s and 1950s. The advent of ultrasound, with its greater ease of application and deeper penetration, has affected the modality preference for pain relief in deeper tissues. Additionally, the number and potential severity of injuries with improper use have left many therapists wary of shortwave diathermy application. Further research into the direct affects of shortwave diathermy on pain receptors, tendon extensibility, and muscle spindle activity appears warranted. The more recent advances of solid state circuitry, enhancing the magnetic field's effect on deeper tissues, should also be further examined in relationship to its effects on pain management. Comparative studies of diathermy as opposed to other modalities (hot packs, ultrasound, etc.) still may reveal important differences in pain control for certain specific conditions as illustrated by the McCray study.[10]

MICROWAVE DIATHERMY

Microwave diathermy has been in clinical use since the late 1940s and early 1950s. In comparison to shortwave diathermy, microwave has a much higher frequency with a corresponding shorter wavelength. In patients with ≤0.5 cm of fat, microwave has the ability to penetrate and cause tissue temperature rises at the 5 cm depth. The main reason reported for the efficiency of this penetration is that no energy is lost between the oscillating circuit and transmitting antenna. Furthermore, only 10 percent or less of the electromagnetic energy is lost between the transmitting antenna and the patient, because microwave has the characteristic of focusing the wavelengths produced. Treatment contraindications are the same as for shortwave diathermy.

When deeper tissues are the origin of the painful stimulus, microwave may be the preferred modality over shortwave diathermy, because (1) the depth of penetration is greater and (2) a greater volume of tissue/unit area is absorbing the energy transmitted, diminishing the possibility of burns due to poor heat dissipation.[28] Recent advances in modality design, using frequencies of 915 MHz have diminished the electric field's effects and decreased the change of superficial burns.[29-31] The closer the transmitting antenna is to the patient, the greater the amount of energy absorbed and the smaller the area treated. Microwave diathermy may be preferred over ultrasound when pain relief of muscle spasm is desired, and pressure on superficial mechanoreceptors of the skin due to sound head contact elicits pain.

Farrell and Twomey compared the effects of microwave and abdominal strengthing exercises versus spinal mobilization/manipulation techniques on 48 patients diagnosed with acute low back pain.[32] By evaluating eight pain indicators, significantly less pain was perceived by the group receiving mobilization rather than microwave 1 week after therapy had commenced. By the third week, the researchers reported no significant differences between either group's pain perception.

Microwave is used less frequently in clinical practice than ultrasound therapy. The FCC demands a plus or minus two percent frequency tolerance on all manufactured microwave units presently. The cost of microwave units designed with such accuracy has limited their manufacturing and purchasing in comparison to ultrasound. Further research into the short and long term effects of microwave in comparison to ultrasound would provide practitioners needed data in deciding which modality is more effective in various clinical pictures of pain. As we learn more about the mechanism of pain and how it can be affected, we will be able to select the type of modality for pain management based on evidence rather than supposition.

ULTRASOUND

Ultrasonic waves were first utilized for military purposes in the early twentieth century and first used for medical purposes in the United States in the 1950s. Ultrasound is currently used for a variety of diagnostic and treatment purposes. The discussion of ultrasound in this chapter is confined to the use of ultrasound as it applies to the treatment of painful conditions.

Ultrasound is defined as sound waves at a frequency too high to be detected by the human ear.[33] Generally, acoustic waves with a frequency above 17,000 Hz are considered to be ultrasound. Ultrasonic equipment used in the practice of physical therapy emits waves in the .8 to 1 MHz range. In the production of ultrasound, an electrical current is converted into a mechanical current. To understand how this conversion of energy occurs, one must first understand the reverse peizoelectric effect.

Ultrasound is essentially a sound wave. It has all the characteristics of sound waves except that it cannot be heard. Acoustic waves are longitudinal waves in which the movement of particles or compressions occur in the direction of wave propagation. Acoustic waves travel best in dense solids and poorly in gases. They travel fairly well in degassed liquids but not at all in vacuums. For this reason ultrasound requires a coupling medium to be applied efficiently.

Ultrasound is known to have a large number of physiologic effects, but we will limit our review to those effects which relate to pain control.

Nerve conduction velocity is altered by exposure to ultrasound. Farmer investigated the effect of varying intensities of ultrasound on the conductivity of human motor axons.[34] Each subject's nerve conduction velocity was measured before and after 5-minute ultrasound treatments. The effects of .5, 1, 1.5, 2, and 3 watts per square centimeter (W/cm^2) were compared. Intensities of .5 W/cm^2 and 3 W/cm^2 correspond to increases in nerve conduction velocity. Intensities of 1.0, 1.5, and 2.0 W/cm^2 were associated with a decrease in nerve conduction velocity. Selection of the ultrasonic intensity is an important component of an ultrasound treatment. Theoretically, a reduction in nerve conduction velocity should decrease pain. When the desired therapeutic result includes decreasing nerve conduction velocity, the treatment intensity should be set between 1.0 and 2.0 W/cm^2.

The depth of penetration of a physical agent is generally taken to be the depth at which 50 percent of its energy will penetrate. The depth of penetration of ultrasound is between 3 and 5 cm.[1,12,35] Ultrasound is an effective agent for increasing the tissue temperature of the deep joints.

In a 1967 study, Lehmann et al studied the tissue temperature rise in the thigh following ultrasound in four groups of human subjects:[35] (1) a group with greater than 8 cm of soft tissue in front of the femur receiving ultrasound at an intensity of 1.0 W/cm²; (2) a group with greater than 8 cm of soft tissue in front of the femur receiving ultrasound at an intensity of 1.5 W/cm²; (3) a group with less than 8 cm of soft tissue in front of the femur receiving ultrasound at an intensity of 1.0 W/cm²; and (4) a group with less than 8 cm of soft tissue in front of the femur receiving ultrasound at an intensity of 1.5 W/cm². In the subjects with a soft tissue cover of greater than 8 cm the tissue temperature rise was greater with the 1.5 W/cm² intensity than with the 1.0 W/cm² intensity. In the subjects with less than 8 cm of tissue cover, the tissue temperature rise was greater in the 1.0 W/cm² group than in the 1.5 W/cm² group. An explanation for this unexpected finding may be that bone was heated to intolerable levels prior to soft tissue temperature heating in the thinner subjects. This fourth group was only able to tolerate ultrasound at a 1.5 W/cm² intensity for an average of 2.41 minutes before pain occurred. From this study it is learned that a higher intensity (1.5 W/cm²) is desirable in the treatment when the painful area involves large amounts of soft tissue and that a lower intensity (1.0 W/cm²) is desirable in treatment when the painful area involves a bony area with a small amount of soft tissue cover.

Ultrasound is superior to other forms of deep heat in that is able to penetrate large layers of subcutaneous fat. Lehmann et al studied the efficiency of shortwave, microwave, and ultrasonic diathermy in the heating of the hip joint.[36] Of the three modalities, only ultrasound was able to bring about a tissue temperature rise to a therapeutic level.

Ultrasound may be used safely in the presence of implanted metal.[37,38] Gersten conducted a series of experiments which included the application of ultrasound in the presence of metal.[39] In one experiment, ultrasound was applied to a dog's femur with and without the presence of a metal plate. In most of the tissue surrounding the implant, heating was lower in the presence of a metal implant than with bone at the same depth. Thus, the presence of metal is not by itself a contraindication to the use of ultrasound. Ultrasound has an advantage over shortwave and microwave diathermy in that it may be used to treat painful areas in which a metal implant is located.

Ultrasound may also be used in the presence of implanted prosthetic joints. Lehmann studied the effect of ultrasound on metal, high density polyethylene and polymethyl methacrylate.[37] In six models simulated to represent the clinical use of polymethyle methacrylate, ultrasound selectively heated bone except when the material was directly beneath the muscle layer and was at least 1 cm thick. Ultrasound application can be used to treat painful conditions in the area of a joint implant as long as the ultrasound transducer is moved continuously and innervated bone is in the transducer field.

In recent years, some controversy has arisen in regard to whether or not the application of hot packs interferes with deeper heating by ultrasound.

Lehmann examined the temperature distribution of ultrasound preceeded by hot packs in the human thigh.[40] Ultrasound did not lose its selective ability to heat joint structures when treatment was preceded by 8 minutes of hot packs treatment.

As with most heating modalities, the primary physiologic effect desired is a tissue temperature rise. The application of ultrasound has a few distinct advantages over other physical agents. First, its depth of penetration is greater than with most other agents, and this is particularly advantageous when the pain-producing pathology involves deep structures. Second, ultrasound penetrates subcutaneous fat, and third, ultrasound may be safely used in the presence of metal implants. All of these factors combine to make ultrasound one of the most widely used physical agents today.

Ultrasound has fewer contraindications as compared to other forms of deep heat. Fluid-filled areas of the body such as the eye, the pregnant uterus, and the spinal cord should not be treated with ultrasound. Normally the vertebral bones provide protection for the spinal cord and ultrasound can be used safely in the treatment of facet joint pathology. When the spinal cord is exposed (e.g., laminectomy), however, care must be taken to avoid ultrasound treatment to the area. Other areas that should not be treated with ultrasound include anesthetic areas, the heart, malignant tumors, the epiphysis of growing bones in children, healing fractures, and areas of vascular insufficiency.[16,17] Ultrasound should also not be used in any condition where a tissue temperature rise is contraindicated.

CRYOTHERAPY

Ice has been used throughout history for medical purposes. This section reviews the basic concepts involved in the therapeutic use of cold in physical therapy practice, with emphasis on the use of cold in painful conditions.

The application of cold has many effects. When cold is applied to a person's skin surface for a significant period of time, he or she generally experiences four sensations in sequence: cold, burning, aching, and local numbness or analgesia. Local numbness is often the goal of pain control treatment. Functional loss during a prolonged cold treatment will also occur in a predictable pattern. Loss of light touch and cold, loss of motor power, vasconstriction, and loss of pain and gross pressure will be lost in that order. From this we learn that pain control with a cold treatment will have consequences for sensory, motor, and vascular function.

The application of cold has many uses in modern medical practice. It is used to decrease edema, to reduce inflammation, to help control muscle spasms and spasticity among other uses. It is also a valuable tool in the control of pain. Just how cold functions in the reduction of pain is not exactly known, but it may have many components. Cold has a direct effect on pain receptors and fibers, reduces edema that may cause pain, can decrease an inflammatory reaction that causes pain, and can act as a counterirritant. Cold affects tissues in a variety of ways. It reduces muscle tone when spasticity or muscle spasm are caused by musculoskeletal pathology. It increases joint stiffness when applied for a prolonged time; however, it stimulates muscle activity when used in short doses for muscle re-education. It reduces tissue temperature and consequently causes vasoconstriction of blood vessels.

Cold has been shown to relieve pain.[41,42] Grant treated almost 7,000 patients with ice massage of a duration long enough to cause numbness followed by range of motion exercises in the patient's pain-free range.[42] Some improvement in symptoms was achieved in 95 percent of his patients. The number of patients in this study is impressive; however, no control group was studied.

Lane examined the use of cold and heat for treating low back pain.[41] Cold and heat both seemed to be effective in reducing back pain; however, length of hospital stays differed between the heat and the cold treatment groups. Among those with *chronic* back pain, hospital stays were shorter among those who had been treated with cold instead of heat. Among those with *acute* back pain, hospital stays were shorter among those who had been treated with heat. The quality of pain should be one of the determinants when selecting a thermal modality for use with back pain.

Pain due to overexertion of muscle can be effectively reduced by the application of cold and static stretch.[43] Two types of pain are associated with overexertion. The first type is related to fatigue and resolves within 6 hours after exercise. The second type appears 12 hours after exercise and appears to be associated with ischemia. Prentice studied the influence of cold packs and heat packs, each with proprioceptive neuromuscular facilitation (PNF) or static stretch in the treatment of latent muscle pain on electromyogram (EMG) activity.[43] The treatments were applied 24 hours after injury. EMG activity was measured before and after treatment. It is interesting to note that all of the treatment approaches significantly reduced EMG activity; however, treatments with cold packs and stretching were found to have the most effective relaxation and pain relieving effects.

Edema and inflammation are associated with pain following trauma. Edema formation may be enhanced or reduced depending on how cold is applied. McMaster and Liddle applied crush injuries to the forelimbs of five different groups of rabbits and measured edema at 1, 4, 6, and 24 hours postinjury.[44] The first group received no post injury treatment. The second group was treated with a 20°C ice bath for 1 hour. The third group was treated with a 30°C ice bath for 1 hour. The fourth was treated with three cycles of 20°C water bath for 1 hour on and 1 hour off. The fifth group was treated with 30°C water bath for 1 hour on and 1 hour off. Results showed that the third treatment group, or those who were treated with a 30°C ice water bath for 1 hour, to be the only group that showed a reduction in edema compared to the control group 24 hours following the injury. In fact, all of the other treatment groups showed edema to be greater than in the control group following injury. From this study, it can be concluded that a very intense or very prolonged cold treatment application will actually interfere with edema reduction. When one is attempting to control pain secondary to edema, a mildly cold application of a relatively short duration is indicated.

The influence of cold on the inflammatory response has also been studied. Farry et al conducted an experiment using groups of domestic pigs.[45] In the control groups the limbs were uninjured and in the experimental group the forelimbs were subjected to carefully controlled crush injuries. One limb of each animal was treated twice, 1 hour apart, with an ice bag for 20 minutes. Results showed edema to be increased 48 hours following the ice treatment whether or not an injury was sustained. Results also showed, however, histologic evidence of inflammation reduction in the ice-treated injured limbs compared to the nonice-treated injured limbs. One can extrapolate that cold can be an effective component of the treatment of pain due to inflammation if the edema that occurs following the ice pack removal does not in itself increase pain.

Benson and Cobb investigated the effects of heat and cold on pain threshold.[46] Pain threshold was evaluated using an algesimeter before and after a 20-minute shortwave diathermy treatment to the shoulder and before and after a 15-minute ice towelling treatment to the shoulder. The results showed both shortwave diathermy and ice treatments to greatly increase pain threshold immediately following application, but pain threshold was increased much more with an ice treatment than with shortwave diathermy. Fifteen minutes following treatment, the pain threshold associated with shortwave diathermy was just above zero, and 30 minutes after treatment the pain threshold was no longer elevated. At 15 minutes following ice treatment the pain threshold was significantly elevated although it wasn't elevated as much as it was immediately following treatment. At 30 minutes following the ice treatments, the pain threshold elevation was not significant. From this study, it can be concluded that (1) cold is more effective than shortwave diathermy in increasing pain threshold, (2) the elevation of pain threshold is negligible 30 minutes following an ice treatment and 15 minutes following shortwave diathermy, and thus (3) cold may be superior to shortwave diathermy in reducing pain because the pain threshold elevation is greater and lasts longer following cold treatment than following shortwave diathermy.

Knight and Londeree looked at blood flow in the ankle during and following therapeutic applications of heat, cold, and exercise.[47] The first group had ankle blood flow measured during 45 minutes of lying supine. The second group received a 25-minute hot pack treatment before lying supine for 20 minutes. The third group received a 20-minute cold pack treatment before lying supine for 20 minutes. The fourth group experienced a 45-minute exercise session. The fifth group had a 45-minute hot pack and exercise program. The sixth group experienced a similar cold pack and exercise program. Results of this study showed (1) no cold-induced vasodilation during or following the application of a 7°C cold pack, (2) exercise increased blood flow superior to the application of heat, and (3) the effects of heat and cold did not significantly elevate blood flow beyond that which was achieved by exercise alone.

The results of the previous two studies should be considered when the aim of using a physical agent is to control pain during an exercise program. The authors believe that cold is superior to heat for this purpose because it elevates pain threshold for a longer duration without compromising the benefits of increased blood flow. Pain serves the purpose of protecting a part from injury or further injury. When using cold to increase the pain threshold, one must be especially careful to control the exercise program.

According to the gate theory of Melzack and Wall, a counterirritant can be used to close the gate to painful stimuli from other areas.[2] Melzack et al showed that ice massage to the webb space of the hand could be used to decrease patients' perception of dental pain.[48] Individuals in one treatment group were given ice massage for 7 minutes or until the subject reported numbness, the other was given a tactile massage for 10 minutes. Those in the ice massage group reported their dental pain to be much more reduced than those in the tactile massage group. Melzack et al explained the effectiveness of pain modulation with brief application of cold by their belief that cold is only carried by the large, myelinated A fibers. Stimulation of the large afferent fibers help close the gate to C-fiber pain. If ice massage has similar pain relieving effects as transcutaneous nerve stimulation then it should be able to be used to control the pain associated with many other painful conditions such as low back pain.

Once a therapist has decided to apply cold in the control of pain, a choice needs to be made. From the literature it is difficult to tell which method(s) are most effective in pain control, although methods have been studied as to their efficacy in reducing muscle temperature. McMaster et al evaluated the effect of the application to the skin of chipped ice, frozen gel, chemical ice envelope, and refrigerant-inflated bladders on muscle temperature.[49] Chipped ice and frozen gel were far superior to the other two in reducing muscle temperature with chipped ice being the best. Since cold is associated with decreased muscle tone, it follows that the modality that is the most effective in decreasing muscle temperature should be most effective in decreasing muscle tone. For this reason, we believe ice chips to be the modality of choice when cryotherapy is being used to control the pain secondary to muscle spasm.

Cases of nerve injury have been reported in the literature.[50] Generally speaking this has occurred when ice has been applied for an extended period of time in an area where a major nerve is close to the skin surface. Decreased local metabolism reduces the oxygen supply to the nerves. Neuropraxia can occur even when freezing of tissue does not occur. It is important, therefore that an individual ice treatment be limited to 30 minutes, preferably 20 minutes, even when used following trauma. As in other thermal modalities, cold treatments should not be used for pain in the presence of severe cardiac or respiratory conditions, for patients with circulatory impairments, over an area of anesthetic skin or for patients who have a cold allergy or Raynaud's disease.

SUMMARY

In any discussion of pain and the conventional methods of treatment that have been utilized in the past, the question of modality preference frequently is broached. Which modality works the best for acute pain? What are the effects of heat application on chronic pain? What are the parameters used in measuring the success of pain relief? All too frequently, the decision of modality preference has been based on the factors of personal preference, availability of resources or time limitation. The experienced therapist is adept at intuitively matching the patient's symptoms of pain with an appropriate modality or method of treatment. But he is hard pressed when challenged to defend or justify, in a scientific method, the choices made. Additionally, the use of certain heat modalities, once in favor, are no longer prevalent, while others have enjoyed a resurgence in popularity. The paucity of scientific research into the direct correlation of heat modalities' effects on pain relief, have left the clinician with relatively little guidance.

In recent years, greater emphasis in the investigations of quantitative measurements of pain perception have been accomplished (see Ch. 2). As these investigations provide the practitioner with more practical and efficient tools of evaluation and assessment, a more accurate picture of pain and its response to treatment modalities is emerging. The greater importance placed on the understanding of the examination of the painful patient, is providing the clinician a more precise model on which to base his treatment procedures.

REFERENCES

1. Griffin JE, Karselis TC: Physical Agents for Physical Therapists. 2nd Ed. Charles C Thomas, Springfield, IL, 1982
2. Melzack R, Wall PD: Pain mechanisms: a new theory. Science 150:971, 1965
3. Bonica JJ: The Management of Pain. Lea & Febiger, Philadelphia, 1953
4. Sternbach RA: Pain Patients: Traits and Treatment. Academic Press, New York, 1974
5. Licht S: History of Therapeutic Heat and Cold. p. 11. In Lehmann JF (ed): Therapeutic Heat and Cold. 3rd Ed. Williams & Wilkins, Baltimore, 1982
6. Feibel A, Fast A: Deep heating of joints: a reconsideration. Arch Phys Med Rehabil 57:513, 1976
7. Cailliet R: Soft Tissue Pain and Disability. FA Davis, Philadelphia, 1981
8. Kaltenborn F: Manual Therapy for the Extremity Joints. Olaf Norlis, Oslo, 1976
9. Campbell JA, Laheurta J: Physical methods used in pain measurements: a review. Royal Soc of Med 76:407, 1983
10. McCray R, Patton N: Pain relief at trigger points: a comparison of moist heat and shortwave diathermy. JOSPT 5:175, 1984
11. Guyton A: Basic Human Physiology and Mechanisms of Disease. WB Saunders, Philadelphia, 1971
12. Lehman, JF, deLateur BJ: Diathermy and superficial heat and cold, p. 275. In Kottke FJ, Stillwell GK, Lehmann JF (eds): Krusen's Handbook for Physical Medicine and Rehabilitation. 3rd Ed. WB Saunders, Philadelphia, 1982
13. Downey J: Physiological effects of heat and cold. Phys Ther 44:713, 1964
14. Newton MJ, Lehmkuhl D: Muscle spindle response to body heating and localized muscle cooling: implications for relief of spasticity. Phys Ther 45:2–91, 1965
15. Montgomery P: Compounding effects of infrared and ultraviolet irradiation upon normal human skin. Phys Ther 53:5–489, 1973

16. Lehmann JF, DeLateur BJ: Therapeutic heat. p. 404. In Lehmann JF (ed): Therapeutic Heat and Cold. 3rd Ed. Williams & Wilkins, Baltimore, 1982

17. Hayes KW: Manual for Physical Agents. 3rd Ed. Northwestern University Medical School, Chicago, 1984

18. Guyton AG: Textbook of Medical Physiology. WB Saunders, Philadelphia, 1981

19. Hamilton G: Mobilization of the proximalinterphalangeal joint: the influence of heat, cold and exercise. Phys Ther 47:1111, 1967

20. Borrell RM, Parker R, Henley EJ, et al: Comparison of in vivo temperatures produced by hydrotherapy, paraffin wax treatment and fluidotherapy. Phys Ther 60:1213, 1980

21. Federal Communications Commission. Rules and Regulations, Vol. 2, Subpart A, Section 18.13, US Government Printing Office, Washington, DC, 1964

22. Lehmann JF, deLateur BJ, Stonebridge JB: Selective muscle heating by short diathermy with an inductive coil. Arch Phys Med Rehabil 50:117, 1969

23. Cherry TH: The results of diathermy in pelvic infections. JAMA 86:1745, 1926

24. Gobel RE, Gowers JI, Green GC, Nichols PH: Out-patient physiotherapy: patterns of provision. Rheumatol Rehabil 18:248, 1979

25. Lehmann JF, Brunner GP, McMillan, et al: Modification of heating patterns produced by microwaves at the frequencies 2456 and 900 mc. by physiologic factors in humans. Arch Phys Med Rehabil 45:555, 1964

26. Bisgard JD, Nye D: The influence of hot and cold application on gastric and intestinal motor activity. Surg Gynecol Obstet 71:172, 1940

27. Fischer E, Solomon S: Physiological responses to heat and cold. p. 126. In Licht S(ed): Therapeutic Heat and Cold. 2nd Ed. Waverly Press, Baltimore, 1965

28. Engel JP, Herrick JF, Wakim KG, et al: The effects of microwaves on bone and bone marrow and adjacent tissues. Arch Phys Med Rehabil 31:453, 1950

29. Guy, AW, Lehmann JF: On the determination of an optimal microwave diathermy frequency for a direct contact applicator, IEEE, BME-13.76, 1966

30. Guy AW: Electromagnetic fields and relative heating patterns due to a rectangular aperture source in direct contact with bilatered biological tissue. IEEE, MTT-19:214, 1971

31. Lehmann JF, Guy AW, Warren CG, et al: Evaluation of microwave contact applicator. Arch Phys Med Rehabil 51:143, 1970

32. Farrell JP, Twomey LT: Acute low back pain: a comparison of two conservative treatment approaches. Med J of Aus 1:160, 1982

33. VanWent JM: Ultrasonic and Ultrashort Waves in Medicine. Elsevier, Amsterdam, 1954

34. Farmer WC: Effect of intensity of ultrasound on conduction of motor axons. Phys Ther 48:1233, 1968

35. Lehmann JF, De Lateur BJ, Stonebridge JB, Warren CG: Therapeutic temperature distribution produced by ultrasound as modified by dosage and volume of tissue exposed. Arch Phys Med Rehab 48:662, 1967

36. Lehmann JF, McMillan JA, Brunner GB, Blumberg JB: Comparative study of efficiency of short-wave, microwave and ultrasonic diathermy in heating the hip joint. Arch Phys Med Rehabil 40:510, 1959

37. Lehmann JF, Warren CG, Wallace JE, Chan A: Ultrasound considerations for use in the presence of prosthetic joints. Arch Phys Med Rehabil 61:502, 1980

38. Lehmann JF, Brunner GD, Martinis AJ, McMillan JA: Ultrasound effects as demonstrated in live pigs with surgical metallic implants. Arch Phys Med Rehabil 40:483, 1959

39. Gersten JW: Effect of metallic objects on temperature rises produced in tissue by ultrasound. Am J Phys Med 37:75, 1957

40. Lehmann JF, Sonebridge JB, DeLateur BJ, Warren CG: Temperatures in human thighs after hot pack treatment followed by ultrasound. Arch Phys Med Rehabil 59:472, 1978

41. Lane LE: Localized hypothermia for relief of low back pain? Phys Ther 51:182, 1971

42. Grant AE: Massage with ice (cryokinetics) in the treatment of painful conditions of the musculoskeletal system. Arch Phys Med Rehabil 45:233, 1964

43. Prentice WE: An electromyographic analysis of the effectiveness of heat or cold and stretching for induced relaxation in injured muscle. J Ortho and Sports Phys Ther 3:133, 1982

44. McMaster WC, Liddle S: Cryotherapy influence on post-traumatic limb edema. Clin Ortho and Related Res 150:283, 1980

45. Farry PJ, Prentice NG, Hunter AC, Wakelin CA: Ice treatment of injured ligaments: an experimental model. N Z Med J 91:12, 1980

46. Benson TB, Cobb EP: The effects of therapeutic forms of heat and ice on the pain threshold of the normal shoulder. Rheumatol and Rehab 13:101, 1974

47. Knight KL, Londeree BR: Comparison of blood flow in the ankle of uninjured subjects during therapeutic applications of heat, cold, and exercise. Med Sci Sports and Exer 12:76, 1980

48. Melzack R, Guite S, Gonshor A: Relief of dental pain by ice massage of the hand. CMAJ 122:189, 1980

49. McMaster WC, Liddle S, Waugh TR: Laboratory evaluation of various coldtherapy modalities. Am J Sports Med 6:291, 1978

50. Drez D, Faust DC, Evans JP: Cryotherapy and nerve palsy. Am J Sports Med 9:256, 1981

4 | Movement Dysfunction: A Conceptual Approach to the Management of Low Back Pain

Jerry N. Fogel

Estimates show that as much as 80 percent of the general population will suffer from low back pain at some time in their lives.[1,2] Grieve states that the majority of pain in an individual's lifetime is caused by degenerative changes in the musculoskeletal system, much of it vertebral.[3] Andersson demonstrates that in Sweden, low back pain accounts for the greatest number of days absent from work, and in the United States it is the most frequent cause of reduced activity in persons under 45 years of age[1]. Sparrell and McKean report that the cost of low back pain to employers exceeds $14 billion annually. Kelsey and White cite a Washington State study that concluded that employees absent from work with low back pain more than 6 months have only a 50 percent chance of returning to work. Those out for more than 1 year have a 25 percent chance and if out more than 2 years, the chances of returning to work are negligible.[2] It is apparent from the literature that low back pain is one of society's major problems and solutions must be sought.

The purpose of this chapter is not to report the current state of knowledge or to provide a comprehensive review of the literature regarding back pain. There are numerous texts and articles available for that purpose,[3-8] such as Grieve's *Common Vertebral Joint Problems,*[3] by far the most ambitious effort to date. The intention of this chapter is to present a case for the use of a generic framework or system for the evaluation, treatment, and prevention of musculoskeletal dysfunction and pain, using low back pain as an example of application.

Why a generic approach? Why not treat the patient's diagnosis?

DEFINING THE PROBLEM—THE DIAGNOSIS

It should be noted that the majority of low back pain cases go undiagnosed.[5] It has been suggested that up to 85 percent of all low back pain is treated without a diagnosis[2,9] due to a combination of biomechanical, clinical, and research factors.

Anatomically, there are numerous structures in the lumbopelvic region which have nociceptive (pain sensitive) receptor systems[10] (Fig. 4-1 and Table 4-1). The structures are innervated from the corresponding spinal nerve levels and therefore, if injured, could be represented systematically in the same sclerotomes, myotomes, and/or dermatomes[10] (Fig. 4-2). In addition, Korr suggests that due to the interneuronal connections of the spinal cord, as well as the multilevel innervation pattern, signals can be transmitted to and from structures in a complex fashion outside that of the traditional segmental representation.[11] This has been suggested as a factor in the clinical phenomena of referred pain.[10,12,13] Pain, however, is not a sensation but an unpleasant emotional experience usually precipitated by mechanical deformation or chemical irritation of a somatic structure that has nociceptive nerve endings.[10] This further complicates the relationship between the anatomic involvement and its symptomatic representation. Grieve states that difficulties in diagnosis are compounded by the fact that almost every pathologic change and lumbopelvic anomaly to which back pain has been attributed has subsequently been demonstrated in the symptom-free population.[3]

Biomechanically, the spinal structures work together as a system. Schmorl and Junghanns suggest the term *motion segment* as the functional unit of the spine.[14] A motion segment consists of two adjacent vertebrae, the interposed intervertebral disc, two apophyseal joints, the corresponding ligamentous and muscular structures, the spinal canal, and two intervertebral foramina (Fig.

Table 4-1. Distribution of Lumbosacral Nociceptive Receptor Systems

1. Skin, subcutaneous and adipose tissue.
2. Fibrous capsules of apophyseal (facet) and sacroiliac joints.
3. Longitudinal spinal, interspinous, flaval and sacroiliac ligaments.
4. Periosteum covering vertebral bodies and arches (and attached fasciae, tendons and aponeuroses).
5. Dura mater and epidural fibro-adipose tissue.
6. Walls of blood vessels supplying the spinal and sacroiliac joints, and in vertebral cancellous bone.
7. Walls of epidural and paravertebral veins.
8. Walls of intramuscular arteries within lumbosacral muscles.

(Wyke B: The Neurology of Low Back Pain. In Jayson MIV (ed): The Lumbar Spine and Back Pain. Pitman Medical Ltd, England 1980.)

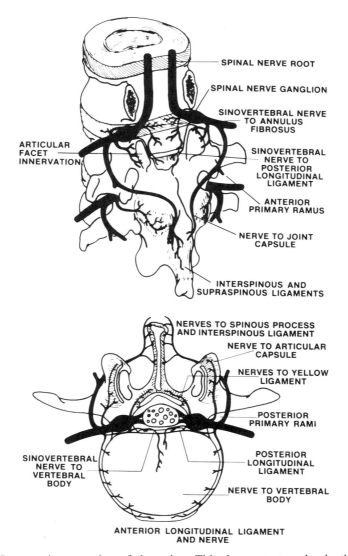

SPINAL NERVE ROOT

SPINAL NERVE GANGLION

SINOVERTEBRAL NERVE
TO ANNULUS
FIBROSUS

ARTICULAR
FACET
INNERVATION

SINOVERTEBRAL
NERVE TO
POSTERIOR
LONGITUDINAL
LIGAMENT

ANTERIOR
PRIMARY RAMUS

NERVE TO JOINT
CAPSULE

INTERSPINOUS AND
SUPRASPINOUS LIGAMENTS

NERVES TO SPINOUS PROCESS
AND INTERSPINOUS LIGAMENT

NERVE TO ARTICULAR
CAPSULE

NERVES TO YELLOW
LIGAMENT

POSTERIOR
PRIMARY RAMI

SINOVERTEBRAL
NERVE TO
VERTEBRAL
BODY

POSTERIOR
LONGITUDINAL
LIGAMENT

NERVE TO VERTEBRAL
BODY

ANTERIOR LONGITUDINAL LIGAMENT
AND NERVE

Fig. 4-1.   Sensory innvervation of the spine. This demonstrates clearly the sensory innervation of practically every anatomic structure in the spine. The annulus fibrosis, the major ligaments, the intervertebral joints and their capsules, the vertebral body, and all the posterior structures are provided with sensory innervation. Thus, virtually any structure can be a potential source of spine pain. (White AA, Panjabi MM: Clinical Biomechanics of the Spine. JB Lippincott, Philadelphia, 1978.)

4-3). One lumbar vertebra, therefore, has six major articulations: two discs and four apophyseal joints. As a result, any biomechanical alteration will stress many structures, multisegmentally, thereby making specificity of provocation or analysis difficult. This system of spinal structures is discussed later in this chapter.

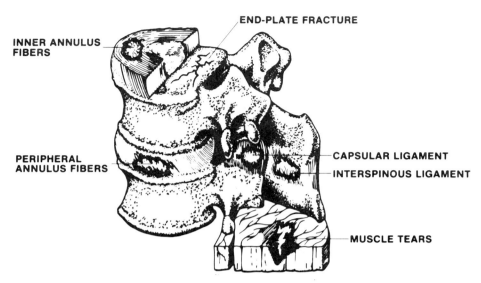

Fig. 4-2.   The structures from some spinal levels are innervated from the corresponding spinal nerve levels and, therefore, if injured could be represented systematically in the same sclerotomes, myotomes, and/or dermatomes. (White AA, Panjabi MM: Clinical Biomechanics of the Spine. JB Lippincott, Philadelphia, 1978.)

Categorization of low back syndromes also contribute to the difficulty in diagnosis. The literature suggests from 20 to 30 major categories of low back pain.[3,10,13,15] This large number of categories poses a dilemma to researchers and clinicians. When testing the efficacy of a treatment procedure or technique or the influence of different etiologic factors on the development of low back pain, the researcher must first decide with which category a study will be conducted. Assigning patients to categories is difficult, for as Grieve states: "There is no clinical sign, nor combination of signs which prove diagnostic of a disc protrusion, other than the signs of a space occupying lesion".[3]

In regard to diagnosis of specific types of mechanical or structural low back pain, radiography has and continues to play a major role. However, the literature strongly suggests that there is little evidence of any significant correlation between radiographic findings and the clinical picture.[3,4,16,17] Park thoroughly summarized the literature to date in regard to radiography and low back pain.[17] He cited a 1969 study by Lawrence using conventional radiograms and a survey on a large population to assess the frequency of disc degeneration and its relationship to back pain. Utilizing conventional criteria for disc degeneration, the results showed a 59 percent sensitivity (41 percent false negative rate and a specificity of 55 percent (45 percent false positive rate). In other words, approximately one half the time X rays revealed degenerative changes when there were no clinical complaints and vice versa. Park also notes a study by Epstein that involved 300 patients with surgically proven prolapsed disc where in analysis of the subjects' radiographs showed that at L5-S1, 64 percent of the

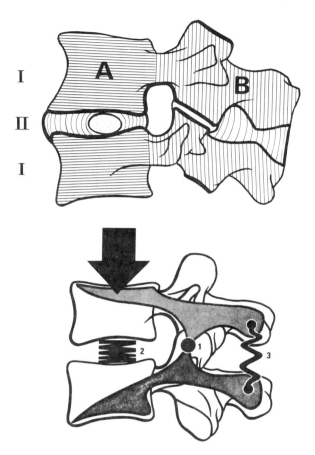

Fig. 4-3. A motion segment consists of two adjacent vertebrae, the interposed intervertebral disc, two apophyseal joints, the corresponding ligamentous and muscular structures, the spinal canal, and two intervertebral foramina (top). One lumbar vertebra, therefore, has six major articulations: two discs and four apophyseal joints. As a result, any biomechanical alteration will stress many structures, multisegmentally, thereby making specificity of provocation or analysis difficult (bottom). (Kapandji IA: The Physiology of the Joints. Vol. 3. 2nd Ed. The Trunk and the Vertebral Column. Librairie Maloine SA, France, 1974. Translated by Churchill Livingstone, Edinburgh.)

radiographs showed normal disc spaces and only 16 percent showed significant decreases in height. At L4-L5, 5 percent were normal and 25 percent showed narrowing. These studies support the view that traditional radiography has little value in the diagnosis of low back pain.

Nachemson summarizes the state of the art clinically and states that regarding diagnosis, "the true cause of back pain remains obscure."[4]

What about the cases where there is a definitive diagnosis? Even in these cases, a diagnosis oriented treatment approach is limited at best. First, there is the assumption that the diagnosis is correct. Then there is an additional assumption that the selected treatment technique or approach is appropriate for that condition. For example, a patient presents with a dull, short-lived ache in the low back on backward bending, becoming a sharp pain of long duration radiating down the left lower extremity on forward bending. Symptoms are worse sitting, better when standing and walking. First conclusion clinicians might draw is that the patient has an acute disc dysfunction. Then, a decision is reached to prescribe extension exercises. The obvious questions should be (1) whether a disc lesion is the only possibility and (2) whether extension is the way to treat this patient, as opposed to traction, flexion, immobilization, or manipulation. What do we know with absolute certainty about this patient? All we know is what we find from our clinical assessment and observations. There is less room for error if we treat what we find (observations) and not what we think it means (interpretations). This is described as the brick wall phenomenon (Fig. 4-4).

Another major issue regarding clinical philosophy is the lesion or culprit notion versus the system inbalance concept. A diagnosis such as herniated disc or facet syndrome suggest that these structures are in dysfunction and when the dysfunction is corrected the problem is resolved. As mentioned earlier, the spine and its supportive structures work as a system. In addition, the spine is also part of the larger musculoskeletal system. Let's examine the impact of each of these two factors.

Kramer states that mechanical back pain is a sequence of biomechanical and biochemical events that affect any combination of structures in the lumbo-pelvic region.[8] At the core of this hypothesis is the concept of the motion segment and its dependence on the intervertebral disc. Kramer states that any alteration in the height or volume of the disc will immediately result in position changes of the apophyseal joints. This produces alterations of movement and

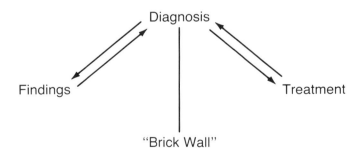

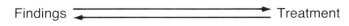

Fig. 4-4. Brick wall phenomena (top). Direct intervention approach (bottom).

abnormal loading. The entire biomechanical system is disturbed by these alterations. The shock-absorbing capability is diminished, muscle function is altered, and unguarded movements occur.[8] Park and Grieve suggest that even mild degeneration changes of the disc have profound effects on the motion segment causing undue stress on any or all of the unrelated structures.[3,17] Ogata and Whiteside also state that disc degeneration is the major factor in the development of low back pain.[18] This concept is further supported by the fact that a healthy disc is so remarkably resistant to forces, especially compression, that the vertebra will usually fracture before the disc undergoes failure.[19-21] If the disc has undergone degenerative changes, its vulnerability to damage is significantly increased.[3-5,8,14,17-20,22-25] This disussion of the first factor demonstrates that if any component of the motion segment is dysfunctional, then the entire motion segment is involved.

The second factor is that of the spine being a component of the musculoskeletal system. This issue is best illustrated by example. Two patients both have diagnosis of herniated L5 discs, confirmed on computed tomography (CT) scans. One has a tight psoas muscle and the other one does not. One has hypermobility of the L4 vertebra, the other patient has a hypomobile L4 segment. Clinically, these patients would be treated differently even with the same diagnosis and symptoms.

Haldeman summarizes this controversy by stating that "any therapeutic procedure aimed at a single etiological factor, in an unselected population of patients with low back pain, could not be expected to help more than a small percentage of these patients".[13] This position is well supported by others in the literature.[3,5,8,14,17,25]

Does a generic or systems approach mean that a clinician must give up his or her techniques, stop subscribing to a particular approach (e.g., Maitland and Norwegian), or necessarily learn new techniques? The answer is no. The systems approach provides a context or framework for the content (methods) currently utilized. For example, if manual therapy, electrical modalities, or therapeutic exercise is used for treatment, the systems approach determines the use and treatment approach that is most effective.

For this approach to be successful, it must be truly fundamental to the clinician's specific approach so as to apply to all patient populations (pediatric, geriatric, athletic, severaly disabled) as well as be the basis for prevention, assessment, treatment, education, and research of musculoskeletal dysfunction and pain.

FUNDAMENTAL BASIS FOR THE GENERIC APPROACH

The generic approach is presented as one form of clinical thought process. It is not meant to be a "cookbook" check list, or a predigested interpretation of what a clinician should do in evaluating and managing a patient. A discussion of its development serves as the introduction to this chapter and some of the basic tenets upon which it is based is offered. This should add the necessary perspective to allow for optimal application.

Few would disagree that one of the most fundamental principles regarding the body is the intimate and direct relationship between structure and function. A change in one will invariably produce a change in the other though this change need not be proportional. This relationship exists at the cellular, tissue, organ, and system level, and at the organism level where the change is expressed as the relationship between health and performance. This aspect is considerably more complex and will be addressed later in this chapter.

Clinically, this relationship serves as a basis for understanding how the body works, what happens when it doesn't work, and what can be done about it. A comprehensive evaluation of the patient would therefore need to assess the (1) structural integrity and balance of the musculoskeletal system and (2) the corresponding function of the same structures and systems. *Function,* however, is a very broad term. A particular context or viewpoint would permit a given group of clinicians with a defined set of abilities to focus on a specific aspect of function. Recently, a context for physical therapists has been proposed called *movement dysfunction.*[26]

Movement dysfunction serves well as a perspective from which to provide service. The musculoskeletal system is the core; the neuromuscular system provides the control; and the cardiopulmonary system supplies the fuel. Movement dysfunction becomes the bond or connecting thread. Consider this sentence taken from a philosophy statement adopted by the House of Delegates at a recent annual American Physical Therapy Conference.[26]

> Physical therapy is a health profession whose primary purpose is the promotion of optimal human health and function through the application of scientific principles to prevent, identify, correct, or alleviate acute or prolonged movement dysfunction.

Note that it addresses the relationship between health (the state of the structure) and function. It then applies this relationship to the perspective of movement dysfunction.

Another paradigm to consider is that of predisposing, precipitating, and perpetuating factors. Very often the clinical focus appears to be on the precipitating factor or event. The precipitating factor frequently is a one-time occurrence, seemingly the straw that broke the camel's back, presenting as the lifting incident, the motor vehicle accident, or a fall. More often than not, this event is almost unrelated to the patient's true problem.

The predisposing and perpetuating factors appear to be the more significant clinical issues to contend with. Consider an example of a person who has "poor" posture with musculoskeletal imbalances and asymetries throughout. As he attempts to lift an object, he "feels something give." What gave? More than likely it was one of the weak links in the system that was affected by that particular task. His poor posture is a predisposing factor. The event (the lift) is past, the pathomechanics of which may or may not be related. His poor posture has now become a perpetuating factor. Meaningful clinical intervention therefore must deal with his poor posture, in addition to the acute tissue trauma.

A final paradigm to consider as basic to a conceptual framework is that of treatment. A simple organizing scheme, based on Farfan's work,[21] is offered.

1. Correct the anatomy: re-establish the appropriate positional and structured relationships, such as correcting a "lateral shift" or "freeing" an impinged nerve.

2. Maintain the correction (healing): allow for appropriate tissue healing. For example, keeping a patient from flexing the lumbar spine (maintaining a lordosis) following a flexion injury or dysfunction would allow for healing of the posterior spinal structures.

3. Rehabilitate the structure or system: address the restoration of function. Extension exercises to restore range of motion (ROM) and stimulate appropriate biomechanical and neuromuscular development should serve to illustrate this point.

As various treatments are considered, I believe they will (or should) all fall into this organization.

A CONCEPTUAL FRAMEWORK (GENERIC APPROACH)

This system divides various clinical factors into two catagories: (1) direct determinants of movement dysfunction and (2) indirect determinants of movement dysfunction.

Direct determinants are defined as those factors which produce an uninterrupted effect or change in movement (function). Indirect factors therefore would be those which produce changes through a chain reaction. In other words, indirect determinants affect the direct determinants, which in turn alter movement. Although assignment of a determinant to a catagory is founded on physiologic rationale, the ultimate criteria were clinically based (Table 4-2.) A reminder, however, that this is *an* organization, not *the* organization.

Table 4-2. Determinants of Movement Dysfunction

Direct determinants
Biomechanical dysfunction of inert structures
Adaptive changes of muscle tissue
Dysfunction of the peripheral neuromuscular mechanism
Inappropriate motor programs
Common indirect determinants
Cardiopulmonary/cardiovascular or metabolic disturbances
Psychological dysfunction
Pain

Direct Determinants

There's an old axiom in teaching that states "tell them what you're going to tell them, tell them, then tell them what you told them". Using this example, I would like to present the conceptual framework briefly in its entirety. Then, with this complete picture in mind, I will examine the specifics and consider their application. Finally, I will consider the framework in relation to the "bigger picture" of low back pain.

The direct determinants begin with two elements defined by a predominantly structural perspective. The last two come from a more physiologic perspective.

The first determinant, biomechanical dysfunction of inert structures, concerns itself with bone, cartilage, ligaments and joint capsules, fascia, tendons, and the fibrous components of skeletal muscle. Some examples of dysfunction might include fractures, sprains and tears, degenerative changes, impingement, contractures, inflammations, and other entities that result in an alteration in biomechanical integrity. Samples of techniques used to assess these entities include palpation, passive accessory motion testing of joints, ligamentous laxity tests, radiographic tests, and neurologic tests which focus on integrity of innervation. Treatments that could relate to this category might include traction, immobilization, orthotics, joint/soft tissue mobilization, and ultrasound.

The second determinant, adaptive changes in muscle tissue, concerns itself with three major areas (1) length-associated changes, (2) fiber size and number, and (3) enzymatic profile. Our discussion will focus mainly on length-associated changes. Clinically, this would present as either "stretch-weakness"[27] or muscle tightness. Examination procedures for example, might include muscle length testing, posture analysis, and computerized dynamometry. Sample treatment techniques include stretching, immobilization, orthotics, and therapeutic exercise.

Dysfunction of the peripheral neuromuscular mechanism, for our purposes concerns itself with abnormal tone produced from any cause outside the central nervous system. Our discussion will concentrate on disturbances in the internal regulatory mechanism including the muscle spindle and the gamma system. Clinically this problem may present itself as a muscle unable to lengthen (allow motion in the opposite direction) and may be demonstrated during active or passive osteokinematic motion testing, gait analysis, or computerized dynamometry. Correction may be attempted through so called "muscle energy" techniques, or icing followed by exercise.

The final direct determinant, inappropriate motor programming, is concerned with the central nervous system and motor control. This problem may be noted clinically following movement analysis when a habitual and less then optimal pattern is observed. Techniques such as Alexander, Functional Integration (Feldenkrais), or Proprioceptive Neuromuscular Facilitation (PNF) have been suggested as mechanisms which may allow the nervous system to choose more appropriate options for movement.

Having now presented the basic framework, a more detailed discussion of each determinant and its application for prevention, assessment, and treatment of movement dysfunction is presented. Also, a brief discussion of the indirect determinants will follow.

Biomechanical Dysfunction of Inert Structures

This category, the broadest of the four, concerns itself with the structural aspects of the musculoskeletal system. Inert, as defined by Cyriax, describes those structures that possess no inherent ability to contract and relax.[28] As stated previously, this includes every musculoskeletal structure except for the muscle tissue component of skeletal muscle. All of these structures are primarily connective tissue. They all evolved from the same developmental origins— the mesoderm. Therefore, their generic compositions will be very similar. For the most part, it is just a matter of different proportions of the same basic materials and as a result, their functions are similar, with the differences resulting from the variations in the proportions of these basic components: the cells, fibers, and ground substance. As the component mix is altered (vary the structure), a new entity is formed, and there is a commensurate change in function. For example, a ligament has a large number of fibers, with considerably less ground substance. Cartilage is essentially the same substance as ligament with the proportions reversed, fewer fibers and substantially more ground substance. Now, the function must be considered. Fibers are predominantly of the collagen type, which have the biomechanical property of tensile strength, or the ability to resist being pulled apart. Ground substance consists primarily of water and proteoglycans (large protein/sugar molecules), thereby endowing the material with compressive strength, or the ability to absorb or transmit compressive forces. It should be clear that a ligament has greater tensile strength while cartilage is more suited to handle compressive forces. The intervertebral disc is comprised of fibrocartilage, thereby possessing significant quantities of both biomechanical capabilities.

The predominant material of the musculoskeletal system has been identified as connective tissue, with the function being noted as biomechanical in nature, dealing with the absorption or transmission of compressive and tensile forces.[19,29,30] This should serve as the foundation for clinical interpretation or intervention. However, using the spine as an example, it is apparent that dealing with the ["generic" material or] structure alone is only part of the picture. The various structures must be considered as they exist in real life, as part of a complex system. A clinical discussion of the complexity of the issue serves to illustrate the implications of the premise.

It is well understood that the curves of the spine increase its ability to handle compressive forces.[19,30,31] In the cervical region, the lordotic curve is created by the increased anterior height of the intervertebral disc (IVD). The thoracic curve is a result of the vertebral body having increased posterior height. The cervical spine requiring high mobility and relatively low weight-bearing requires that the curve be adaptable. In contrast, the thoracic spine requires more stability and must support a moderate load so the curve is bony and therefore less adaptable. The lumbar spine carries the largest load of the three regions, and is moderately mobile. The lumbar curve therefore is a result of both the IVD and, to a lesser extent, the vertebral body, having a greater anterior height.[30]

This paradox of high load, moderate mobility, and an abrupt cessation of motion distal to the lumbar spine are some key structural reasons why the lumbar spine is vulnerable when compared to the other spinal regions.

It has already been mentioned that the spinal structures work together as a system with the motion segment as its functional unit, and that this makes specificity of provocation or analysis difficult. It has also been mentioned that central to the integrity and the performance of the motion segment is the state of the IVD. This presents a major problem. The disc is biomechanically and biochemically predisposed to degeneration.[3,8,14,18,19,22,24,29] The result is that the motion segment is predisposed to dysfunction. But is degeneration a natural process that is inevitable, or a series of events that occur more frequently than necessary? The literature indicates that the disc is strongly predisposed to degenerative changes but that the biomechanical and biochemical factors can be influenced significantly to alter the inevitable outcome.[8,29] The maintenance of the integrity of spinal structures, especially the disc, is through intermittent normal use.[8] As mentioned earlier, normal use for connective tissue is compression and tension. Clinically, it seems essential to assess, enhance, and maintain the normal mechanics and mobility of the various spinal motion segments.

To accomplish this end, a clinician must be able to assess segmental spinal mobility and not be satisfied with only overall trunk ROM. The "give" in the tissues may be analyzed using such methods as traction and distraction and through end-feels of passive movements of both joint and soft tissue. A biomechanical analysis should be performed to determine the distribution of forces, not just of the lumbar-pelvic region, but the entire kinetic chain. This could be a simple structural/postural examination and observation of movement; or a more sophisticated examination such as motion analysis using computers with technology such as force plates, accelerometers, and high speed videotaping with digitization.

The rules for this determinant are consistent with the general rules of treatment by Farfan mentioned previously. If the dysfunction involves acute tissue irritation, a primary concern would be to decrease the inflammatory process, thereby minimizing further tissue damage. However, this is not where the intervention ends. The involved structures must be restored to their normal integrity or they will not function correctly and will become a "weak link" in the system, an accident waiting to happen. This restoration includes tissue quality, length, mobility (or stability), and nutritional integrity. In the spine, this level of specificity is not often attainable. But it can be performed at some individual structures, and the others can be assessed as part of the motion segment. I believe this to be the true benefit of sophisticated manual technique.

For example, thrust manipulation is very controversial as to whether it is or is not restoring dislodged disc material. However, its utilization as a technique for assessing or altering motion and thereby assessing or restoring mechanics seem to be much more to the point, and certainly less controversial.[25,32,33]

Any modality or technique can now be employed, but now within a context, measured against criteria other than subjective complaints. For example, the spine needs intermittant compression and decompression to maintain nutritional and thereby biomechanical integrity of the discs.[8,29] Manual traction could be used to assess this capability. If there is too little "give" in the longitudinal axis, further investigation of the related segments and structures is the next logical step. Intervention can be in the form of (1) passive joint or soft tissue techniques, (2) active mobilization, (3) positional techniques, or (4) modalities to alter the physiology of the related tissue. Maintenance programs can include exercise or prophylatic inversion (partial or full). For example, if shortening of a connective tissue structure was responsible for the problem, a method which takes it into its plastic range and results in elongation must be used. Understanding and utilizing biomechanical principles of (1) creep (gradual deformation due to prolonged low loading), (2) speed of loading characteristics (materials often have defined patterns of behavior depending whether the load is abrupt or gradual), and (3) pattern of development (collagen for example is produced according to the rate, direction, and intensity of stress applied) allow for a more direct, accurate assessment and intervention of the involved structures. This seems to be better understood when dealing with areas such as the knee or foot, but often seems conspicuously absent from low back pain management.

Due to the number of structures included in this determinant, the examples may seem almost endless. This certainly doesn't support its utilization in a cookbook approach. If the principles are understood and the technical competence is available, a more effective and consistent clinical intervention is possible, with enhanced potential for prevention and carry over. Creative applications are frequently being developed in this area. Samples include (1) using inversion, exercise, or aquatics to prevent degenerative and/or osteoporotic changes, (2) advances in clinical technique for manipulating deep connective tissues such as fascia to significantly alter postural alignment and movement, and (3) the use of immobilization, orthotics, and ergonomics to alter the state of these inert structures in everyday life. Specific application of biomechanical principles apply to clinical findings of other structures as well. For examples, on neurologic examination of a patient it is noted that there is sensory and/or motor deficit, suggesting spinal nerve compromise. By altering the patient's position (sitting, supine) causing the foramen to open or close, and repeating the neurologic testing specific information regarding the cause and segmental location of the entrapment might be uncovered. If the clinical picture remained unchanged, for example, a nonmechanical origin should be ruled out prior to proceeding. Other possibilities could be a severe structural problem such as stenosis or osteophytes. If the neurologic picture changes, then the same process could be used to deduce what the issues are and what needs to be altered, such as the mobility/stability of a given spinal segment interfering with the foraminal opening.

A tissue is a tissue, regardless of where it is located. A spinal ligament is no different than one found in the knee. Once the tissue biomechanics and the implications of its regional location are understood, this determinant of movement dysfunction provides the first consideration in clinical analysis and intervention.

Adaptive Changes in Muscle Tissue

In the last decade, advances in muscle biology have re-established muscle as a significant factor in movement dysfunction. Now the focus is less on issues of force development and more on the integrity and appropriateness of function (with function being used in a broader context). Clinically, it is important to know more than just how strong a muscle or muscle group is. In addition to their function as primary movers, muscle must be looked at as force attenuators, postural adjustors, and joint stabilizers.

As previously stated, adaptive changes can be organized into three areas: (1) length-associated changes, (2) number and size of fiber, and (3) enzymatic profile.

The focus of this section concentrates on length-associated changes. The other aspects of muscle mutability are also significant but clinically, length-associated changes have been more associated with postural dysfunction and low back pain.[27]

Length-associated changes in muscle, in its clinical presentation, were described by the Kendalls originally over 50 years ago.[27] In addition to polio victims, they observed these changes in patients with faulty musculoskeletal alignment. They catagorized these muscle adaptations as either lengthened or shortened. Kendall explains:

> Muscle weakness or shortness may cause faulty alignment, and faulty alignment may give rise to stretch-weakness or adaptive shortness of muscles. The appearance of the fault is the same in either case, making it impossible to distinguish cause and effect when dealing with established postural faults. Stretch-weakness may be defined as the effect on muscles of remaining in a lengthened condition, however slight, beyond the neutral (physiological rest) position. The concept is related to the duration of the faulty alignment rather than to the severity of it. It does not refer to overstretch which means beyond the range afforded by muscle length. In standing, the ideal alignment may be taken as the neutral position. Persistent postural deviation from this alignment may result in stretch-weakness. Such weakness frequently is found in the middle and lower trapezius muscles in persons with kyphosis and forward shoulders, and in hip abductor muscles on the side where the hip is high or prominent.

Important to an understanding of adaptive shortening of muscles is this basic physiological concept as stated by Ralston, "After a muscle has been caused to shorten by stimulation, there is no appreciable spontaneous lengthening of the muscle during relaxation. Muscles are caused to lengthen in the intact body by the pull of antagonistic muscles, by the action of gravity and the like. The lengthening of inactive muscle is a passive, not an active process." Consequently, unless the opposing muscle is able to pull the part back to neutral position, or some outside force is exerted to lengthen the short muscle, there will be a tendency for the shortened muscle to remain in a somewhat shortened condition.

Recent studies by muscle biologists have attempted to explain this clinical occurrence. Gossman et al noted that with prolonged immobilization of a muscle in a lengthened position, there is an increase in the number of sarcomeres and a decrease in the length of each sarcomere. When immobilized in a shortened position, there is a decrease in the number of sarcomeres and an increase in sarcomere length. (Fig. 4-5) This appears to be true regardless of muscle

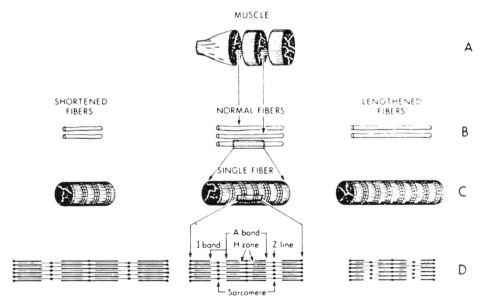

Fig. 4-5. The structure of normal muscle (center) and the relative changes that occur when a muscle undergoes changes due to a shortened position (left) or lengthened position (right). (A) Skeletal muscle composed of single fibers (cells). (B) Single fibers. (C) Single fiber enlarged to show myofibrils; note decreased and increased sarcomere numbers in the shortened and lengthened fibers, respectively. (D) Myofibril enlarged to show contractile proteins of the sarcomere (actin and myosin myofilaments); note increased and decreased sarcomere length in the shortened and lengthened fibers, respectively. (Gossman MR, Sahrmann SA, Rose SJ: Review of length-associated changes in muscle: experimental evidence and clinical implications. Reprinted from Physical Therapy 62:1799, 1982 with permission of the American Physical Therapy Association.)

activity or neuronal integrity. Apparently, these changes can occur very rapidly, possibly within 24 hours. There is also a shift in the length-tension relationships, with the clinical possibility that manual muscle tests may give misleading data depending on whether in the ROM the test is performed.[34]

Kendall also observed that muscle imbalances often occur in well defined patterns.[27] These observations were further developed by Janda[35,36] who notes that postural muscles tend to have increased tone and are frequently short. Phasic muscles tend to have less tone and are more commonly lengthened. He notes this to occur in patterns of postural antagonists. For example, the iliopsoas is one of the most commonly found shortened muscles. Concurrently, there is a stretch-weakness of its phasic antagonist, the gluteus maximus. This scenario could be used to explain an inhibition or stretch weakness of the "lower abdominal" muscles accompanying a tight or short erector spine muscle group. There is a resultant decrease in hip extension, an increased lumbar lordosis with side bending and rotation, and a unilateral or asymetrical anterior pelvic tilt. This results in altered mechanics of the lower extremities and the trunk. Grieve adds to this clinical picture the element of "residual tone".[3] In an extensive review of the literature, he noted that repetitious activity or movement patterns were highly related to the incidence of musculoskeletal dysfunction, especially low back pain. He stated that residual tone in the frequently used muscles predisposed them to adaptive shortening. The antagonistic muscles would be frequently called on to lengthen thereby allowing the required motion to occur. That stimuli, plus inhibition from the shortened, active group result in an adaptive lengthening. Krämer contends that these postural abnormalities create abnormal loading of the disc, thereby contributing to the degeneration/dysfunction scenario discussed in the preceeding section.[8] Radin observed that the inability of a muscle to lengthen plays a significant role in the development of osteoarthrosis and cartilage degeneration, as well as predisposition to fractures and bony failure.[37]

Muscle length is a significant factor in the patient with low back pain. Once this is acknowledged, assessment, treatment, and prevention become clearer.

First, muscle length testing must be performed. Here is where specificity of technique becomes essential. Each function of a muscle must be accounted for in the test. For example, the iliopsoas is often tested by performing the "Thomas Test" (supine, opposite knee to chest, the involved lower extremity hanging over the table). This test essentially checks for hip extension (or hip flexor length). The iliopsoas, however, flexes the hip, sidebends the lumbar spine to the same side, rotates the lumbar spine to the opposite side, abducts the femur, externally rotates the femur, and pulls anteriorly on the lumbar spine possibly causing increased lordosis. To truly assess this muscle length, all these motions should be tested (Table 4-3).

Primary treatment must start with specific stretching of the short musculature.[38] Exercise of the weak or lengthened muscles will accomplish little if the length of their tight antagonists is not restored. This can be addressed by using both passive stretching and self-stretching techniques. Using hold-relax techniques will allow the clinician or patient to get past the neurologic component (see next determinant), followed by a static prolonged stretch to biomechanically alter the involved tissue components (muscle and its connective tissue).

Table 4-3. Muscle Length Findings on a
Typical Low Back Pain Patient

Shortened muscles	Lengthened muscles
Iliopsoas	Gluteus maximus
Hamstrings	Lower abdominals
Sartorious	Internal rotators
Rectus fermoris	Middle trapezius
Upper abdominals	Lower trapezius
Low back extensors	Rhomboids
External rotators	
Pectorlis minor	
Serratus anterior	
Upper trapezius	
Sternocleidomastoid	
Levator scapulae	
Latisimus dorsae	
Tensor fascia latae	
Quadratus lumborum	

(Adapted from Janda V: Muscle Function
Testing. Butterworths, London, 1983, © V.
Janda.)

Use of taping, supports, or other external devices may be useful to immobilize
(or restrict to a shortened range) the lengthened muscles. This is especially true
for the rhomboids and mid and lower trapezius.[27] Resistive exercises could then
be used to allow the muscles to adapt to their new length. This adaption is at
three levels: biomechanical, neuromuscular, and motor programming. Excellent clinical references of techniques for muscle length testing and treatment
are available.[27,38]

Another consideration of treatment is that of enzymatic profile or more
commonly, fiber type. Consideration must be given to the predominant function of a muscle (i.e., low intensity and long duration activity vs. high intensity
and short duration activity) when assessing or treating muscle. Suppose a
patient needed function restoration to the erector spine group in the lumbar
region. Based on fiber type, active extension exercises against gravity or resistance would be less than optimal treatment. Activities which called for their use
as dynamic stabilizers or segmental postural adjusters such as rhythmic stabilization (emphasis on timing, not resistance), balancing on a rocker board, or any
activity with alternate reciprocal limb movement might be more productive.

An axiom that continues to manifest itself with each topic is balance. In
this case, if there is a stimuli to a muscle or muscle group, such as flexor tone or
postures, then an extension stimuli must be introduced to counter any adaptive
tendencies (Fig. 4-6).[39]

Dysfunction of the Peripheral Neuromuscular Mechanism

In the third determinant of movement dysfunction, the problem is more
physiologic than structural in nature concerning itself with the integrity of the
peripheral neuromuscular regulatory mechanism. Knowledge in this area is
evolving rapidly with resulting changes in our understanding of the mechanisms
involved. This discussion will therefore concentrate on behavior. There seems

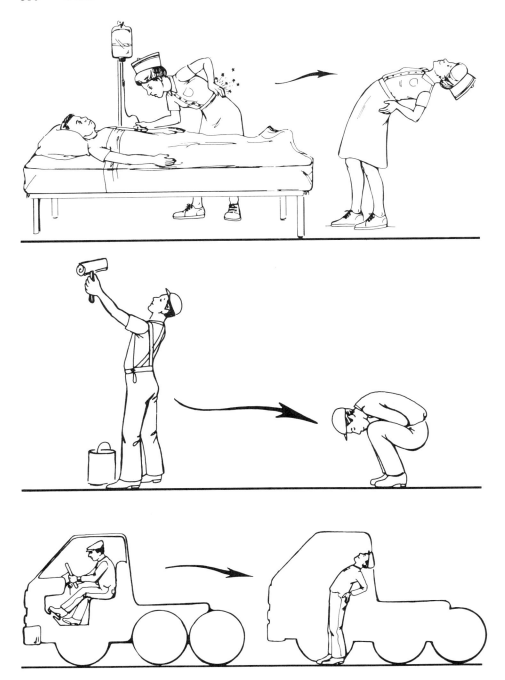

Fig. 4-6.   Interrupt or change stressful positions frequently. (Saunders HD: For Your Back: Self-Help Manual. Minneapolis, 1985.)

to be considerably less discussion regarding what happens in response to a given stimuli than to why it happens. With that in mind, clinical discussion can concentrate on observed behavior and simple physiologic descriptions which may be used to improve understanding.

Often clinicians say that their patients have "abnormal tone," are "guarding," or "in spasm." Unfortunately, these terms are either used interchangeably or with an assumed understanding of their meaning. In addition, this clinical finding is treated either in isolation (not as a behavioral expression of some specific stimuli) or as the expression of some vague occurrence such as "spasm due to pain."

Recently these terms have been defined by the Orthopaedic Section of the American Physical Therapy Association.[40] *Tone* is defined as the tension in a muscle or muscle group resulting from both active (contractile) and passive (inert) mechanisms. Structurally, both aspects have been discussed in the prior two determinants. In this section, the peripheral neurologic component will be addressed.

Abnormal tone would therefore be any state of tonus that was clinically or physiologically inappropriate. That may seem obvious, yet many clinicians use the term *abnormal tone* to represent spasticity or flaccidity exclusively.

Spasm is defined as an involuntary muscular contraction, a purely reflexive phenomenon. *Cramp* is defined as a painful muscle contraction brought on by voluntary use of that muscle or muscle group. *Guarding,* or *splinting,* is noted as generalized increased tone as a protective response to pain, dysfunction, and stress. While the exact physiology of these phenomenon are still unclear, clinically they appear as distinct entities. For example, generalized relaxation exercises or biofeedback essentially decrease tone throughout the system due to a decrease in sympathetic output. This may have somewhat lasting effects on guarding. However, spasm would return, assuming it even changed in the first place, as long as the causative irritating stimuli was still present. Another example would be the treatment for cramp. Passively stretching the muscle will usually quickly relieve a cramp.[28] However, this approach may initially aggravate and even reinforce spasm.

There is still the issue of normal. The "normal" tone of someone who was very anxious would probably be increased. Would this person be considered hypertonic? The tone is increased compared to resting levels but expected, considering the situation. Therefore, it seems clinically more useful to think of tone in terms of appropriate (expected), functional (performed) and deleterious (eventual changes in a system).

Why is tone an issue? Inbalances of tone contributing to the degeneration/ dysfunction scenario have already been discussed. The role of tone in proprioceptive feedback to the central nervous system (CNS), as well as an effector occurrence regarding motor control, is discussed in the next determinant. The clinical focus here is the phenomenon of peripheral neuromuscular "bias" and its role in the direct limitation or aberration of movement.

Let's consider an easily visualized example. A person has restriction in the ability to sidebend the head and neck to the left. Upon examination it is noted that there is a palpable muscle contraction of the right lateral flexors on left sidebending. One possible explanation for this is that the muscle spindles' regulatory mechanism in the right lateral flexors is "set" too high, which results in the muscle spindle being stimulated too early in the movement, causing a contraction and not allowing the muscle to lengthen. This is an oversimplified explanation used for conceptual purposes.

In attempting to correct this situation in terms of movement, what are the options? Active left sidebending only stretches the right sided muscles causing them to fire. Passive left sidebending will more than likely not help as both the alpha and gamma (muscle and spindle) systems are stimulated. Passive right sidebending, however, should take the tension off the muscle and spindle. Theoretically, this turns down the gamma "bias." Passively moving into left sidebending after waiting a moment should cause the muscle to lengthen. Exercise or movements could now take place at the lengthened range of the right lateral flexors to allow the spindle to "reset" at a more appropriate level. This schematic representation has been proposed by Korr.[11,41] It has been used to offer an explaination for the clinical observations of various practitioners. Jones (in Rex and Mitchell[32]) used this scheme to explain his counterstrain (functional technique) of moving the body part where it "wanted to go". Denslow (in Korr[11,14]) described the "osteopathic lesion" by the existence of the tonal disturbance. Mitchell, another osteopath, developed a system of "muscle energy" techniques on the same principle.[32,42] Feldenkrais used passive shortening or "kinetic mirroring" to alter specific tonal patterns.[43] This scenario might be applied as a possible explanation of Maigne's "no pain, contrary movement" approach of passively moving the spine into the opposite, nonpainful, nonrestricted direction prior to attempting to move into the involved range.[44]

Janda observed asynchroneous and inappropriate firing patterns in muscles of the trunk and lower extremity of low back pain patients on movements such as hip extension in prone lying.[35] This state of hyperexcitability in certain muscles might represent a factor in Janda's observations. Tone as cause or result of a clinical problem is not the issue, but the presence of tone is. The reader can refer to the prior discussion of predisposing, precipitating, and perpetuating factors.

The clinical usefulness of this determinant is first the recognition of tone and tonal behavior. Then if intervention is necessary, will it be local or systemic? Treatment intervention can be electrical, thermal, mechanical, or chemical. However, there must be an effort to restore an appropriate balance to reset the spindle to normalize peripheral neuromuscular regulatory activity. If the tone or the abnormal muscle spindle bias has been masking other stimuli, such as an irritated joint structure, then that would need to be addressed prior to balancing the system.

Inappropriate Motor Programming

The fourth direct determinant of movement dysfunction concerns motor programming. Though predominantly a physiologic distinction, this determinant depends heavily on the three prior determinants. Two points are discussed. First, the inert structures, muscle tissue, and peripheral neuromuscular mechanisms all provide afferent input to the CNS through the peripheral receptor system.[10,30] This provides the major source of information used by the CNS when producing movement. Second, the CNS can only use what is practically available. For example, if there is an ankylosis (fusion) at L4-L5, obviously there will not be any motion at that segment regardless of the motor program. If there is an inability to lengthen the iliopsoas due to either an increased gamma bias or adaptive shortening of the muscle and connective tissue, that motion will be compensated for in the motor program. The CNS will always choose the most efficient option. From the CNS's perspective, a compensatory pattern is more efficient.

In recent clinical practice, the issue of motor programming in low back pain patients is often (1) essentially omitted, correcting the tissue dysfunction and/or reducing the pain, and then allowing the patient to return to the "old" nonfunctional movement patterns or (2) severely misapplied by attempting to "teach proper body mechanics" in place of facilitating optimal movement patterns. The trend, however, seems to be toward integrating "movement technique" into clinical practice.

The following is a common clinical scenario of a patient who presents with subjective complaints of low back pain. On forward bending the pain is increased and spreads into the right buttock. Upon backward bending, the pain is centralized in the low back, with no complaints of buttock pain. The patient then starts on an "extension" regimen of exercises and must avoid flexed postures (maintain lordosis). As this patient progresses through treatment the pain eventually subsides. Eventually flexion activities are added to the routine. If progress continues without further incidence, the patient continues the program as preventive treatment. Two concerns are apparent. First, treatment addresses the tissue of provocation, with little concern for the status of other structures that contribute to the clinical picture. Second, even if the structures have been restored to a functional state, what is to prevent the CNS from "misusing" these structures again with a less than optimal motor program. Therefore, once the first three determinants are balanced (restored to appropriate function) the CNS must be allowed to perceive or experience the new afferent information so that a more efficient movement pattern can be chosen.

The second issue, that of "teaching body mechanics," has two major concerns. First, there is the assumption that there is a correct way to move. Take for example "back school" instruction. Lifting is a major focus in these courses. However, Grieve contends that there is little or no scientific evidence that supports the theory that instruction in lifting has been successful in reducing the severity or frequency of low back pain, even though this is universally believed to be so.[3] In addition, he states that there is no natural way of lifting which is universal and therefore biologically correct. The second concern is that of "telling" someone how to move. Movement is an experiential phenomona comprised of complex relationships between afferent input, subcortical filtering, and cortical initiation, memory, and awareness. It seems presumptuous to assume that by telling someone how to move, they will learn the movement. This may be why mat exercises (such as PNF) have been relatively successful with low back patients. These activities have facilitated proprioceptive activity from the skin, joint, and muscles providing the CNS with necessary information.

There are many methods which may assist the CNS in achieving the necessary information for motor programming improvements including PNF, neurodevelopmental technique (NDT), Alexander technique, and dance therapy. There is one, however, that appears to have an extremely significant role. Awareness Through Movement, developed by Feldenkrais,[43] is an extremely noninvasive method which allows a patient to discover his or her habitual movement patterns, thereby opening up a spectrum of movement options. Because the patient moves within his or her own limitations, it can be used with patients who previously may have been judged to be too acute to participate in movement activities. Clinically, it can be used at any point in the treatment sequence. If applied early, many of the findings may resolve rapidly, leaving only those that need specific intervention (probably within the other three determinants). If used later in the sequence, it can be used to incorporate all the structural changes into normal activity.

Clinically, we have all seen the difficulty of inadequate carryover. To ensure adequate carryover, the corrections and increased abilities must be integrated as part of everyday use.

Summary

The clinical application of each determinant has been suggested. As a system, it should serve to organize thoughts, clinical findings, and techniques. If a patient has a disturbance of movement, the process of analysis can be organized, assessing the role of each determinant, and their inter-relationships. Clearly, ultrasound is not going to contribute if the problem is one of central motor control. On the other hand, if a band of fascia is contractured, ultrasound may serve well in altering the tissue, prior to mechanical intervention.

Another attribute to the framework is that it is founded on the anatomy and physiology of the body, something we may safely assume will stay constant. Therefore, as the body of clinical knowledge develops, the new information, techniques, and technologies may be used within the framework. In addition, it addresses assessment, treatment, and prevention. Prevention would be based on the balance of the four determinants. Since the system is based on the structure and function of the body, it is applicable to all possible client populations, from pediatric to geriatric, from sports to industry, from symptomatic to the severely disabled.

The Indirect Determinants

A brief discussion is offered regarding these three issues (see Table 4-2). Both pain and psychological considerations are indirect for the same reason. They affect movement by affecting one of the other systems, predominantly the two neurologic determinants. They do influence the two structural determinants as well, through a biochemical mode. Clinically, pain and emotional influences must be considered in the larger picture of case management. They do not serve well as indicators of change since they are not directly tied to anatomy or physiology.

Cardiopulmonary, cardiovascular, or metabolic disturbance is a similar yet dissimilar case. These are obviously directly tied to anatomy and physiology, but not to movement. All four direct determinants depend upon these systems, therefore any disturbance would indirectly alter movement.

LOW BACK PAIN: THE "BIGGER PICTURE"

There are numerous additional issues to consider when discussing a topic as broad in its presentation and as pervasive in our society as low back pain. Topics such as advances in technology, increasing demands on the medicolegal system, shifts in health focus (such as prevention, ergonomics, and fitness), and competition in the health care marketplace for the patient and the dollar are important issues that could be discussed; however, these are beyond the scope of this chapter. Yet, if some current examples such as functional capacity evaluations, work hardening programs, and dynametric technologies, are considered it becomes apparent that our framework still serves as our base. These methods of evaluating or treating are just assessing function at a larger level—the performance level. As noted earlier, the relationship between health and performance is a complex one with all the determinants, direct and indirect, coming into play in their broadest application.

A final thought regarding clinical practice in general. Facts change, yet clinicians will always retain the ability to think. They should always question, always challenge, both others and themselves. Remember the big picture includes the camera.

REFERENCES

1. Andersson GBJ: Epidemiologic aspects on low back pain in industry. Spine 6:53, 1981
2. Kelsey JL, White AA III: Epidemiology and impact of low back pain. Spine 5:1333, 1980
3. Grieve GP: Common Vertebral Joint Problems. Churchill Livingstone, Edinburgh, 1981.
4. Nachemson A: The lumbar spine: an orthopedic challenge. Spine: 1:59, 1976
5. Nachemson A: A critical look at conservative treatment for low back pain. In Jayson MIV (ed): The Lumber Spine and Back Pain. Pitman Medical Ltd, England, 1980
6. Jayson MIV (ed): The Lumbar Spine and Back Pain. Pitman Medical Ltd, 1980

7. Finneson BE: Low Back Pain. 2nd Ed. JB Lippincott, Philadelphia, 1980

8. Krämer J: Intervertebral Disk Diseases: causes, diagnosis, treatment and prophylaxis. Year Book, Chicago, 1981

9. Burkart S: Continuing education course: Scientific and clinical approach to treatment of low back pain. Chicago, March 1982 (Presently at U of WVa)

10. Wyke B: The neurology of low back pain. In Jayson MIV (ed): The Lumbar Spine and Back Pain. Pitman Medical Ltd, 1980

11. Korr I: The facilitated segment. In Kent B (ed): International Federation of Orthopaedic Manipulative Therapists Proceeding, 1977; distributed by IFOMT, Haywood, CA

12. Cyriax J: Textbook of Orthopaedic Medicine. 10th Ed. Vol. 2. Balliere Tindall, London, 1980

13. Haldeman S: Why one cause of back pain? In Buerger AA, Tobe JS (eds): Approaches to the Validation of Manipulative Therapy. Charles C Thomas, Springfield, IL, 1977

14. Schmorl G, Junghanns H: The Human Spine in Health and Disease. Grune & Stratton, New York, 1971

15. Anderson JAD: Back pain in industry. In Jayson MIV (ed): The Lumbar Spine and Back Pain. Grune & Stratton, New York, 1976

16. Glover JR: Prevention of back pain. In Jayson MIV (ed): The Lumbar Spine and Back Pain. Grune & Stratton, New York, 1976

17. Park WM: Radiological investigation of the intevertebral disc. In Jayson MIV (ed): The Lumbar Spine and Back Pain. Pitman Medical Ltd, 1980

18. Ogata K, Whiteside LA: Nutritional pathways of the intervertebral disc. Spine 6:211, 1981

19. White AA, Panjabi MM: Clinical Biomechanics of the Spine. JB Lippincott, Philadelphia, 1978

20. Farfan HF: Mechanical Disorders of the Low Back. Lea & Febiger, Philadelphia, 1973

21. Farfan HF: Normal function and biomechanics of the lumbar spine. In Kent B (ed): Int Fed Orthop Man Ther Proc, 1977; distributed by IFOMT, Haywood, CA

22. Ritchie JH, Fahrni W: Age changes in lumbar intevertebral discs. Can J Surg 13:65, 1970

23. Bateman JE: Spine research project progress report: application and use of inverchair traction. Orthopaedic and Arthritis Hospital, Toronto, Canada, Dec 1981

24. Beard HK, Stevens RL: Biochemical changes in the intervertebral disc. In Jayson MIV (ed): The Lumbar Spine and Back Pain. Pitman Medical Ltd, London, 1981

25. Stoddard A: Manual of Osteopathic Technique. Hutchinson & Co, London, 1980

26. Minutes of the 39*th* Annual Session of the House of Delegates of the American Physical Therapy Association. Kansas City, MO, June 12-14, 1983

27. Kendall FP, McCreary EK: Muscles: Testing and Function. Williams & Wilkins, Baltimore, 1983

28. Cyriax J: Diagnosis of soft tissue lesions. In Textbook of Orthopaedic Medicine. Vol. I. William & Wilkins, Baltimore, 1975

29. Beresford WA: Intervertebral disc and mechanisms of degeneration. In Kent B (ed): International Federation of Orthopaedic Manipulative Therapists Proceedings. Hayward, CA, 1977

30. Williams PL, Warwick E: Gray's Anatomy. 36th British Ed., WB Saunders, Philadelphia, 1980

31. Kapandji IA: The Physiology of the Joints. Vol. 3. Churchill Livingstone, Edinburgh, 1974
32. Rex LH, Mitchell FL Jr: Osteopathic Muscle Energy. International Federation of Manipulative Therapists, Pre-Congress Course. Vancouver BC, June 18-22, 1984
33. Haldeman S: The importance of neurophysiological research into the principles of spinal manipulation. The Research Status of Spinal Manipulative Therapy. DHEW publication No (NIH) 76-998, Washington DC, 1975
34. Gossman MR, Sahrmann SA, Rose SJ: Review of length-associated changes in muscle: experimental evidence and clinical implications. Phys Ther 62:1799, 1982
35. Janda V: Die Bedeutung der muskularen Fehlhaltung als pathogenetischer Faktor vertebrangener Storungen. Arch Phys Ther 20:113, 1968
36. Janda V: Muscle Function Testing. Butterworths, London, 1983
37. Radin EL: Aetiology of Osteoarthrosis. Clin Rheum Dis 2:509, 1976
38. Evjentth O, Hamberg J: Muscle Stretching in Manual Therapy. Vol. I & II. ALFTA Rehab. ALFTA, Sweden, 1984
39. Saunders HD: Evaluation, Treatment, and Prevention of Musculoskeletal Disorders. Beacon Press, Minneapolis, 1985
40. Fogel JN: Orthopaedic Physical Therapy Terminology. Orthopaedic Section APTA Inc. LaCrosse, WI, in press
41. Korr I: Muscle spindle and the lesioned segment. In Kent B (ed): International Federation of Orthopaedic Manipulative Therapists Proceedings. 1977; distributed by IFOMT, Haywood, CA
42. Mitchell FL JR, Moran PS, Pruzzo NA: An Evaluation and Treatment Manual of Osteopathic Muscle Energy Procedures. Mitchell, Moran, and Pruzzo Associates, Valley Park, MO, 1979
43. Feldenkrais M: Awareness Through Movement. Harper & Row, New York, 1977
44. Maigne R: Orthopedic Medicine: A New Approach to Vertebral Manipulations. Charles C Thomas, Springfield, IL, 1972

5 | Approaches to Dealing with Musculoskeletal Pain

Joseph McCulloch

To begin outright with a discussion of various approaches to the treatment of pain would presume that therapists, who treat patients with musculoskeletal pain, already have an accurate "diagnosis" on which to base the treatment. In reality, this is seldom the case. How often is it that the patient arrives at the clinic with a referral for treatment of "low back pain," a statement of the patient's symptoms rather than a diagnosis. Therapists should not be greatly concerned by this since it is signs and symptoms which will guide the therapist as he or she selects treatment techniques and monitors the patient's progress. What should be of concern, however, is that an accurate determination be made of which structure or structures are actually responsible for the patient's pain.

Just as there are numerous schools of thought on the treatment of musculoskeletal pain, there are equally as many thoughts as to what significance pain should play in the diagnosis of musculoskeletal dysfunction and the assessment of the patient's response to treatment. It would appear rather radical, in a publication on pain, to state that pain should be ignored when monitoring patient progress. Though it is not my belief that pain is insignificant, the therapist must learn to place things in a proper perspective and constantly remind him or herself that pain is often an intermittent symptom of dysfunction. Allowing absence of pain to be the primary determinant of goal achievement puts the therapist in a compromising position: the therapist may unintentionally be providing a disservice by discharging the patient from care even though the dysfunction, which precipitated the pain, may have only been partially treated. Just as the disappearance of a toothache is not an indication that the tooth is okay, relief of musculoskeletal pain should likewise not necessarily mean that further treatment is not indicated.

Since proper examination, assessment, and reassessment are paramount to proper treatment, it would be derelict not to address this issue prior to discussing techniques of management. The approach which I will use was developed from many sources and personal experiences. However, the general concepts of the hands-on assessment techniques are modeled after those of Dr. James Cyriax, who has probably done more to advance the art of musculoskeletal assessment in physical therapy than any other practitioner to date. Obviously the discussion needs to be brief and the reader who wishes to pursue the topic in greater depth should refer to Dr. Cyriax's work.[1]

EVALUATING MUSCULOSKELETAL PAIN

A comprehensive history and subjective examination should be performed before any objective tests. An account of the patient's symptoms will be of great benefit to the therapist in gaining an understanding of the patient's problems and subjective complaints of pain. Many therapists tend to rely on a history previously gathered by the referring practitioner or another therapist. This should be avoided for two reasons. First, people use terminology and phrase questions differently. A much greater understanding of the patient's situation can be gained if the therapist asks his or her own questions. This does not mean that the patient's medical record should not be read. It should be decided, however, unless the nature and severity of the problem dictate otherwise, to put off reading the chart until after the examination. This will better ensure that the patient will obtain an unbiased assessment of the problem. A second, but no less important, reason for taking the patient's history is rapport. Taking the time and showing the attention necessary to obtain a good history, demonstrates to the patient your genuine concern and willingness to listen. This concern does a great deal to develop the patient's sense of confidence in the therapist's abilities. An assured patient is usually a cooperative one.

The history gathering session should focus on the first episode of dysfunction or pain and follow through to the present with emphasis on the mechanism of injury and how symptoms have changed with time and treatment. A schematic of the history taking process is presented in Figure 5-1.

The subjective examination is a logical extension of the history taking process. This portion of the examination allows the patient to describe or interpret the current or most recent symptoms. It will be information from this part of the examination that will be of use to the therapist in planning for the objective examination and monitoring the patient's response to various examination and treatment techniques.

The subjective examination ascertains the area, depth, and behavior of the patient's symptoms. In so doing, the therapist must constantly be aware of the

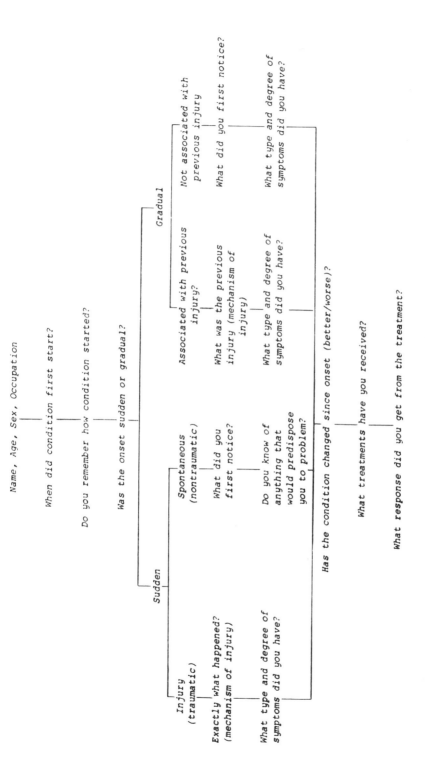

Fig. 5-1. Schematic for history taking.

problem of referred pain, which is perceived at some spot other than its true site. Referred pain is considered by many to be an error in perception and is usually noted not to travel any further than the limits of the dermatome with which it is associated.[1-3]

The therapist should also ask how the symptoms of the patient's current problem manifested themself over the past several days. How the patient's pain changes, in response to various activities, will help determine the severity of the problem. Again, a schematic is provided to illustrate the questioning process (Fig. 5-2). After determining the behavior of the symptoms, the therapist should note any further relevant information, such as the patient's general health, weight loss, radiographic findings, and current medication. Based on information obtained from the history and subjective examination along with the therapist's observations of the patient, plans should be made for the objective examination. The therapist should also have a sense of how gently the patient should be handled during the objective examination.

Movement dysfunction is what physical therapy is all about. Unfortunately, it is more often than not, pain which makes the patient seek help. Since pain, in lesions of the musculoskeletal system, is caused primarily by tension being applied to injured structures, the best way to localize or diagnose the problem is to apply tension to the tissues in various fashions. The therapist can then record the effect of the maneuvers on the patient's pain. The patient must be cautioned that the therapist is looking for situations which alter the existing pain; and any new pains that develop should be reported by the patient.

Before applying stress to moving parts, one should first understand the distinction between contractile and noncontractile substances. Classifying structures as contractile or noncontractile is not as simple a task as it may appear. In manual therapy circles the term *contractile* is extended to mean not only muscle tissue but also any structures that form part of the muscle complex; namely the muscle belly, its tendons and their insertions on the bone. Pain from a dysfunctional contractile substance may be elicited by stretching the structure in the opposite direction of its function or by active contraction. Applying resistance to an active contraction should maximally stress the damaged tissue and result in pain. Pain from a resisted contraction can also be provoked when a fracture lies close enough to the functioning muscle to cause torque of the fracture site or when an inflamed gland, bursa, or abscess is situated directly beneath the muscle belly and is compressed during a contraction.

By the process of elimination, the structures which do not possess any inherent ability to contract and relax are termed noncontractile or inert. Joint capsules, ligaments, bursae, fasciae, dura mater, and nerve roots are noncontractile structures. Noncontractile structures can be stressed by the patient actively moving a joint through a range of motion or by having it passively moved. The importance of the concepts of contractile and inert structures will become evident as the examination process is discussed.

The first objective test, usually performed in a musculoskeletal assessment, has the patient actively carry the joint through its range of motion.

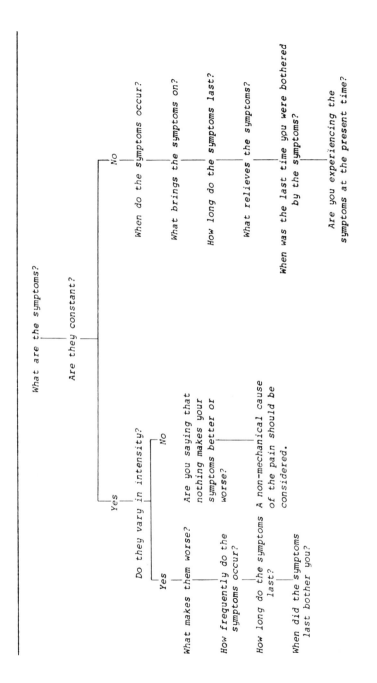

Fig. 5-2. Schematic for subjective examination.

Active motion is used to evaluate four things: the patient's willingness to move, the minimum movement available at the joint, the relative muscle power, and whether an irritable condition is present. Though active movement does not offer any clear information on what is causing the pain, it does indicate to the therapist how aggressively the joint can be examined.

The concept of irritability possibly needs some explanation. In manual therapy, a condition is termed *irritable* when a patient performs an activity which produces pain that lingers after the patient returns to the starting position. Irritable conditions serve as a warning to the therapist and influence the choice and manner of application of the treatment technique.

Once the patient has actively moved the joint, it is then safe for the therapist to perform passive range of motion, which will provide information concerning the state of the inert tissues. As the end of the available motion at the joint is reached, the therapist then pushes a little further and senses, through palpation, what the joint feels like. This motion is appropriately termed the *end feel* of the joint and is best classified as an examination movement. Every joint has its own normal end feel. Finding other than what is expected for the joint and motion in question is considered abormal. The various end feels and their diagnostic significance are listed in Table 5-1.

It should be noted that the terminology used to classify joint movement is not universally accepted. With the exception of the end feel movements, the active and passive movements previously discussed can be best classified as

Table 5-1. End Feel

When passive movement is tested at a joint, various sensations are imparted to the examiner's hands as the extremes of motion are approached. Their names and significance are discussed below.

1. *Soft tissue approximation*—This is a soft and spongy sensation such as one might feel at the end of elbow or knee flexion. This is a normal sensation.

2. *Bone to bone*—This is often termed a cartilagenous end feel and is like that sensed at the extremes of elbow extension. The examiner senses an abrupt halt to motion. If this sensation is felt prematurely in a range of motion, further forcing of the joint, in that direction, serves no purpose.

3. *Capsular*—The examiner senses a firm arrest of movement with a slight give. This type of end feel is like that which occurs normally at the extremes of shoulder external rotation. When this motion occurs before the expected full range is reached, a nonacute arthritis is felt to be present.

4. *Spasm*—When subacute or acute arthritis is present, the examiner often senses a sudden hard end feel resulting from a muscle contracting strongly and suddenly.

5. *Springy block*—This end feel is indicative of internal derangement. The sensation imparted to the examiner is like that one might feel when trying to close a door with a piece of hard rubber placed between the door and the frame.

6. *Empty*—This is a boggy, soft or mechanically nonlimiting end feel that occurs in association with significant pain. The patient states that further motion is not possible yet the examiner is able to gain further motion. Such conditions as acute bursitis, neoplasm, and extra articular abscess produce this type of end feel.

classical movements, which categorize standard techniques generally understood by all therapists.

The movements, about to be discussed, are most appropriately termed
examination movements. Although active and passive movements are used in
examination and treatment, the examination movements are specifically considered in association with manual therapy techniques. There are three types of
examination movement, one of which is the end play or end feel movements
already discussed. The second type of examination movement is component
movement. Component movements are those joint movements that are components of the active movements of flexion, extension, abduction, adduction, and
rotation. An example of component motion is the conjunct rotation or spin of
the tibia on the fixed femur during active knee flexion and extension. The other
type of examination movement is the joint play movement described by Mennel.[4,5] Joint play movements are passive ranges of motion which can not be
performed under voluntary control and yet their integrity is considered essential for full pain-free range of motion of the joint to occur. An example of a joint
play motion is the ability of the joint surfaces of the metacarpophalangeal joints
to be separated longitudinally. This motion is termed *long axis extension* or
distraction and can obviously not be actively performed. It is felt, however,
that if this motion is not present a full range of motion at the joint will not occur.

The objective examination is concluded by a neurologic and palpation
examination and any other special tests which may be indicated for the joint or
joints in question. These types of tests can be found in any standard orthopedic
text and will not be discussed here.

PRINCIPLES OF TREATMENT

This section is divided into three separate areas of treatment—mobilization techniques, traction techniques, and massage—to provide the therapist
with a general guide to treatment. Any number of the techniques may be used in
conjunction with others and though not specifically addressed, the possible
benefits of combining medicine with physical therapy should not be forgotten.

Mobilization Techniques

Mobilization is a graded manual therapeutic technique performed on articular structures, which have demonstrated on examination to be in dysfunction.
There are several schools of thought concerning how articular dysfunction
manifests itself and what effect mobilization has on the problem.

It has long been recognized that chiropractic functions on the belief that
subluxations in the spinal column interfere with nerve function, resulting in
disease. Manipulations of appropriate areas therefore are supposed to remove
this pressure and relieve symptoms. Cyriax took a similar approach to the
treatment of dysfunction by attributing a great many problems to displaced disc

tissue. His mobilizations, though general in nature, were designed to reposition the disc. He did not, however, subscribe to the philosophy of manipulation for the treatment of problems such as diabetes and heart disease.[1]

A second school of thought centers around the role of pain in dysfunction. Maitland, an Australian physical therapist, uses *articulatory* techniques involving oscillatory movement of specific joints to treat dysfunction and pain. A great deal of emphasis is placed on gentleness and assessing the patient following each maneuver. A schematic summary of Maitland's grading system is presented in Figure 5-3.

Robert Maigne, a French physician, also places an emphasis on the role of pain in treatment. Maigne subscribes to the principle that a technique designed to relieve pain and increase motion should not cause pain; if it does, that procedure should not be followed and if motion is limited in a certain direction, it should be freed by moving the joint in the direction which allows the greatest mobility.[6]

A third school of thought places emphasis on the normalization of joint mobility. Kaltenborn,[7] Paris[6], Mennel[4,5], and other practitioners, who subscribe to this school, state that normal motion should (1) take place smoothly, regardless of speed (2) be full range, and (3) be pain free. Pain is considered to be a secondary phenomenon which will disappear when normal joint function is restored.

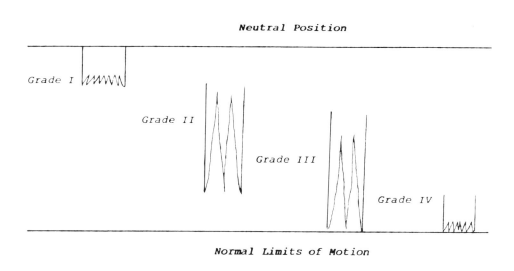

Fig. 5-3. Grades of mobilization.

Regardless of the philosophic orientation of the therapist, primary consideration should be given to individualization of the treatment program. Therapists should avoid the tendency of wanting to subscribe to the latest treatment technique, or to a specific school of thought, unless it can be clearly demonstrated that the techniques will benefit the patient. As stated previously, it is my opinion that an eclectic approach to evaluation and treatment is best.

When considering mobilization as a potential treatment of choice in musculoskeletal dysfunction, one must be aware of the severity and irritability of the condition. Unfortunately, when physical therapists first became exposed to mobilization techniques they looked upon them as a panacea for all of the patients who did not respond to conventional therapies. Often, little attention would be given to the acuteness of the condition and whether it was immobilization, and not mobilization, which was most indicated. While it is difficult to generalize on a subject of this complexity, several suggestions or guides to treatment are given, organized by the stage of dysfunction.

Basically we can look at musculoskeletal dysfunction, and its associated pain, as being grouped into a four stage process. The first stage can be termed the *emergent stage*. The emergent stage is that period of time immediately following a musculoskeletal injury. During this early stage, muscle guarding has usually not occurred and the patient will often gain relief by self ranging of the joint and by applying gentle distraction. This is especially true if a compressive type injury has occurred. When the injury occurs to an area where the patient cannot provide his own distraction, such as the cervical spine, then this should be supplied gently by a therapist. Once acute swelling, pain, and muscle spasm begin to appear, further ranging may prove difficult to perform and should be avoided at the risk of further damaging the implicated structures. In many acute sprains and strains, rest and immobilization are necessary to initiate the healing process. This immobilization may require the use of such supportive devices as slings, traction, or lumbar rolls. Other techniques such as acupressure, transcutaneous electrical nerve stimulation (TENS), and cryotherapy may prove beneficial and are discussed in greater depth in other chapters. The emergent stage may last 24 to 48 hours.

The *acute stage* is a logical extension of the emergent stage and can start as soon as a determination has been made that gentle range of motion, within the limits of pain, will not be harmful. It is desirable that healing of fibrous structures be directed in such a fashion that maximal mobility of the joint be allowed to occur with maximal stability being present. Work performed by Burri et al[8] demonstrated that when rabbit legs were casted for 3 weeks after sectioning the medial collateral ligament, fibroblasts tended to lie unevenly in all directions. This was in direct opposition to rabbits who were allowed free mobility. These rabbits developed scars with lengthwise arrangement of fibroblasts. Applying this principle to humans in a controlled manner will hopefully direct the laying down of fibrous tissue to provide the maximum stability and mobility. To accomplish this task, therapists should provide gentle grade I oscillations and distractions to the joint. Grade I mobilizations are small amplitude movements which are applied at the beginning of the available range and should not be painful. Two to three oscillations per second is usually comfortable to the patient.

As the patient becomes accustomed to the techniques and reflex muscle guarding decreases, the therapist should attempt to work further into the available range. Grade II oscillations and distractions can be employed, which are larger amplitude motions within the range. This is obviously dependent upon the acuteness of the condition and may not be attempted until later in the acute stage, which often lasts several days. Adjunctive measures addressed earlier may be continued throughout this stage.

Numerous manufacturers have developed machines which provide patients with passive motion throughout a selected range. Many units are designed specifically for the knee joint, while others allow greater diversity. The units can be set by the therapist to provide the patient with continuous range of motion in an attempt to prevent or correct limitations of joint movement. These units are often applied immediately postoperatively and have proven very beneficial in minimizing soft tissue contractures which often develop.

The third stage, the *recovery stage,* is characterized by reduction in pain and improvement in function. During this stage, tissues have healed well enough to tolerate more aggressive therapy. Grade III oscillations, which are large amplitude oscillations up to the end of range, may be employed. In addition, many patients can tolerate stretching of shortened connective tissue structures. If complications from edema have ceased to exist, heat can be included to facilitate the stretching process. Though postural problems should be addressed from the beginning, most patients have difficulty actively working with postural problems until this stage, unless it has been previously demonstrated that a specific posture offers pain relief. Many patients at this stage still have a minor, but nonetheless painful, restriction of motion. These individuals often gain benefit from grade IV oscillations. Grade IV oscillations are defined as small amplitude oscillations at the end of the range. When a grade IV technique is employed with a series of gentle stretches designed to free a restriction, the term *articulation* is often used.

Unfortunately, many patients do not recover readily and completely from musculoskeletal injuries. This lack of recovery is sometimes a result of inadequate or nonexistent conservative treatment. These patients are classified in the fourth stage called *chronic dysfunction.* These patients require a thorough evaluation to rule out objective pathology and often require a more specialized approach to treatment such as might be found in a pain rehabilitation program. Patients who have not developed a handicapping pain, however, often obtain good results from mobilization procedures. These persons are usually found to have some limitation in joint function which, when appropriately treated, leads to improvement or disappearance of their pain. All grades of techniques are utilized with these individuals, depending on the severity of the problem at the time. These patients also benefit greatly from programs which aim at correcting postural abnormalities.

Regardless of the stage of dysfunction or technique used, the patient should be reassessed following each technique. It is only by this constant reassessment of signs and symptoms that the therapist can ascertain the benefit of the technique.

Traction Techniques

Traction is a technique in which a distractive force is applied to the body in an effort to separate joint surfaces or bone fragments. Joint distraction, as a technique of mobilization, has already been addressed and traction applied for the purposes of realigning bone fragments is outside the scope of this text. Attention therefore will be directed to the traditional and nontraditional methods of providing spinal traction.

Saunders[9] describes the effects of spinal traction as being sixfold: (1) distraction or separation of vertebral bodies, (2) distraction and gliding of facet joints, (3) tensing of ligamentous structures of the spinal segment, (4) widening of the intervertebral foramen, (5) straightening of spinal curves, and (6) stretching of spinal musculature.

Traditionally, traction has been applied to the spine by a pulley system or other mechanical device which delivered a tractive force in a vertical or horizontal direction. Traditional forms of traction include continuous static and intermittent traction. When continuous traction is employed, low tractive forces are used. This is done in order to prevent patient discomfort due to the long duration of treatment. An example of this type of traction is the continuous lumbar traction applied to patients on bed rest. Usually the forces are less than 50 pounds and generally believed to be ineffective in actually separating lumbar spinal segments. The main mechanics by which continuous traction appears to relieve pain is by keeping the patient on bed rest.

Sustained or static traction consists of a stronger tractive force which is delivered for 20 minutes to 1 hour. When applied to the lumbar spine, this type of traction is more effective if adequate countertraction is used. When applying static cervical traction, the weight of the body itself serves as the countertractive force. When the traction is applied to the lumbar area, however, the trunk usually requires stabilization by attaching a harness to the thorax and the traction table. Intermittent traction is a third type of traditional traction which is similar to sustained traction but, owing to its intermittent nature, allows a still greater tractive force to be delivered to the patient with less discomfort.

Attempts have been made for years to determine the magnitude and duration of tractive force necessary to be effective in pain relief. The literature reveals a great deal of variance in both of these parameters. Judovich[10] was one of the first to define a minimum necessary force. He found that the earliest measurable separation, in the cervical spine, occurred at approximately 25 pounds. The tractive force required to produce measurable separation in the lumbar spine is much greater than that of the cervical spine. Some clinicians such as Cyriax[11] have advocated the use of 100 to 200 lbs of traction for $\frac{1}{2}$ to 1 hour. Colachis and Strohm[12] found that one of the major effects of lumbar traction was an increase in the mean total posterior separation of the intervertebral units. While no significant total separation of the vertebrae may occur, pressure on nerve roots could be relieved by this posterior gapping. This concept is further addressed at the end of this section.

Within the last 20 years, other methods of providing spinal traction have come into vogue. While many of these techniques are not new to medicine, they do represent a renewed interest in less common traction techniques or nontraditional techniques.

Manual therapists have long advocated that therapists provide more direct hands-on care to the patient and rely less on machines and gadgetry. While all of the nontraditional techniques do not fit this philosophic orientation, several do, and are discussed first. Paris[13] has long advocated the use of two manual therapy traction techniques: manual traction and positional traction. *Manual* traction is a technique which the therapist applies by grasping the segment to be treated and manually applying a tractive force. This force, which may last from seconds to minutes, has as its advantage the fact that the therapist can feel the patient's reaction and adjust the tractive force accordingly.

Positional traction, on the other hand, is a technique in which the therapist places the patient into various positions utilizing pillows, sandbags, or blocks. The positioning, which can often be taught to the patient, is best used in patients with unilateral spinal involvement. By incorporating a lateral bending component into the maneuver, pressure can theoretically be removed from a compromised spinal nerve root.

Another nontraditional traction technique is *gravity assisted lumbar* traction. This technique involves suspending the patient from a specially constructed vest and allowing the weight of the pelvis and lower extremities to provide the tractive force.[14] More recently, a system of *gravity* traction known as inversion therapy, has gained notoriety.[15] Various techniques of suspending the body in a heads down position have been developed. Earlier models used inversion boots, which attached to the ankle. The patient then attached the boots to an overhead bar and hung upside down. Though not specifically designed as a form of spinal traction, claims were made that the system helped to reverse the compressive forces applied to the spine daily. Other systems have since been developed which place the hips into flexion and allow much of the weight to be borne by the anterior thigh. While the potential benefits and possible hazards of this type of traction are not completely understood at present, it must be stated that if one wishes to obtain spinal traction via an inversion system, the latter technique is preferable as it would minimize unnecessary forces being applied to the lower extremity joints.

The preceding discussion has dealt with a variety of traction techniques, some more common than others. Before leaving this subject, however, consideration needs to be given to exactly why it is felt that spinal traction is of benefit in treating musculoskeletal pain. While it is widely accepted that nerve root compression can lead to pain, it is also felt that movement and entrapment of the nerve root are also essential for pain to develop.[16,17]

Some pain of spinal origin has been attributed to capulitis and osteoarthritis, which are associated with erosion of articular cartilage. In addition, *nipping* of the synovial membrane of facet joints has been implicated.[18] This theory has been challenged by Cyriax[1] who states that synovial tissue is devoid of a nerve supply and is therefore not capable of responding in this fashion. He does not, however, address the possibility of other innervated structures being stressed by tension applied through the synovial membrane.

The fact that pain can arise from ligamentous and muscular structures has not been questioned. One should question, however, the logic behind using traction to treat an injury to either of these structures. Possibly, if one subscribes to the belief that muscle spasm is an entity that requires treatment, then the stretch applied by spinal traction may be indicated. Forceful spinal traction, however, has no place in the treatment of ligamentous sprain.

Massage

Massage, as a therapeutic tool in the treatment of musculoskeletal pain, requires little introduction. Recorded use of massage dates back to 1800 BC when it was used by a yoga cult in India. It is believed, however, to have its origin in earlier Chinese cultures.[19]

The development of massage parlors and weight reduction clinics, that advocate massage as a substitute for exercise, has lead to many medical professionals abandoning its use. Despite this trend, massage remains a powerful therapeutic tool and is advocated highly by those practitioners who still use it with good results.

There are numerous classical massage techniques which have been taught in physical therapy schools for decades. These techniques are effleurage, petrissage, tapotement, and generalized friction. Other less familiar techniques have only recently begun to be taught in American schools. Included in this category are such techniques as deep friction massage, connective tissue massage, and acupressure.

As stated earlier, Cyriax believed that the primary aim of treatment for nonspecific inflammation of moving parts should be the formation of a strong and mobile scar.[2,20] Much of the rationale behind early passive motion was that the therapist could influence the laying down of fibrous tissue. When this early guided motion is not permitted to occur, the patient is often left with an unwanted, painfully adherent scar. It is in these instances that a deep friction massage is beneficial. Since the technique of deep friction massage is designed to move tissue and not blood, Cyriax states that the massage should be given at right angles to the tissue being treated.[20] Deep friction is indicated in the treatment of muscular, ligamentous, and tendonous lesions; the indications are different for each, however.

The primary function of muscle tissue is contraction. When this contraction occurs, the muscle belly broadens. Following minor ruptures or repeated strains, transverse deep friction assists in the mobilization and separation of adhesions which occur between muscle fibers.

When ligamentous sprains occur, hemorrhage is often an associated finding. Once the acute episode has past and edema has subsided, transverse friction is indicated to disperse any coagulated blood or effusion which might be present. Obviously, the least amount of effort necessary to accomplish the task is employed. Passive and active range of motion is used following the massage, in an effort to facilitate normal movement.

When applying deep friction massage to tendonous injuries, consideration must be given to whether or not the tendon is incorporated in a sheath. Tenosynovitis exists when there is a dysfunction in the gliding mechanism of ensheathed tendons. Pain is usually the presentation when the roughened surfaces attempt to glide against each other. As a rule, tenosynovitis occurs as a result of overuse. One would therefore question the logic of using deep friction as a mode of treatment. Cyriax states, however, that it is this very condition that responds quickest to deep friction. He hypothesizes that the original problem is caused by longitudinal stresses and that the transverse massage likely works to smooth the gliding surfaces.[20]

Tendonitis is the term reserved for strains of tendons that do not possess a tendon sheath. The strain usually occurs at the tendoperiosteal junction and often leads to scar formation. Transverse friction is indicated in these instances to break up this scarring.

In 1929, Elisabeth Dicke introduced a new approach to massage termed *Bindegewebsmassage*. The approach emphasized the use of specific reflex zones in treatment. Dicke considered that organic disturbances followed vascular channels and were influenced by arterial reflexes. It is also believed that dysfunction in many body parts occurred as a result of these reflexes. Dicke developed an extensive list of conditions which she felt were amenable to this type of treatment.[19]

Bindegewebsmassage is still used today but under the term *connective tissue massage*. This English term was first used in 1926 by Maria Ebner. Ebner has probably done the most current work with this subject and was primarily responsible for clarifying some of the more confusing aspects of Dicke's work.

Ebner terms connective tissue massage as a manipulation carried out in the layers of the connective tissues.[21] She states that connective tissue is continuous throughout the body and present in all structures. It is believed that abnormal tension in one part of the connective tissue network is manifested as pathology in other structures and tissues. Though this concept is not widely accepted, it must be stated that those who use this treatment approach report excellent results. Frazier compared various procedures including epidural injections, steroids, TENS, acupuncture, and connective tissue massage in the treatment of reflex sympathetic dystrophy. He concluded that, in spite of the use of numerous sophisticated treatment approaches, none were any more effective than connective tissue massage.[22] This, however, represents only one study. More controlled research is still warranted to provide better documentation of this technique as a therapeutic approach in the treatment of musculoskeletal pain.

Several nonclassical massage techniques, and the theoretic mechanisms by which they afford pain relief, have been presented. As discussed earlier, musculoskeletal pain is best treated when the dysfunction itself, and not pain, is treated. In general, this is what occurs when massage techniques are used in the treatment of musculoskeletal pain. While there are those who still treat the pain directly by instinctively rubbing the painful area, they usually find that the pain relief is short lived. When the massage is directed at correcting the cause of the pain, such as removing edema or mobilizing scar tissue, the results are frequently much longer lasting and often provide permanent pain relief.

SUMMARY

This chapter has attempted to present an overview of the treatment of musculoskeletal pain. Emphasis has been placed on correctly assessing the problem and designing a treatment approach which addresses the dysfunction and not the pain itself. The roles of mobilization, traction, and massage in the treatment of musculoskeletal dysfunction have been discussed. While none of the approaches have been advocated as a panacea or the only method by which musculoskeletal dysfunction can be treated, the role of each in a comprehensive approach to the patient has been presented.

REFERENCES

1. Cyriax J: Textbook of Orthopaedic Medicine. Bailliere Tindall, London, 1982
2. Cyriax J: Massage, Manipulation and Local Anaesthesia. Hamilton, London, 1941
3. Lewis T: Pain. Macmillan, New York, 1942
4. Mennel JM: Joint Pain. Little Brown, Boston, 1964
5. Mennel JM, Zohn DA: Musculoskeletal Pain: Diagnosis and Physical Treatment. Little Brown, Boston, 1976
6. Paris SV: Extremity Dysfunction and Mobilization. Institute Press, Atlanta, 1980
7. Kaltenborn F: Manual Therapy of the Extremity Joints. Olaf Norlis Bokhandel, Oslo, 1976
8. Burri C, Helbing G, Spier W: The Knee: Rehabilitation of Knee Ligament Injuries. Springer, New York, 1978
9. Saunders HD: Orthopaedic Physical Therapy: Evaluation and Treatment of Musculoskeletal Disorders. WB Saunders, Minneapolis, 1982
10. Judovich BD: Herniated cervical disc: a new form of traction therapy. Am J Surg 84:646, 1952
11. Cyriax J: Conservative treatment of lumbar disc lesions. Physiotherapy 50:300, 1964
12. Colachis SC, Strohm BR: Effects of intermittent cervical traction on vertebral separation. Arch Phys Med Rehab 47:353, 1966
13. Paris SV: Course Notes: The Spine. Atlanta Back Clinic, Atlanta, 1981
14. Burton C: Low Back Pain. 2nd Ed. Lippincott, Philadelphia, 1980
15. Nosse L: Inverted spinal traction. Arch Phys Med Rehab 59:367, 1978
16. Hinterbuchner C: Traction. In Rogoff JB(ed): Manipulation, Traction and Massage. 2nd Ed. Williams & Wilkins, Baltimore, 1980

17. Cailliet R: Neck and Arm Pain. FA Davis, Philadelphia, 1964
18. Crisp EJ: Discussion on the treatment of backache by traction. Pro R Soc Med 48:805, 1955
19. Tappan FM: Healing Massage Techniques: A Study of Eastern and Western Methods. Reston, Reston VA, 1978
20. Cyriax J: Clinical application of massage. In Rogoff JB(ed): Manipulation, Traction and Massage. 2nd Ed. Williams and Wilkins, Baltimore, 1980
21. Ebner M: Connective tissue massage. Physiotherapy 64:208, 1978
22. Frazier FW: Persistent post-sympathetic pain treated by connective tissue massage. Physiotherapy 64:211, 1978

6 | Foot Pain*

Gary C. Hunt
Andrew Novick

The significance of a properly functioning foot can not be refuted. Since the foot takes body weight repeatedly with variable force, it tends to be a common site of pain. One only has to observe the awkward gait pattern resulting in excessive energy consumption to appreciate the affects on one's life style. The often quoted remark "when your feet hurt, your entire body hurts" may be trite but succinctly tells a revealing story. Since the body is a multijointed structure it seems reasonable that when one segment hurts movement patterns in other areas will be affected. Numerous studies have indicated the prevalance of foot problems occurring in all age groups. Many texts written on the foot have dealt with major deformities with little emphasis on foot biomechanics. A large number of problems may also develop from biomechanical deviations which over time may produce very significant disabling limitations. Frequently these mechanical deviations coupled with systemic diseases produce devastating results.

This chapter identifies common sources of foot pain with a special emphasis on biomechanical foot faults. Etiologic factors including altered foot biomechanics as they relate with other biologic systems and specific disease processes are discussed. Rationale for specific management approaches based on an assessment of history and subjective and objective data is outlined.

KINEMATICS

The foot has three major functions during gait. It must be a shock absorbing mechanism to dissipate compression forces, a loose adapter to accommodate to the walking surface, and a rigid lever to provide a stable base of support

---

* Written in authors' private capacity. No official support or endorsement by the United States Department of Health and Human Services is intended or should be inferred.

during push-off.[1] These events occur during the stance phase of gait, which comprises 62 percent of the gait cycle. Swing phase accounts for the remaining 38 percent, with the duration of the total gait cycle lasting approximately one second.[2] A complete gait cycle begins with the heel strike of one foot and ends with the successive heel strike of that same foot.

The lower limb presents with a slightly externally rotated position at heel strike. The foot correspondingly shows a slightly supinated position, measuring 1 to 2° of calcaneal inversion from the vertical reference perpendicular to the floor.

Commencement of floor contact initiates a period of internal rotation of the limb, which continues through 15 percent of the gait cycle (Fig. 6-1). This internal rotation in the transverse plane acts upon the subtalar joint, which transmits this rotation into pronation of the fixed foot. During subtalar pronation, the talus undergoes adduction and plantarflexion as the calcaneus shows frontal plane eversion.[3] It is pronation that allows the foot to function as a shock absorber and a loose adapter. Pronation ceases when the lower limb

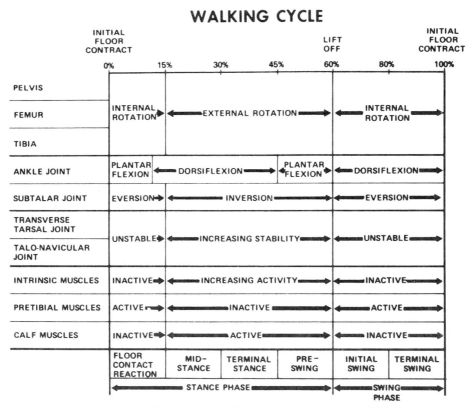

Fig. 6-1. Kinematic and electromyographic events during the walking cycle. (Mann RA: Biomechanics of the foot. In American Academy of Orthopaedic Surgeons, 2nd Ed. CV Mosby, St. Louis, 1985.)

terminates internal rotation and shows a maximal position of 4° calcaneal ever-sion.[3] Subtalar pronation allows the midfoot to become flexible due to the parallel alignment of the oblique and longitudinal midtarsal joint axes. The ankle joint begins stance in an approximately neutral position, then undergoes plantarflexion through the first 20 percent of stance to achieve floor contact. The ankle begins to dorsiflex after reaching a maximum of 15° plantarflexion, just before internal rotation and pronation have ceased. The pretibial muscles and the posterior tibialis contract eccentrically to control the movements of plantarflexion and pronation.[4]

The remaining 75 percent of the stance phase is characterized by a change in direction of lower limb and foot motion. The limb undergoes progressive external rotation, moving through a range of 12° during this period.[5] The subta-lar joint transmits this rotation to the foot creating supination. The talus dorsi-flexes and abducts in conjunction with frontal plane inversion of the calcaneus. Supination progresses such that at midstance, the calcaneus assumes a near vertical alignment, and by heel off, 2° of calcaneal inversion is measured.[3] The foot now functions as a rigid lever to provide stability as weight is transferred over the fixed foot. Subtalar supination creates a locking of the midtarsal joint due to the convergent reorientation of the longitudinal and oblique axes. Tight-ening of the plantar fascia occurs at this stage of gait secondary to the "windlass action" of the foot. This results from extension at the metatarsopha-langeal (MTP) joints, which places a tensile force on the plantar fascia. The resultant tightening of the fascia elevates the longitudinal arch adding further stability to the midfoot.[4] The ankle joint continues to dorsiflex until 75 percent of stance as the tibia is advanced forward over the fixed foot, reaching a maximum of 10°. At heel-off, ankle plantarflexion occurs which continues until the termination of the stance phase when a maximum value of 20° is achieved. The intrinsic muscles of the foot are active during this period to provide added stability to the longitudinal arch and toes.[4,6] The posterior calf muscles are active to control tibial advancement whereas the pretibial muscles become inactive during the remaining 75 percent of stance.

PHYSICAL EXAMINATION

Examination of the lower limb and foot requires identifying anatomic alignment, measuring motion, and testing muscle strength. A complete exami-nation is extensive and includes the entire leg. However, only those areas having the greatest impact upon proper biomechanical function are discussed. Normal findings are reported to establish a reference.

Prone

Assessment of lower limb alignment begins by observing the relationship between the lower leg and hindfoot. A line bisecting the distal one third of the lower leg is visualized or physically drawn as a reference. A second line bisect-

Varus   Neutral   Valgus

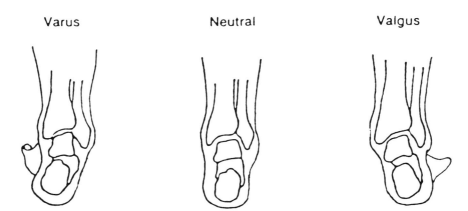

Fig. 6-2.   Nonweightbearing alignment of hindfoot.

ing the calcaneus is drawn by carefully palpating the medial and lateral margins of the posterior tubercle of the calcaneus. The subtalar joint is then placed in neutral position, determined by palpating the medial and lateral aspect of the talar head for congruency. The two bisected lines should form one contiguous line while in subtalar neutral. Deviation of the calcaneus in a position of inversion is termed *subtalar,* or *rearfoot, varus* with the position of calcaneal eversion termed *rearfoot valgus* (Fig. 6-2).

Alignment of the forefoot to hindfoot is established by examining the relationship between the bisection of the calcaneus with the plane of the metatarsal heads. The subtalar joint is placed in neutral position and maintained. Pressure is then applied under the fourth and fifth metatarsal heads in an upward and outward direction, which is tangent to rotation about the oblique axis of the midtarsal joint, and results in midtarsal pronation. This continues until all slack is taken up at the midtarsal joint such that further midfoot pronation would initiate subtalar pronation, reflected by a change in the congruency of the talar head. The bisection of the calcaneus and the plane of the metatarsal heads should show a perpendicular orientation. An inverted forefoot posture is called *forefoot varus,* with valgus denoting an everted alignment (Fig. 6-3).

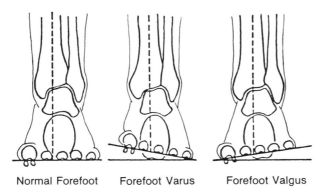

Normal Forefoot   Forefoot Varus   Forefoot Valgus

Fig. 6-3.   Nonweightbearing alignment of forefoot.

Subtalar mobility is determined by measuring passive motion of the calcaneus. Calcaneal eversion is measured by grasping the midfoot/forefoot and maximally pronating the subtalar joint. The bisection of the calcaneus should show 10° of eversion measured from the reference line of the distal one third of the leg (Fig. 6-4). Inversion should measure 20°. Ankle dorsiflexion is measured by attaining maximal motion while being careful to avoid pronation of the subtalar joint. Full functional motion with the knee extended is 8 to 10°.

Stance

In the stance position, the ideal alignment of the lower limb is as follows:

1. The line bisecting the distal one third of the lower leg is vertical, and therefore perpendicular to the floor.
2. The line bisecting the calcaneus is vertical when the subtalar joint is in neutral position.
3. The plane of the metatarsal heads coincides with the transverse plane, such that in subtalar neutral, all five should lie on the supporting surface.
4. The leg in the sagittal plane should be vertical with the heel and forefoot on the floor.
5. The lower limb in the transverse plane should be in neutral position or slightly toed-out, not more than 5 to 10°.[7,8]

It should be emphasized that is the "ideal" position and not often found. A postural deviation that could alter this alignment is the presence of excessive

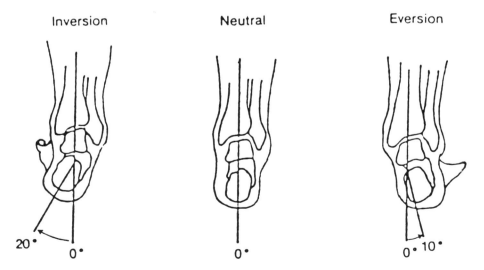

Inversion   Neutral   Eversion

20°   0°   0°   0° 10°

Fig. 6-4. Calcaneal frontal plane motion.

tibia vara. The testing position to assess the degree of tibia vara requires the patient to be weightbearing on one leg only, allowing toe-touching with the contralateral leg for balance. This posture best reproduces the functional position of the lower limb during single limb stance, and will clearly demonstrate the amount of compensatory pronation necessary at the subtalar joint. The measurement is taken by relating the bisection of the distal one third of the leg to the supporting surface.

Now by comparing the measurements of tibia vara and calcaneal eversion, one can decide if the magnitude of subtalar pronation is sufficient. Ideally, the amount of calcaneal eversion should at least equal the tibia vara measurement in order to allow the foot to comfortably rest flat on the floor. If inadequate calcaneal eversion exists, one will often find a forefoot valgus or plantarflexed first ray as a compensation to obtaining forefoot contact.

In assessing foot pain, the entire lower extremity chain must be examined in order to rule out problems in the knee, hip, or spinal segments that might produce foot dysfunction.

FOOT PRESSURE STUDIES

Many foot problems develop secondary to forces imposed upon the foot. The difficulty in measuring these forces has caused considerable frustration for the clinician. The use of a force plate gives a general picture of various forces but often more specific information such as pressure is necessary. Pressure is a force per unit area and assessment can be critical particularly in dealing with tissue injury. At the present time, technology has not been able to provide a cost effective system to measure these pressures. Attempts have been made using pressure/temperature sensitive crystals[9] and pressure transducers.[10] Scranton et al[9] looked at the pressure patterns during walking, jogging, and running and suggested that the foot functions according to the individual's gait demands. In walking he found a smooth hindfoot, midfoot, metatarsal heads, and toes progression. He observed that the great toe and lateral toes provide a great deal of support. In jogging, the foot appears to slam down and then the forefoot functions to initiate push-off. In running, he observed the forefoot-hindfoot-forefoot pattern and suggested that the foot was acting as a decelerator for impact and later providing a means of propulsion.

During static stance, Morton[11] identified that an individual's weight is equally shared between the forefoot and heel with the first metatarsal head taking twice as much as any of the other metatarsal heads. However, subsequent studies emphasized that this pattern can be quite varied. Arcan and Brull[12] used a force plate with an optical pressure system and found that the heel supported 63 percent of body weight and that the forefoot supported 37 percent. Stokes et al[13,14] and Schwartz et al[15] emphasized that the pattern of pressure in ambulation was different from static stance.

During dynamic load, Stott and co-workers[16] found that 50 to 60 percent body weight was found under the heel, followed by 2 to 15 percent in the midfoot, and 30 to 50 percent in the forefoot. They found that standing load patterns do not correlate with walking load patterns and that the metatarsal bones do not necessarily carry loads in proportion to their size. The midfoot pattern seemed to vary with the amount of pronation or supination of the hindfoot. Schwartz et al[15] further pointed out that variation in foot pressure patterns were caused by:

1. Different foot postures
2. Walking velocity
3. Weight
4. Use of footwear
5. Changes in heel height

In their studies, Schwartz and co-workers[15] found that the third metatarsal head supported as much as the heel. As velocity increased, so did the maximum forces in the foot. With increased heel height they found minimal change in the heel but increased pressure under the first metatarsal and decreased pressure under the fifth metatarsal with no change under the third metatarsal.

STRESS FRACTURES

The occurrence of stress fractures has certainly become more common since the interest in running has increased. A stress fracture is actually a site of fatigue microdamage where remodeling of bone is occurring in response to increased force. It is the point of failure in a normal adaptive process. Since normal functioning muscle has been identified as a shock absorbing mechanism, it is understandable that when muscles cease to function properly the absorption of force is increased in other structures. One of these other structures is bone. In the foot the most common stress fractures occur in the second and third metatarsals.[17] The importance of repetitive stress in producing tissue destruction has been discussed in the literature and it is that critical level of stress that the clinician would like to recognize before dysfunction occurs.[18] A certain level of stress is necessary in order to further develop a system and when this stress is reduced the system becomes weaker. This is evident in the musculoskeletal and cardiovascular systems. With increased levels of exercise (stress) these systems become stronger. Scully and Besterman[19] identified that in one military basic training program, 4.9 percent of the recruits developed stress fractures which adversely affected the program. After initiating a new program which included a reduced physical activity period during every third week of training, the incidence of stress fractures reduced to 1.3 percent. In another of their controlled training studies similar results followed. In those who participated in the usual training regimen, the incidence of stress fractures was 4.8 percent. In the group which reduced their activity every third week, the incidence was 1.6 percent. The conclusion was based on the explanation that bone needs the opportunity to remodel in response to applied stress and that reduced physical stress on every third week allowed the normal physiologic responses to occur. They also emphasized the importance of muscle fatigue and stiff soled combat shoes in contributing to stress fractures.

Of significance also is the transfer of force proximally where joint structures in the lower extremity and spine may be affected. As pointed out by Cavanaugh and La Fortune,[20] vertical peak forces in sprinting approach 550 percent body weight. People with cavus foot structure and limited subtalar joint mobility tend to have problems with shock absorption.[17] Light et al[21] identified a deceleration transcient at heel strike which travels up the human skeleton during normal walking and appears to be dampened with the use of crepe rubber shoes and viscoelastic material within the heel of the shoe. They also discussed the potential shearing forces within the spinal facets and sacroilliac joints.

Scranton et al[22] pointed out the high incidence of fibular stress fractures at the region immediately above the tibiofibular syndesmosis. They believe that this fracture occurs secondarily to the axially rotated motion of the fibula as it descends during stance and is pulled by the flexors of the foot as they contract to support the arch and provide push-off. Fractures have also been identified in the distal and proximal tibia. The mechanical relationship of subtalar joint motion and transverse rotation of the lower extremity cannot be overlooked. Inman[23] pointed out that the subtalar joint acts as a torque convertor, allowing the absorption of torque at the ground interface. With individuals who demonstrate high inclined subtalar axes, this function becomes quite critical. For example, by mechanical analysis one can recognize that the high arched foot will produce greater transverse lower extremity rotation than the low arched foot for an equal amount of foot pronation/supination. What this means functionally is that if a person has a high degree of tibia vara and a high arched foot, the lower extremity will need to internally rotate further in order to get the foot flat to the ground. If the range of calcaneal eversion is insufficient, which is often the case in high arched feet, than the internal torque will be absorbed within the knee or distally in the tibia/fibula. It seems reasonable that repetitive stress, without rest, may eventually lead to a stress fracture in the leg. From a mechanical point of view, this situation can be helped by a varus heel wedge with a strong shoe counter. Forefoot wedging may also be necessary depending on the forefoot-to-hindfoot relationship.

It has also been recognized that people who have had fractures of the tibia and who were treated with casting have had problems with inadequate subtalar motion following cast removal.[24] X-rays revealed no osseous subtalar joint pathology so that limitation was felt to be due to soft tissue restriction. Though motion is small in the subtalar complex, attempts to achieve adequate motion through mobilization techniques should not be ignored.

The important point to remember is that more than just vertical forces act on the foot, and therefore multiple mechanisms to handle these forces must exist. When any of these mechanisms are insufficient, then problems secondary to mechanical stress usually result. These factors are discussed as they relate to common hindfoot, midfoot, and forefoot problems.

Hindfoot

The hindfoot consists of the calcaneus and talus, and thus the subtalar joint complex provides the major movement. Since the hindfoot provides one of the main weight supporting structures, it is subjected to considerable stress and is a common site of foot disorders.[25]

The ability of the foot to maintain its shape under load has been a topic of discussion throughout the literature. Hicks[26] and Lapidus[27] have proposed that the foot behaves as a truss and as a beam at times. A truss is a mechanical structure where a tie-rod prevents the ends of its rigid members from becoming further apart and there is no bending within it rigid members. The hindfoot (calcaneus and talus) and forefoot (five metatarsals, navicular, cuboid, and cuneiforms) make up the rigid members, and the plantar fascia is the tie-rod (Fig. 6-5). The height of the truss influences the amount of tension within the tie-rod. In a high arched structure the bending strain is decreased in its members but the stress is increased at the ends of the tie-rod. Conversely as the tie-rod lengthens, stress at the attachments is less but the bending strain of the members is greater. If this were transferred to the foot, one might expect that bending strains would be greater in the metatarsals of a low arched foot and that plantar fascial tension at the calcaneal attachment would be increased in the high arched foot. The reader is referred to the work by Hicks[28] for further details. Another interesting point is that as the center of body mass shifts anteriorly in the standing posture, tension in the plantar fascia as well as the Achilles tendon significantly increases.[29] Due to variation of foot types, one might expect that some feet will rely more heavily on the truss mechanism and some will rely more on the beam mechanism.

Plantar Heel Pain

Heel pain is one of the most common symptoms in the foot. A variety of causes estimated to account for about 15 percent of all adult foot complaints have been identified including the following:

1. Heel spurs
2. Painful fat pad
3. Neuritis
4. Plantar fascitis

Fig. 6-5. Foot as a truss: (a) rigid posterior member, (b) rigid anterior member, (c) tie rod

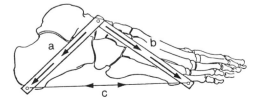

  5. Periosteitis
  6. Bursitis
  7. Syphilis
  8. Calcaneal stress fractures
  9. Those associated with systemic disorders
  10. Tarsal coalition
  11. Peripheral vascular disease

As one can see it seems imperative that a proper diagnosis be made in order to establish a reasonable management program. McCarthy and Gorecki[30] performed a cryomicrotomy study of 30 human feet to identify the structures associated with heel spurs. The human heel tissue is quite diverse and thus many structures may have the potential for producing symptoms (i.e., nerves, blood vessels, muscles, tendons, ligaments, and fascial planes). Their findings suggest that several levels of tissue are associated with heel spur formation and are summarized in the following discussion.

Connective tissue slips from the Achilles tendon were found to interdigitate with the calcaneus and then continue into the plantar fascia. On the medial side, the spur location was found to be intimately associated with the origin of the flexor digitorum brevis muscle and thus was positioned superior to the plantar fascial calcaneal attachment. Also in close proximity was the plantar accessorius and abductor hallucis muscles. Only on the lateral section was the plantar fascial calcaneal attachment associated with the spur. Numerous references in the literature have documented that the presence of a heel spur does not correlate with symptoms, and this seems reasonable in light of the variety of pain sensitive tissues under stress in this region.[31-33] It should also be clear from McCarthy and Gorecki's study that the spur is not entirely related to tension within the plantar fascia but is closely related to the short flexors in the foot. Common to most studies describing heel pain related to the spur is excessive subtalar joint pronation. As Perry[34] pointed out, subtalar pronation is a passive movement in gait and is controlled eccentrically by the posterior tibialis and soleus and later in stance by the toe flexors. There are two distinct force patterns in the heel: (1) compression during loading and (2) increased tensile force on the Achilles tendon and plantar fascia during the latter part of stance.

At initial contact a considerable amount of force is applied to the heel, and the anatomic structure of the heel helps to absorb the impact. The heel pad is constructed such that the fat cells are contained in compartments bounded by fibrous tissue. This fat pad gradually diminishes with age and as a result so does its shock absorbing capabilities. In patients with atrophic heel pads, synthetic material with similar viscoelastic properties should be placed in the shoe to supplement the remaining shock-absorbing tissue in the heel pad. Such materials are readily available in various sporting goods stores. Other treatment approaches that have been successful include polypropylene heel cups and custom fabricated foot orthoses with deep heel cups.[30,35,36]

The so called windlass action occuring during late stance as the MTP joints dorsiflex causes a tightening of the plantar fascia in an attempt to make the foot more rigid for an efficient lever system (Fig. 6-6). This supports the truss theory in that the height of the truss is raised by tightening the tie-rod (plantar-fascia) and a more rigid structure is obtained.

Heel pain caused by tensile forces on the soft tissue structures usually includes a nonradiating pain in the medial plantar aspect of the heel with no associated history of severe trauma. The individuals are usually obese and have either been on their feet for prolonged periods or have probably recently increased their activity. As stated previously, the presence of a heel spur does not correlate with symptoms. It is felt that the heel spur is a reflection of bone remodeling in response to tensile stress placed upon it.

It may well be that one might find low arched feet having heel spurs as a result of increased tension caused by the pull of the short toe flexors and not by tension in the plantar fascia. Remember in low arched feet the tension in the plantar fascia is decreased while the bending strain is greater in the metatarsals. Mann and Inman[37] studied the activity of the short toe flexors in a walking gait and found that in normal subjects, these muscles usually start to contract at about 35 percent of the gait cycle and continued to the end of stance. However, in people with "flat feet", the muscles began to contract much sooner in the gait cycle, anywhere from zero to 25 percent of the gait cycle. They concluded that intrinsic and short toe flexor muscles of the foot play a significant role in attempting to stabilize the midtarsal and subtalar joints in people with pronated feet. This excessive muscular activity may be responsible for medial plantar heel pain and the associated heel spur. Since these muscles are working overtime, fatigue from overuse may also result in arch pain or cramping. Attempts to control subtalar pronation are usually helpful if foot orthotic devices are indicated. However, one must be careful in prescribing foot orthotics if the excessive pronation is occurring due to deviations outside of the foot itself. Some disastrous results have occurred when foot orthoses have been prescribed when the pronation was due to transverse plane deviations (e.g., femoral anteversion and tibial torsion) or sagittal plane deviations (limited ankle joint dorsiflexion). In the former deviation, the knee is usually adversely af-

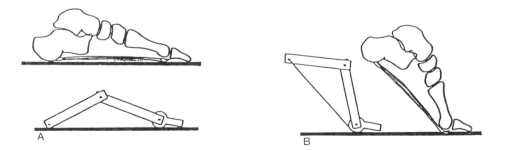

Fig. 6-6.   Windlass action: (A) relaxed plantar fascia during footflat (B) taut plantar fascia during heeloff. (Redrawn from Hicks JH: The foot as a support. S Karger AG, Basel. In ACTA Anatomica 25:180, 1955.)

fected with increased torque occurring, while in the latter, the problem is excessive pressure under the navicular resulting in more arch pain.

In patients with high arched feet, the tension in the tie-rod (plantar fascia) is greatest and it is this situation where the heel spur and pain may be related to the plantar fascia. In this case when the windlass action is tested in the clinical examination, pain is produced at the medial calcaneal fascial attachment. If the pain is not produced, some tissue other than the plantar fascia is probably inflamed (e.g., origin of the short toe flexors).

Katoh et al[38] used forceplates, foot switches, and videotape to study patients with plantar fascitis and painful heel syndromes. They compared the use of heel cups by measuring a variety of parameters and concluded that those with painful heel pads improved their parameters with heel cups while those with plantar fascitis did not.

Graham[39] evaluated a series of patients with painful heels. Routine roentographic examinations were negative. Bone scans were performed on 43 feet and 97.7 percent were found to be positive. Another roentgenogram was taken at a 45° angle superior to the transverse plane and fatigue fractures were observed. Bony condensation or collapse was found to occur on the medial facet of the calcaneus which appeared to be related to the pull of the flexor digitorum brevis and compression of the concave surface of the calcaneus. Conservative treatment consisted of either a heel cup or molded Plastazote inserts backed with foam rubber, and the patients were instructed to gradually increase their activity. Eighty-five percent reported satisfactory pain relief within 6 months.

The successful management of plantar heel pain obviously depends upon a proper diagnosis. In some instances, ill-defined migratory heel pain may be due to an early thrombophlebitis[40] or may be associated with a systemic disease process.[31] In either case, appropriate medical management is absolutely necessary. From a mechanical point of view, however, plantar heel pain may be due to excessive subtalar pronation resulting in elongation of the foot with tensile stress on the soft tissue attachments to the calcaneus. In this particular situation, attempts to decrease the tensile force of the soft tissue structures are usually helpful. Taping techniques to relieve arch strain are effective approaches as initial treatment.[7,41] The use of orthotic devices to control excessive pronation due to either rearfoot or forefoot deviations in the frontal plane are also usually successful.[42] However, as mentioned previously, when excessive pronation is due to mechanical deviations either in the transverse or sagittal planes, care must be taken in using foot orthotic devices due to causing problems in more proximal structures.[43] Generally, shoes with strong heel counters and crepe soles provide good heel control and shock absorption. Various materials added to the inside of the shoe may help to decrease the impact during gait.[44]

Posterior Heel Pain

Haglund's syndrome is a common cause of posterior heel pain.[45] It is characterized by painful soft tissue swelling at the level of the Achilles tendon insertion. Associated with it is a prominent calcaneal bursal projection which can be measured with lateral radiographs. The syndrome occurs in all ages and is usually associated with limited subtalar joint pronation. The heel counter of the shoe, if too rigid, may rub and cause discomfort over time. Management should include relieving pressure on the heel by adapting the heel counter.

Sever's disease is a syndrome which is found in young, active children between the ages of 8 and 12 years old. Pain is experienced at the superior/posterior margin of the calcaneus. It is caused by an increased pull of the Achilles tendon on the calcaneal epiphysis causing an inflammatory process. Treatment is conservative consisting of a $\frac{1}{8}$ to $\frac{1}{4}$ inch heel lift and a reduction of activity until the symptoms resolve.[46]

Tendon Injuries

Disabling pain may be associated with overuse in the tendons crossing the ankle and subtalar joints. Paratendinitis of the Achilles tendon is pain described over the tendon about 4 to 5 cm proximal to the insertion on the calcaneus.[47] Pain arising from the retrocalcaneal bursa can be distinguished from Achilles paratendinitis in the fact that the bursal pain is elicited by squeezing the area just anterior to the Achille's tendon. The etiology of pain in both areas appears to be related to mechanical causes either coming from training errors or biomechanical imbalances. The treatment initially is rest and control of the inflammation. From a mechanical point of view, heel lifts and supportive heel counters are beneficial. Excessively soft heel pads or soft soled shoes should be avoided as they may aggravate the problem. Weakness or decreased endurance of the gastroc–soleus complex should also be suspected.

Common among many individuals and especially runners is pain located posterior to the medial malleolus. The source of this pain may come from at least three different sources: the posterior tibial tendon, flexor hallucis longus tendon, or flexor digitorum longus tendon. During the first part of stance phase, the first posterior leg/foot muscle to contract is the tibialis posterior. It functions eccentrically to control calcaneal eversion during weight acceptance. If this motion occurs too rapidly or excessively then increased stresses are imparted on the tibialis posterior tendon resulting in overuse and pain. This may occur in runners who are rearfoot strikers as opposed to midfoot or forefoot strikers and may also occur quite frequently in patients with rheumatoid arthritis. In fact rupture of the tibialis posterior tendon has been identified in some patients with a history of chronic pain in this area.[48]

One should realize that the flexors hallucis and digitorum longus are intimately related anatomically and these tendons may also be the source of inflammation. Sprinters or ballet dancers will often experience pain in the flexor hallucis longus tendon since they are apt to be on their toes more than other athletes. In situations where the flexor digitorum longus is overused, symptoms may result in the same anatomic area. An example of this latter case has been found in individuals who wear wooden clog sandals where the toe flexors function to grip the front of the sandal. In any case, the inflamed tendon must be identified through clinical assessment and then a management approach established. With posterior tibial tendinitis, methods to control the rate or magnitude of subtalar joint pronation are usually helpful. This may include the use of medial heel wedges, foot orthotic devices, or shoe modifications.

Managing the flexor hallucis longus tendon problem is more challenging because of stress applied to the tendon when the heel is off the ground with the first metatarsophalangeal joint maximally extended. Weakness of the muscle may be responsible or it may be complicated by gastroc/soleus weakness. Foot orthotic devices do not seem to have any significant benefit. With overuse of the flexor digitorum muscle, relief of symptoms is usually obtained by changing shoes. Again, however, other areas that may be weak could potentially cause these muscles to be overworked and therefore careful assessment of muscle function is important.

Midfoot

Midfoot problems primarily include the talonavicular, calcaneocuboid, and cuneiform-metatarsal articulations. Obviously, the hindfoot (talocalcaneal) complex is intimately related functionally with the midfoot and thus many problems involve both areas. Mann et al[17] state that the most common midfoot complaint is medial longitudinal arch pain which may be related to painful fascitis, myalgia, and/or intermetatarsal ligament pain. The cause of this pain is usually excessive subtalar joint pronation and in the runner may be aggravated by softer running shoes with poor rearfoot stability. Management approaches should concentrate on changing these areas.

Midfoot pain may be associated with inadequate mobility of the midtarsal and subtalar joints. Tarsal coalitions which are cartilaginous or osseous unions of two or more tarsal bones have been described and may account for this stiffness and pain syndrome.[49] The resulting pain is often vague and insidious in onset and referred to the talonavicular joint, but may also be deep in the subtalar joint. The onset may be precipitated by minor trauma or by walking over uneven ground. A common observation is spasm within the peroneals.[50] The coalitions may or may not be evident with x-ray since some are cartilaginous. Conservative treatment is usually aimed at supporting the foot with the use of Thomas heels, medial heel wedges, and accommodative arch pads. In some instances surgical removal of the coalition is necessary in order to improve normal hindfoot and midfoot function. Peroneal muscle spasm has also been observed in patients with rheumatoid arthritis.[51] Anatomic studies performed by Kyne and Mankin[52] identified that the pressures within the subtalar joint increase with progressive subtalar supination and decrease with pronation.

Theoretically, if subtalar joint pathology exists and if increased pressure within the joint causes pain, then the foot might assume a more relaxed position. As a result, the posterior tibialis may relax reflexly and the peroneals may shorten or go into spasm to allow subtalar pronation. Again accurate diagnosis is imperative and perhaps early intervention with adequate rearfoot control might prevent the osseous collapse and dysfunction.

Dorsal midfoot pain located at the medial cuneiform/first metatarsal joint is a common finding and can be quite disabling. A dorsal exostosis at this joint probably results from compressive forces and causes a problem with shoe fitting. The extensor hallucis longus tendon which crosses the joint dorsally can become inflamed if the shoe lacing pattern causes excessive pressure or friction. Adaptive modifications to the tongue of the shoe or lacing pattern, or a shoe with better conformity to the shape of the midfoot can alleviate this problem.

Kohlers disease is a condition where avascular necrosis of the epiphysis of the navicular bone occurs and is usually seen in children between the ages of 3 and 5 years. Pain is experienced on weight bearing. Conservative management includes shoes with stable heel counters, a Thomas heel, and a soft accommodative arch support. The syndrome is usually self limiting and causes no significant problems.[46]

Forefoot

Forefoot pain can be the end result of numerous biomechanic faults, including hindfoot malalignments, limited motion, and weakness of muscles and associated soft tissue structures. Metatarsalgia is a general term often used to describe such painful conditions of the forefoot. A number of the most common causes of forefoot pain is discussed, including the clinical appearance, etiology, and management.

Forefoot Varus Pronation Syndrome

Forefoot varus, a malalignment of the forefoot in relation to the hindfoot, can lead to numerous areas of pain in both the lower limb and foot (see Fig. 6-3). With the subtalar joint in neutral position, the plane of the metatarsal heads presents with an inverted, or varus, attitude in relation to the hindfoot bisectional reference. This results in lack of medial stability during stance due to elevation of the first metatarsal from the floor. The mechanism of compensation is usually excessive subtalar and oblique midtarsal joint pronation. This compensatory pronation is evident by excessive and prolonged calcaneal eversion during stance and possibly an increase in lower limb internal rotation in the transverse plane. Other clinical signs and symptoms include hallux valgus, callus formation under the second, third, and fourth metatarsal heads, claw toes, plantar fascitis, and medial malleolar or lowerleg pain. The hallux valgus is encouraged by both the ground reaction forces pushing laterally on the medial border of the great toe, and by the cumulative dorsiflexion and eversion of the first metatarsal and great toe associated with pronation.[53] Callosities under the middle three toes are likewise influenced by several factors. Hypermobility of the first ray results from subtalar and oblique midtarsal pronation, allowing the vertically directed ground reaction forces to push this mobile first ray upward. This leaves the second, third, and fourth metatarsal heads vulnerable to shearing forces[54] that are further enhanced by hypermobility of the entire forefoot. The foot should normally be supinating at this point in gait creating a stable base of support for push-off. Excessive pronation, however, allows for an overtly flexible forefoot due to the parallel alignment of the midtarsal joint axes, resulting in excessive motion under the metatarsal heads.

Length of the metatarsals is another significant factor. The second metatarsal is usually longer than the first and in conjunction with the orientation of the second metatarsal head lying more caudal than the first, allows for ground contact with the second metatarsal head to occur before the first.[55] Hypermobility of the first ray then ensures that force under the second will be abnormally high and prolonged. Compensatory pronation has further effects on MTP joint function by causing the foot to utilize the metatarsal break axis instead of the transverse axis of the first and second MTP joints. Normal transfer of weight through the first and second rays, utilization of appropriate levers of the foot, and generation of adequate push-off forces will therefore be altered and lead to excessive stresses under the second, third, and fourth metatarsal heads.

The cause of forefoot varus is thought to be a rotational deformity of the talus. It assumes a varus attitude in the fetus, then a progressive valgus rotation of the talar head and neck normally occurs. Proper alignment is achieved by 15 to 18 months, having completed the 35 to 40° of torsion.[3,7] Delayed or incomplete talar rotation will leave the head and neck in a varus orientation, resulting in a forefoot varus secondary to this abnormal midtarsal joint orientation.

Management principles are directed toward eliminating the need for compensatory pronation. Medial stability of the foot will not be achieved until the first ray makes firm contact with the supporting surface. An orthosis is fabricated with sufficient medial posting to allow first ray contact while the subtalar joint is ideally in neutral position (Fig. 6-7). This medial buildup of orthotic material essentially brings the supporting surface up to the medial foot, thereby

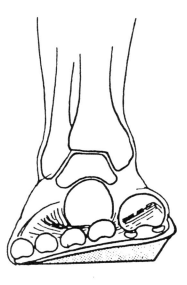

Fig. 6-7. Forefoot varus with medial forefoot post. (Redrawn from Mann RA: Conservative treatment and office procedures. In Mann RA (ed): Surgery of the Foot. 5th Ed. CV Mosby Co, Saint Louis, 1986.)

accommodating the malalignment. The posting is often described as being just proximal to the metatarsal heads, having full thickness medially and tapering off laterally. However, in the absence of palpable pain under the metatarsal heads, the patient can usually tolerate posting directly under the heads provided the orthosis is either fabricated from a semirigid polyethylene material, or a thin layer of compressive shock absorbing material is added on top of a more rigid orthosis. Care must be taken to prevent excessive compression by the orthosis under the shaft of the first metatarsal as it plantarflexes due to active contraction of the peroneus longus or from lowering of the medial foot during pronation. The length of a rigid orthosis must also be considered such that it does not interfere with extension at the MTP joint. Cinematographic studies confirm that orthotic devices restore abnormal parameters of foot function during gait and running to more normal values.[56-58] The affected parameters include more vertical heel orientation at midstance, reduction in maximum pronation, reduction in total rearfoot movement, and decreased maximum pronation velocity. Force platform studies reveal that transverse torque about the long axis of the tibia, termed Mz, normally is in an internal direction at heel strike and reverses at midstance to show an external rotation torque.[59] This shift from internal to external torque never occurs in the pronating foot due to a failure of adequate resupination. Use of an orthosis can restore the normal Mz torque curve. Short term measures may be achieved by taping or padding. Taping techniques, such as the "figure 8" or low dye methods with the foot maintained in a supinated attitude will provide support for the medial structures and relieve tensile stresses on the plantar fascia.[60] Measures to accommodate the associated consequences of excessive pronation are discussed in the appropriate following sections.

Hallux Valgus

Hallux valgus is characterized by an excessively abducted and everted posture of the great toe. A slight degree of valgus is normal at the first MTP joint, with an acceptable range measuring 9 to 17°.[61] The clinical appearance may also include an overriding second toe as it elevates secondary to an acquired hammertoe deformity and pressure from the abducting great toe. The remaining toes may develop claw toe deformities with callus formation under the second, third, and fourth metatarsal heads and on the dorsal aspect of the proximal interphalangeal joints. An inflammatory bursitis can develop over the medial aspect of the first MTP joint, due to shearing of the soft tissue over the prominent, medial osteophyte. This inflamed bursa is often termed a bunion, and is a consequence of repeated trauma and fibrosis.

Hallux valgus may be caused by a number of factors. As previously discussed, an excessively pronating foot with the resultant hypermobility and instability at the first MTP joint and the presence of lateral forces acting on the hallux may push the toe into a valgus attitude.

A predisposing factor closely associated with hallux valgus is metatarsus primus varus. This condition reflects an overtly adducted posture of the first metatarsal. Alignment of the first metatarsal is determined by using the second metatarsal as a reference and measuring the angle between them. A slight degree of first ray varus is normal, with a range measured between 5 and 9°.[61] Determination of a varus alignment can also be made by examining the angle formed between the first and fifth metatarsals. Values between 23 and 29° are considered normal.[61] The first metatarsal may also be adducted in conjunction with the lesser metatarsals in the presence of forefoot adductus. The hallux itself can further accentuate this varus alignment, once the process has begun, due to the ground reaction forces. These act backward through the abducted great toe and have a medially directed component which pushes the metatarsal head further into adduction.[62]

A consequence of hallux valgus is lateral displacement of the extensor hallucis longus tendon due to weakening of supportive soft tissues.[63] This results in yet another abductory force exerted on the great toe secondary to the more lateral pull of the tendon. Further muscle imbalances may occur due to lateral subluxation of the sesamoids, thereby reorienting more laterally the pull of the intrinsic musculature into which they are imbedded.[64] Inappropriate footwear may contribute additional abductory stresses on the hallux. These include shoes having pointed toes, which do not provide adequate space and essentially squeeze the toes together. Shoes without laces or straps must rely on this abnormally high forefoot compression to maintain the shoe on the foot.

Treatment is aimed at reducing the forces which encourage deviation of the great toe. Since excessive pronation may lead to this deformity, measures to control compensatory pronation as outlined in the section on forefoot varus should be considered.

Proper footwear is a basic requirement in the management of hallux valgus. The shoe should have laces to provide both an adequate entry into the shoe, and once donned, the ability to tighten the shoe to maintain stability. The forepart of the shoe, the vamp, and toe-box, should be rounded to prevent squeezing of the toes and minimize laterally directed forces against the great toe. The toe-box should have sufficient vertical height to prevent pressure on the dorsal aspects of the lesser toes from the inside surface of the upper material. This is especially important when deformities of these toes are present. Adequate height may also be necessary to accommodate insertion of an orthosis into the shoe, particularly if the orthosis contains large amounts of posting material.

A splint may be worn to conteract the abductory forces on the great toe. It is fabricated from any sufficiently rigid plastic material and is designed to push the toe medially into adduction (Fig. 6-8). This is achieved by obtaining proximal stability against the medial forefoot, which then creates a torque about the distal component and results in the adductory force on the lateral aspect of the great toe. A similar medial force can be achieved by taping a piece of stockinette, or similar material, to the medial aspect of the great toe and forefoot. The material is initially stabilized on the toe, then a sufficient stretch is applied to the material to create appropriate tension which pulls the hallux into adduc-

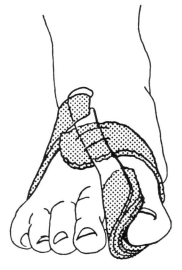

Fig. 6-8. Plastic hallux valgus splint. (Berkemann, West Germany) Distributed by Alimed Inc., 297 High St., Dedham, MA 02026.

tion.[60] The proximal end is then taped to the forefoot for stability. Pain over the medial prominance of the MTP joint may require padding to relieve excessive pressure from the shoe. This is achieved by a crescent shaped pad fabricated from a semirigid or soft foam material placed proximal to the first MTP joint. For more severe cases, a doughnut shaped pad is constructed.[60] Management of the acquired lesser toe deformities and limited motion of the first MTP joint is discussed in the appropriate following sections.

Hallux Limitus/Rigidus

Hallux limitus is marked by a decrease in great toe extension at the first MTP joint. Further progression leading to total loss of motion is termed hallus rigidus. Once the limitation prevents the minimum 60 to 65° of great toe extension necessary for gait, abnormally high stresses are transmitted to the first MTP joint, leading to pain and resulting compensations in an attempt to unweight the area. One such compensation is excessive supination where weight bearing forces are consequently shifted to the lateral aspect of the forefoot. Clinically, callus formation under the fourth and fifth metatarsal heads may be seen in response to these increased pressures. The patient will show deficits in gait from heel-off to toe-off corresponding to the degree of pain associated with great toe extension during this period. As restricted mobility progresses into more advanced stages, additional clinical features appear. These include the formation of an osteophyte over the dorsal aspect of the first metatarsal head due to prolonged exposure to compressive forces, and development of a callus at the plantar aspect of the interphalangeal (IP) joint of the hallux resulting from compensatory hyperextension.[64]

The underlying pathology is that of osteoarthritis which may be caused by one specific traumatic event or a cumulative result of prolonged stresses over a number of years. The first MTP joint undergoes a progression of events from initial episodes of joint swelling to later stage developments of osteophyte formation, erosion of articular cartilage, and fibrosed joint capsule.[63]

Excessive compensatory pronation in conjunction with hypermobility of the first ray is one cause of repeated stress. During excessive pronation, the hypermobile first ray is pushed dorsally, particularly in the presence of an everted calcaneus.[64] Extension of the hallux, however, requires plantarflexion of the first metatarsal so that the proximal phalanx can rotate upward over the cartilaginous surface of the metatarsal head. The abnormal elevation of the first ray therefore alters normal mechanics and leads to the increased compressive and shearing forces at the MTP joint, especially along its dorsal aspect.[36] Osteophyte formation is therefore most likely to occur along the dorsal borders of the joint. Excessive compressive forces can also result from improper footwear. Shoes that are too short may exert a posteriorly directed force on the tip of the great toe, thereby compressing the joint and limiting MTP extension.

Treatment is directed toward minimizing stresses to the first metatarsophalangeal joint. Proper footwear is again of great importance. The shoe must have adequate length to prevent the distal contact of the hallux and the resultant posterior forces. The toe box should possess proper depth to eliminate pressure on the dorsal aspect of the MTP joint in the presence of protruding osteophytes. If pressure on osteophytes persists, the leather upper can be spot-stretched to provide further room or a doughnut shaped pad can be placed dorsally over the joint to redistribute pressure. An extra-depth shoe with deerskin uppers may provide additional softness. The extra-depth may also be necessary to accommodate an orthosis, as previously discussed, if control of excessive pronation is required to alleviate stresses to the MTP joint.

A rocker bottom sole applied with the apex of the curvature just proximal to a line between the first and fifth metatarsal heads can provide two needed functions (Fig. 6-9). First, it helps to unweight the first metatarsal head by redistributing the weight bearing forces proximally. Second, it provides a degree of functional extension distally in the foot and thus minimizes motion in the shoe. This serves to reduce the extension stresses imparted to an immobile joint during heel-off and imitates to some degree, the normal lever system of the foot. The apex of the rocker sole simulates the MTP joint in this lever system model.

Acute episodes of pain can be managed by placing a metatarsal pad proximal to the head of the first metatarsal, thereby redistributing pressure to the metatarsal shaft. This can be incorporated with the more commonly used pad for the second, third, and fourth metatarsals by fabricating a medial extension.[60] When pain under these three middle metatarsal heads is absent, the pad can be extended distally to be directly under the heads. This functionally elevates the first ray and further lessens contact with the supporting surface.

Joint mobilization in conjunction with modalities such as ultrasound, heat, or ice may restore functional joint range of motion in the early stages.

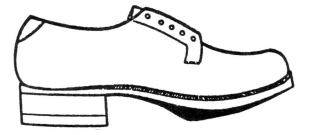

Fig. 6-9. Shoe with rocker bottom sole (Redrawn from Zamosky I: Shoe modifications in lower-extremity orthotics. p. 54–95. Bulletin of Prosthetics Research. Fall 1964.)

Hammer Toes/Claw Toes

These two distinct deformities have many features in common, including the appearance of the MTP and proximal interphalangeal (PIP) joints, similar etiologies, and management principles.

Hammer toes are deformities characterized by hyperextension of the MTP joints and flexion at the PIP joints (Fig. 6-10). The distal interphalangeal (DIP) joint may be slightly extended or remain in a normal alignment.[36] Claw toes show a similar alignment at the MTP and PIP joints with the DIP presenting with flexion, resulting in the characteristic clawed appearance. Accompanying this extended position of the proximal phalanx is planterflexion or depression of the metatarsals. This configuration leads to increased points of pressure under the metatarsal heads, the dorsal surface of the PIP joints and under the DIP or tip of the distal phalanx with resultant callus formation.

These two deformities can be the result of several underlying causes. Maintenance of normal balance in lower leg and foot musculature, especially the intrinsics, is vital in prevention of the deformity. Tension in both the extensor digitorum longus and brevis muscles in a weightbearing position produces extension of the MTP joints and flexion of the PIP and DIP joints.[6] Forces generated by the flexor digitorum longus and brevis result in flexion of the PIP joints, with extension simultaneously occurring at both the MTP and DIP joints due to ground reaction forces pushing upward on the flexing distal phalanx. Combined actions of the flexors and extensors, therefore, produce the same effect in weight bearing, that being extension of the MTP and flexion of the PIP

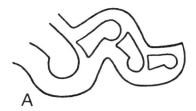

A

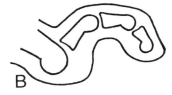

B

Fig. 6-10. Toe deformities: (A) hammer toe, (B) claw toe. (Redrawn from Helfet AJ, Gruebel Lee DM (eds): Disorders of the Foot. JB Lippincott Co, Philadelphia, 1980.)

joints. These forces are normally checked by the intrinsic musculature. Tension developed in both the interossei and lumbricales in a nonweightbearing posture produces flexion of the MTP joint while the lumbricales additionally cause extension of the PIP and DIP joints, the opposite actions of the previously mentioned flexor and extensor muscles. When weightbearing, the interossei and lumbricales provide a flexion stabilizing force at the MTP joint and an extension stabilization at the PIP and DIP joints. These stabilizing forces neutralize the deforming properties of the flexor and extensor groups and maintain the toes in a straight alignment.[6] Weakness of the interossei and lumbricales can therefore lead to hammer toes. The deformity itself will render the interossei ineffective by causing the tendon to move dorsally and eliminating its ability to mechanically create flexion at the MTP joint.[62]

Assisting the intrinsic muscles to stabilize the proximal phalanx are the plantar aponeurosis and plantar joint capsule.[65] Prolonged stretching of these structures will reduce the amount of tensile forces they generate, thereby placing a greater burden upon the intrinsics and altering the normal balance of sagittally directed forces about the MTP joint. Overstretching is likely to occur with sustained, passive MTP extension, such as when wearing high heeled shoes.

Inappropriate footwear may lead to the development of hammer toes. Shoes that are too short may push posteriorly on the distal phalanx. The toes respond to this force by moving in the direction of least resistance, MTP extension and PIP flexion, thereby functionally shortening the toe.

Shoes should be of sufficient length to prevent these posterior compressive forces on the tip of the toes and also possess adequate depth to minimize compressive forces over the dorsally protruding PIP joints. The extra-depth shoe may also be necessary to accomodate insertion of a metatarsal pad.

The metatarsal pad will provide three functions. It redistributes the vertical ground reaction forces proximally to the shafts of the metatarsals and unweights the prominent, depressed metatarsal heads. Second, it imparts a passive force to the plantar aponeurosis, which increases tension within its fibers. This enhanced tensile force acts upon the proximal phalanx to provide flexion stabilization. Wearing a shoe with a negative heel will likewise increase tension within the plantar aponeurosis.[65] Lastly, the metatarsals are pushed dorsally out of their plantarflexed posture, which will further assist in repositioning of the toes downward.

Orthodigital splints, may be worn to counteract the deforming forces with passive, external pressure. The pads are fabricated from a semirigid or soft material and grooved to fit around the toes. One component is placed on the dorsal aspect of the proximal phalanx to provide a downward force. A second component can be placed on the plantar aspect of the middle phalanx to push upward.[60] Force is transmitted to the splints from the inside of the shoe itself, which in turn acts upon the toes. Taping may be substituted in place of the splints to achieve the same external forces. The tape is secured to the plantar aspect of the forefoot, passes between the base of the toes, is then wrapped around the dorsum of the proximal phalanx, and is finally reattached to the sole.

Two other techniques to assist in management of this deformity include the use of toe caps to pad and protect the tip of the toe from irritation and strengthening exercises for the lumbricales and interossei.

Plantarflexed First Ray

A plantarflexed first ray is characterized by a more caudal position of the first metatarsal head in relation to the plane of the lesser metatarsal heads (Fig. 6–11). All five normally lie on the same plane, being perpendicular to the bisected calcaneus. This deformity can be either flexible or rigid, with the rigid condition responsible for the clinical symptoms. Mobility of the first ray can be determined by passive plantarflexion and dorsiflexion, normally showing a range of 10 mm in each direction in reference to the stabilized second metatarsal head. Maintenance of a caudal position with a dorsally directed pressure under the first metatarsal head denotes a rigid plantarflexed first ray. Callus formation under the first metatarsal head is likely to develop in response to excessive shearing stresses. Position of the calcaneus during stance is likely to show inversion, from rearfoot and/or midfoot malalignment, or forced subtalar supination secondary to ground pressure pushing upward under the rigid first ray. This compensatory supination may lead to the development of callus under the fifth metatarsal head.

Plantarflexion of the first ray occurs as an additional compensatory mechanism in the presence of subtalar varus, forefoot varus, or tibia vara. In the absence of adequate subtalar joint pronation to fully compensate for these biomechanic faults, the medial forefoot remains unstable due to continued elevation of the first ray. Contraction of the peroneus longus ensues to pull the

Fig. 6-11. Plantar flexed first ray.

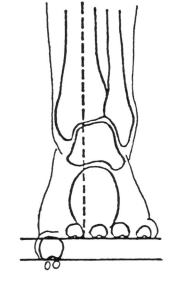

first metatarsal caudally, acting through its attachment at the base of the metatarsal. This results in contact between the metatarsal head and supporting
surface, assuring stability. Prolonged first ray plantarflexion in the presence of
inflammation secondary to repeated trauma or diseases such as rheumatoid
arthritis, may result in a fibrosed, rigid plantarflexed deformity. Other causes
include neurologic deficits which lead to muscular imbalances within the foot or
lower leg and a congenitally plantarflexed first ray.

An orthotic device can be an effective means of accommodation to the
deformity with the degree of posting material dependent upon foot alignment. If
the first ray is rigidly plantarflexed in the absence of varus at the tibia, rearfoot,
or forefoot, the orthosis should contain posting under the second to fifth metatarsal heads. This maintains the normal alignment of these metatarsals in relation to the hindfoot and provides contact with all metatarsal heads to occur
functionally on the same plane, and eliminates the forced supination incurred
by ground reaction forces pushing dorsally under the protruding metatarsal
head. When varus deformities of the tibia or subtalar joint are present, the
orthosis should contain rearfoot posting to obtain rearfoot stability. Since the
forefoot is now in a varus attitude in relation to the supporting surface, secondary to the rearfoot varus, forefoot posting should be under the middle three
metatarsal heads. Maximum thickness is required under the second, tapering
off as the post continues laterally. A plantarflexed first secondary to forefoot
varus only would require forefoot posting similar to that just described. Rearfoot posting would not be necessary as the hindfoot is in a normally balanced
alignment.

Continuing pain under the first and fifth metataral heads can be managed
by the previously mentioned means to relieve pressure, such as with metatarsal
pads or a rocker sole.

Morton's Neuroma

Morton's neuroma is characterized by pain between two adjacent metatarsal heads, rather than directly under them. The symptoms are usually localized
to a specific point on the plantar aspect of the forefoot, with radiation outward
to encompass the toe cleft or less commonly proximally to the distal leg.[66] Pain
may be accompanied by parasthesias, which are both exacerbated during gait.
The symptoms may also be elicited with manual mediolateral compression of
the forefoot or with flexion/extension at the lesser MTP joints. A dorsally
directed compressive force under the involved metatarsal heads in conjunction
with the manual compression may result in a painful, audible "click."[36] Patients may experience relief during ambalation by removing their shoes,
thereby eliminating mediolateral compressive forces on the forefoot.

An understanding of the underlying etiologic factors requires a brief anatomic review of the associated nerves. The planter nerves arise from the tibial
nerve, bifurcating into a medial and lateral branch shortly after entering the foot
behind the medial malleolus. The medial branch terminates into digital nerves

which supply sensation to the medial $3\frac{1}{2}$ toes, with the remaining $1\frac{1}{2}$ innervated by the lateral plantar nerve. Below the third and fourth metatarsals lies a communicating branch, providing direct communication between the medial and plantar nerves and an additional source of innervation to the cleft between the third and fourth toes.[67]

Morton's neuroma, or plantar digital neurites, can result from one of many proposed pathologies, all of which lead to thickening and fibrosis of the digital nerve. One such cause may be the repeated trauma of walking, leading to a localized inflammation of the digital nerve, with resultant fibrosis and enlargement. This is of particular importance in the hypermobile, excessively pronating foot, where shearing forces are exaggerated.[36] Inflammatory reactions may occur in the accompanying vascular supply, leading to arteritis and resultant ischemia to the digital nerves. Ischemia may likewise result from external compressive forces and fibrosis. Enlargement of the intermetatarsophalangeal bursa, secondary to inflammatory changes, provides yet another source of digital nerve compression. Adhesions may also develop between the nerves and bursa, which is positioned caudally to the deep transverse metatarsal ligament and is situated close to the digital nerves.[67]

The most common site of involvement is the cleft between the third and fourth toes. One explanation may be the presence of the communicating branch between the two plantar nerves, found only at this segment. Also implicated as a cause is the apparent hypomobility of the fourth metatarsal in the frontal plane.[68] It shows more equal amounts of inversion and eversion than the remaining metatarsals, having a ratio of 1.4:1 of inversion to eversion. The neighboring third metatarsal, on the other hand, shows the greatest frontal plane mobility, having a ratio of 2.5:1.

Treatment is designed towards reducing compressive forces between the metatarsals. An orthosis with appropriate medial posting to lessen compensatory pronation will lead to reduced shearing forces under the metatarsals. A metatarsal pad, either incorporated into the orthosis or by itself, can decrease forces by elevating the middle three metatarsals and providing support proximal to the heads.

Proper footwear is of basic paramount importance in proper management. Shoes should have both a rounded toe box and laces, to eliminate the excessive mediolateral compression often found in shoes having pointed toes or those overly tight in the forefoot necessary to maintain the foot in the shoe.

ARTHRITIS

Joints within the foot may become clinically involved as a consequence of numerous rheumatic diseases, including rheumatoid arthritis, Reiter's syndrome, psoriatic arthritis, and gout. Manifestations of these disorders result in deformities similar to those described earlier, particularly those of hallux valgus, hallux rigidus, clawed toes with depressed metatarsal heads, and an excessively pronated foot. However, these disease processes may lead to foot syndromes unique to the specific disorder, as a result of solitary lesions or combinations of sequellae. Rheumatoid arthritis is discussed in detail and the remaining three briefly mentioned in regards to symptomatology within the foot.

Rheumatoid Arthritis

Rheumatoid arthritis causes the most severe clinical manifestations of all the rheumatic diseases.[69] Involvement of the feet occurs in 70 to 85 percent of all rheumatoid patients.[70,71]

Rheumatoid arthritis is characterized by inflammation of the peripheral joints. Symptoms early in the course of the disease include morning stiffness, secondary to mild inflammation and sustained immobility. Progression of the disease leads to joint pain upon movement or compression, swelling of the joint and surrounding soft tissue, and fatigue.[70,72] The inflammatory process affects the synovium, particularly along its peripheral attachments of the joint, where the inflammation is most severe. Large villi of granulation tissue called pannus develops at these joint margins and either enters the subchondral bone at this juncture[72] or spreads across the joint surface before eventually communicating with the subchondral bone.[70] The result of both of these processes is erosion of articular cartilage and underlying bone. The surrounding soft tissue, including the joint capsule and ligaments, become stretched and weakened. They consequently lose their ability to exert appropriate stabilizing forces on the surrounding bone ends necessary to maintain proper alignment. Altered configuration of the articular surfaces results in abnormal joint contact and altered joint reaction forces between the bone ends, thereby further reducing the stabilizing forces of the joint. These two factors allow for development of initially flexible deformities within the bony architecture due to either overpowering internal forces generated by associated muscle imbalances, particularly those whose tendons have deviated, or from external forces, such as improper footwear and ground reaction forces. Further progression of the disease shows chronic inflammation, resulting in osteoporosis, weakening and perhaps rupture of muscle tendons, fibrous infiltration into the normally present collagen fibers within the muscle leading to eventual contracture, and marked hypomobility or ankylosis of contiguous bone segments due to fibrosis.[70,72]

Rheumatoid arthritis involves all segments of the foot, most commonly the forefoot.[73] The MTP joints represent the most frequent site of both clinical symptoms and radiologic change within the entire foot.[74] Involvement of the great toe MTP generally leads to hallux valgus or hallux limitus/rigidus. Other, less frequent deformities may occur, such as chisel toe or hallux elevatus. Chisel toe is characterized by an extension deformity of the distal phalanx over the proximal at the IP joint, usually occuring as a compensatory mechanism for a hallux rigidus.[75] Hallux elevatus presents as an extension deformity of the proximal phalanx over the metatarsal at the MTP joint in response to plantarflexion of the first metatarsal.[75] This may lead to a lack of ground reaction with the great toe and result in a functional loss of the anterior lever between the MTP and great toe normally seen with heel-off. This loss of level function also occurs with hallux valgus.[62] Manifestations at the lesser MTPs commonly results in claw toe deformities. This hyperextension of the proximal phalanges is associated with plantarflexion of the lesser metatarsals and spread of the forefoot due to weakening of the intermetatarsal ligament.[74] The forefoot also tends to abduct in the presence of this laxity.[71] The fat pads normally aligned under the metatarsal heads to relieve compressive and shearing forces are dislocated anteriorly due to forces exerted by the extended proximal phalanges, and this results in excessive forces directed towards the now exposed, prominent, metatarsal heads. These compressive forces are exaggerated in the presence of fibrotic ankylosis, as the ability to absorb and disperse these stresses is reduced or eliminated.

Manifestations of the midfoot may lead to hypermobility of and breakdown of medial stability. Integrity of the talonavicular joint, and to a lesser degree the naviculocuneiform joints, is necessary to control the medial displacement of the talus during pronation.[74] This stability is normally provided by ligamentous, capsular, and muscular support. These structures become weak and lax when involved, leading to collapse of the medial longitudinal arch, medial bulging of the midfoot due to excessive talar movement, and subluxation across the talonavicular and calcaneocuboid joints.[70,74] The result is a typically flatfooted appearance which becomes rigidly fixed when exposed to prolonged inflammation. Often accompanying the rigid flatfoot is peroneal muscle spasm, particularly of the peroneus brevis,[71] termed peroneal spastic flatfoot deformity.

Involvement of the subtalar joint gives rise to a valgus deformity of the hindfoot, and may be the initiating factor in the development of rigid flatfoot.[71] Two distinct mechanical events impart valgus forces to the hindfoot. The first concerns the points of application of weight bearing forces acting upon the calcaneus. Body weight is transmitted through the distal tibia and talus to the superior surface of the calcaneus. The point of contact between the calcaneus and the floor, however, occurs lateral to this talocalcaneal force. This noncontiguous vertical alignment between these two opposing forces results in a torque imparted upon the calcaneus, forcing the calcaneus into a valgus position.[34]

Second, this eversion torque is enhanced by internal rotation of the lower limb, which acting through the subtalar joint, also produces a valgus position of the calcaneus. Stretching and weakening of the medial stabilizing structures, including ligaments, joint capsules, and surrounding musculature, results in the inability to counteract these valgus forces. Equilibrium between opposing forces is therefore lost and the calcaneus is thrust into valgus. This deformity, as those previously mentioned, will become fibrosed in the presence of prolonged inflammation. The primary outcome will be marked limitation of subtalar range of motion (ROM), blocking functional calcaneal motion during gait and eliminating the ability of the foot to dissipate weightbearing stresses. Secondary alterations in lower limb function will result by preventing transmission of transverse plane rotation of the leg into the foot.

Manifestations at the ankle joint initially present as pain which progresses to decreased ROM and fibrosis. The condyles of the talus may collapse under the weightbearing forces, further limiting mobility and attenuating pain.[70] The resultant loss of plantarflexion prevents loss of loading response following heel strike, and in conjunction with forefoot involvement, limits the amount of vertical ground reaction forces generated by the forefoot during push-off. The outcome is a flat-footed, apropulsive gait. Limitation of dorsiflexion inhibits proper advancement of the tibia over the fixed foot during stance phase. A related consequence which influences the amount of available ankle ROM, although not affecting the joint proper, is erosion of the calcaneus at the Achilles tendon insertion.[74] Both active contraction during plantarflexion and passive stretching when dorsiflexing increase tensile stresses at this osseotendinous junction, eliciting pain and consequently inhibiting motion.

Comprehensive studies reveal many additional abnormalities associated with rheumatoid gait. Examination of kinematic parameters shows decrease in stride length, cadence, and velocity.[76] These clinically present as a slow gait pattern with short steps and decreased speed of the advancing leg. The duration of double-limb support increases, so that weightbearing forces can be shared among the two feet for a prolonged period of time. This serves to delay the onset of single-limb stance and decreases its duration, thereby minimizing the amount of time required for one foot to bear the entire load.

The center of pressure (CP), defined as the point of application of weightbearing forces on the plantar aspect of the foot, normally follows a path along the midline of the foot.[77] It shows a rapid, forward velocity immediately upon heel strike, which continues until the CP assumes a location under the metatarsal heads. Here the speed markedly decreases, attaining values as low as 6 m/sec.[77] This changing pattern of CP velocities shows the significance of the metatarsal heads in acceptance of weightbearing forces. In the rheumatoid foot, several changes of the CP are observed. The path of the CP deviates somewhat laterally, assuming a forefoot location between the second and third metatarsal heads rather than between the first and second.[76] Velocity of the CP showed a reversed relationship, presenting now with a slow speed in the rearfoot and a rapid velocity in the forefoot. This pattern ensures that weightbearing forces will be predominantly imparted to the heel while reducing the amount of time the load must be borne by the rigid, painful, metatarsal heads. The amount of force is a function of time, which is the area under a force/time curve (the integral of force against time), is termed the impulse and reflects these changes in CP velocity. The prolonged application of weightbearing forces under the heel in the rheumatoid foot, secondary to a slower velocity, is reflected by a larger heel impulse.[76] Correspondingly, a reduced impulse is calculated under the first and second metatarsal heads and toes due to the increased CP velocity.[76]

Many of the manifestations of rheumatoid arthritis result in deformities similar to those discussed in the section on biomechanic faults. Treatment principles, therefore, are likewise similar. However, the prevalence of fibrosis with subsequent rigidity in the presence of long standing inflammation presents unique clinical problems.

Proper management begins with appropriate footwear. Shoes must provide adequate depth in the toe box to accomodate a splayed forefoot, depressed metatarsal heads, clawed toes, and medial bunion of the first MTP often accompanying hallux valgus. Further depth is required if an orthosis becomes incorporated into the treatment plan. Excessive pressure along the mediolateral margins of the forefoot or on the dorsum of the PIP joints with clawed toes may be minimized with shoes having soft upper material, such as deerskin leather. Additional relief can be achieved by stretching the upper material, either the entire forefoot material at once with one of several types of shoe stretchers, or by using a ball and ring stretcher to relieve one isolated spot over a bony prominence. Cutting a small "X" in the upper material relieves pressure even further. This is particularly important when vasculitis becomes part of the clinical picture. It involves the small to medium sized vessels, and with the resultant reduced blood flow, necrosis and ulcerations can occur over bony prominences subjected to intense or prolonged pressure.[72] A communicating sinus can result, providing possible entry to bacteria and potentially leading to osteomyelitis. Alternatives to extra-depth shoes in the acute phase, or in the presence of multiple deformities, include Plastazote shoes or sandals. The shoes are lightweight footwear fabricated from soft Plastazote material, and covered with nylon material or leather. They incorporate a Velcro closure for easy fastening and are rather deep to accomodate the foot and orthosis. Sandals are provided when even further relief of compression is desired. A Plastazote sandal is commercially available having the qualities of the soft Plastazote material, Velcro closure straps, and complete elimination of pressure over the medial aspect of the first MTP. Custom molded sandals can easily be fabricated in the clinic by heat molding two to three layers of soft, orthotic material over the patient's foot. A softer layer directly next to the skin, such as Plastazote #1 or Aliplast 6a, is backed by a firmer material, such as Plastazote #2 or Aliplast XPE. Neoprene crepe is than added as the soling material and Velfoam straps adhered to provide easy, comfortable fastening (Table 6-1).

Orthotic intervention must address several concerns. Protruding matatarsal heads, often rigid and associated with anterior displacement of the plantar fat pad, become painful when subjected to vertical compression forces. Fibrosis reduces flexibility of the foot, thereby eliminating the method by which weightbearing forces are normally dissipated throughout the soft tissues. A low durometer material, such as Spenco, PPT, Plastazote #1, or Sorbothane can provide a substitute means of absorbing these compressive forces. Early in the disease course, this may be the only orthotic intervention necessary. A total contact orthotic can distribute weightbearing forces throughout the entire plantar aspect of the foot, reducing areas of excessive pressure concentration, such as those under the metatarsal heads. Selection of appropriate materials should allow for both adequate support and comfort. A low durometer material can now be used to cover the top of a more rigid orthosis for additional softness. Posting of the orthosis in the rheumatoid foot should be done with care. Attempts at realigning the hindfoot into a more balanced position of subtalar neutral often lead to failure. This is in part due to effects on intra-articular

Table 6-1. Product Manufacturers

Product	Manufacturer
Plastazote (#1 and #2)	Bakelite Sylonite Ltd. Bessemer Rd. Hertfordshire, England
Velcro	Velcro USA, Inc. Manchester, New Hampshire
Aliplast 6a Aliplast XPE	Alimed, Inc. 68 Harrison Ave. Boston, Massachusettes 02111
Velfoam	Smalley and Bates, Inc. 220 Little Falls Road Cedar Grove, New Jersey 07009
Spenco	Spenco Medical Corporation P.O. Box 8113 Waco, Texas 76710
PPT	The Langer Group 21 East Industry Court Deer Park, New York 11729
Sorbothane	IEM Orthopedics, Inc. 251 West Garfield Road Aurora, Ohio 44202

pressure within the subtalar joint. Joint pressure in the presence of effusion is least in a position of eversion, and increases threefold when inverted.[71] Therefore, reducing the valgus attitude with medial rearfoot posting results in elevated intra-articular pressure and pain. It is appropriate to accomodate the foot in the deformed position and use medial posting to hopefully minimize further valgus deviation. At best, the orthosis can be fabricated to slightly back the rearfoot away from the end of eversion range, thereby reinstating some degree of ROM. Metatarsal pads may provide a benefit to the rheumatoid foot only when mobility of the metatarsals is adequate. When hypomobile or rigidly fixed, the metatarsals are unable to displace far enough in a dorsal direction in response to the dorsally directed force of the metatarsal pad. The result is both an increase in localized pressure directly under the metatarsal shafts and an increase in tensile stresses within the surrounding, fibrosed, soft tissues. A rocker sole can provide additional benefits. As mentioned previously, the action of rolling over the curved, soling material reinstates the lever mechanism of the foot and restores functional ROM in the absence of ankle dorsiflexion or great toe extension. Proper placement just proximal to the metatarsal heads allows for a decrease of weightbearing forces directly under the painful, exposed, metatarsal heads, and redistributes these stresses to a more tolerable area of the foot. Placement of the rocker sole should follow a line between the first and fifth metatarsal heads, simulating a compromise between the metatarsal break and transverse axes of the MTP joints. Perhaps yet another benefit can be the affect on CP velocity. Force platform studies show that a similar shoe modification, the metatarsal bar, causes an increase in velocity of the CP across the forefoot.[77] This results in a shorter time interval which weightbearing forces are transmitted across the forefoot, thereby reducing the impulse.

Reiter's Syndrome

Reiter's syndrome is the combination of urethritis and conjunctivitis in association with arthritis. Arthritic symptoms typically show an acute onset with an asymmetrical distribution. Joints commonly affected include the MTP and PIP joints, and calcaneus at the attachment of the plantar fascia and/or insertion of the Achilles tendon.[78,79] Less frequently, involvement of the ankle and DIP joints may occur.

Changes within the synovium are similar to those of rheumatoid arthritis, beginning with edema in the early stages, then progressing to include pannus formation and villous hypertrophy.[78] Clinical symptoms include joint pain, swelling, decreased ROM, and increased warmth to touch. Underlying manifestations include erosion of articular cartilage, diffuse osteoporosis, and calcaneal osteophyte formation secondary to periostitis and continued traction forces of the plantar fascia and Achilles tendon.[78,79] Soft tissue swelling is also common, particularly in the forefoot and ankle. A "sausage-like" appearance of the toes, secondary to inflammation and resulting edema, may also be seen.

Psoriatic Arthritis

Psoriatic arthritis entails the onset of arthritis in the presence of psoriasis. Three distinct patterns of involvement have been identified, one of which involves the feet most frequently. Joint involvement is usually asymmetrical, and in the foot shows a predisposition for the DIP joints. Clinically, these joints are swollen and painful, with psoriatic lesions present on the toenails.[78] The toes, as in Reiter's syndrome, have a sausage-like appearance. Radiographically, a "pencil-in-cup" deformity is seen in the phalanges. This involves a resorption of the distal end of the bone resulting in a thin, pencil-like appearance, articulating with the eroded, proximal bone end, which becomes widened and resembles a cup.[78]

Gout

Gout is a syndrome manifested by hyperuricemia, either due to a primary, biochemical imbalance or as a secondary consequence from a pre-existing disorder.[80] Sodium urate crystals form and become deposited in the articular cartilage, bone, and surrounding soft tissues.[69,80] The area most commonly affected, occurring in up to 70 percent of all cases, is in the MTP joint of the great toe.[70] The initial episode usually presents with a very acute onset and severe pain. This generally subsides completely within several days, but if the formation of uric acid crystals continues, a condition of chronic gouty arthritis emerges.[70,80] Deposited crystals initially induce an inflammatory response, eventually leading to pannus formation, erosion of articular cartilage, and erosion of underlying bone.[80] Tophi develop later in the course as deposition of urates continues into the surrounding soft tissues.[69]

Neurovascular Pain

Pain in the foot can often times be difficult to diagnose and as a result be very difficult to successfully manage. According to some clinicians, if localization of foot pain is difficult or vague to describe, one should consider the peripheral vascular or nervous system as the source of the problem.[81] Common to most descriptions of this pain is a burning quality.

Entrapment of the medical plantar nerve in the tarsal tunnel or long arch of the foot has been identified in persons who run long distances and who excessively pronate. The symptoms have been described as burning heel pain, aching in the arch, and decreased sensation in the sole of the foot just behind the great toe.[82] This cause of nerve pain has been successfully treated with conservative methods including mechanical control.

Other causes of nerve pain have been linked to demyelinization. Calvin et al[83] suggested that sites of demyelinization may become foci of spontaneous impulse initiation which occur due to mechanical stimulation. The neuralgic pain results from minor demyelinization in peripheral nerves without evidence of substantial conduction defects. Such a situation would result from a variety of peripheral nerve disorders where segmental demyelinization is a common feature. Such an example is diabetes mellitus, wherein patients often complain about burning, tingling sensations in their feet.[84] It is well accepted that foot problems in the patient with diabetes mellitus result from both neurologic and vascular compromise and pose a challenge for any clinician. Adequate management of this population necessitates good medical follow-up with control of the disease process and continual education regarding foot hygiene, including preventative medicine and proper footwear.

Sudeck's atrophy or reflex sympathetic dystrophy can be incapacitating. The main problem is overactivity of the sympathetic nervous system with associated vascular instability in the foot. There are three basic characteristics: (1) severe pain throughout the foot, (2) hyperesthesia (sensitivity), and (3) hyperpathia (all sensation is perceived as pain).[85]

Sympathetic changes are noted in the foot which cause blushing and capillary stasis with piloerection and the development of thick coarse hair. Some have described it as the "hairy swollen foot." Approximately 30 percent develop excessive sweating and as a result the syndrome has also been labeled the "leaking foot." Other signs include, shiny, atrophic skin, and osteoporosis. Sudeck's atrophy should be suspected in any patient who complains of severe pain in the foot which starts 1 to 3 weeks after mild injury. Many patients who have experienced this problem have also demonstrated high anxiety personalities. The problem often takes up to 2 years to resolve, and this can also contribute to the anxiety level. A variety of medical management approaches have been attempted with variable results. Since the main problem is over activity of the sympathetic system, approaches to affect it would seem appropriate. Dooley and Rasprak[86] studied the effects of electrical stimulation as applied to various portions of the nervous system in an effort to diminish pain and to modify several functions of the nervous system. As part of the study, they observed an increase in warmth of the extremities with some of the techniques. Digital extremity arterial pulse pressure was measured while applying electrical stimulation over the cervical-thoracic spine (sympathetic area), lumbar spine, and peripheral nerves. The results indicated that significant increases were obtained only with the cervical-thoracic spinal stimulation. They concluded that electrical stimulation produced arterial dilation of the extremities by affecting the fibers in the posterior roots of the spinal cord and also by stimulating the sympathetic fibers. The relief of pain and increased arterial blood flow suggests that electrical stimulation helps to reduce sympathetic tone. If this is true then patients afflicted with Sudeck's atrophy may respond to electrical stimulation techniques to alter sympathetic function.

Arterial spasm has also been identified as a cause of disabling foot pain and efforts to alter the sympathetic system with sympathectomies have improved the condition.[87] In addition, another syndrome with foot pain and spontaneous movements of the foot was reported and it also responded favorably to sympathetic blocks.[88] There seems to be a common thread between these vascular dysfunctions and Sudeck's atrophy—the sympathetic system.

CONCLUSION

Foot pain can be totally devastating and affect one's life to the point that nothing else matters. The understanding of how the foot functions and interacts with other body segments is absolutely essential in order to solve foot complaints. The interplay of the neuromuscular, musculoskeletal, and vascular systems determine how the body will be able to function. The successful management of most of these problems require that the clinician understand how these systems function and affect each other. Only through further questioning and study can we expand our knowledge in the area of foot dysfunction and pain.

REFERENCES

1. Mann RA: Biomechanics of the foot. p. 257. American Academy of Orthopedic Surgeons' Atlas of Orthotics: Biomechanical Principles and Application, CV Mosby, St. Louis, 1975
2. Mann RA, Hagy JL, Simon SR: Biomechanics of Gait: A Critical Visual Analysis. Gait Analysis Laboratory, San Francisco, 1975

3. Hlavac HF: Major considerations in the clinical evaluation of the lower limb. p. 321. In Sgarlato TE (ed): A Compendium of Podiatric Biomechanics. California College of Podiatric Medicine, San Francisco, 1971

4. Mann RA: Surgical implications of biomechanics of the foot and ankle. Clin Orth Rel Res 146:111, 1980

5. Morris M: Biomechanics of the foot and ankle. Clin Orth Rel Res 122:10, 1977

6. Jarrett BA, Manzi JA, Green DR: Interossei and lumbricales muscles of the foot. J Am Pod Assoc 70(1):1, 1980

7. Hlavac HF: The Foot Book. World Publications, Mountain View, California, 1977

8. Wernick J, Langer S: A Practical Manual for a Basic Approach to Biomechanics. Langer Laboratories, Deer Park, NY, 1973

9. Scranton PE, Hootman BD, McMaster JH: Forces under the foot: a study of walking, jogging, and sprinting force distribution under normal and abnormal fee. p. 186. In Bateman JE, Trott AW (eds): The Foot and Ankle. Brian C Decker, Thieme-Stratton, Inc, New York, 1980

10. Bauman JH, Brand PW: Measurement of pressure between foot and shoe. Lancet, 7282:629, 1963

11. Morton DJ: The Human Foot. Columbia University Press, New York, 1935

12. Arcan M, Brull MA: A fundamental characteristic of the human body and foot, the foot ground pressure pattern. J Biomech 9:453, 1976

13. Stokes IAF, Hutton WC, Mech ME, et al: Forces under the hallux valgus foot before and after surgery. Clin Orth Rel Res 142:64, 1979

14. Stokes IAF, Stott JRR, Hutton WC: Force distributions under the foot: a dynamic measuring system. Biomed Eng, 9(4):140, 1974

15. Schwartz RP, Heath AL, Morgan DW, Towns RC: A quantitative analysis of recorded variables in the walking pattern of normal adults. JBJS 46A:324, 1964

16. Stott JRR, Hutton WC, Stokes IAF: Forces under the foot. JBJS 55B:335, 1973

17. Mann RA, Baxter DE, Lutter LD: Running symposium. Foot and Ankle 1:190, 1981

18. Brand PW: Pressure sores: the problem. p. 19. In Kenadi RM, Cowden JM (eds): Bedsore Biomechanics. University Press, Baltimore, 1976

19. Scully TJ, Besterman G: Stress Fracture: a preventable training injury. Military Medicine 147:285, 1982

20. Cavanaugh PR, La Fortune MA: Ground reaction forces in distance running. J Biomech 13:397, 1980

21. Light LH, McLellan GE, Klenerman L: Skeletal transients on heel strike in normal walking with different footwear. J Biomech 13:477, 1979

22. Scranton PE, Rutkowski R, Brown TD: Support phase kinematics of the foot. p. 195. In Bateman JE, Trott AW (eds): The Foot and Ankle. Brian C Decker, Thieme Stratton Inc, New York, 1980

23. Inman VT: The Joints of the Ankle. Williams & Wilkins, Baltimore, 1976

24. McMaster M: Disability of the hindfoot after fracture of the tibial shaft. JBJS 58B:90, 1976

25. Draganich LF, Andriacchi TP, Strongwater AM, Galante JO: Electronic measurement of instantaneous foot: floor contact patterns during gait. J Biomech 13:875, 1980

26. Hicks JH: The three weight: bearing mechanisms of the foot. p. 19. In Evans EG (ed): Biomechanical Studies of the Musculoskeletal System. Charles C Thomas, Springfield, IL, 1961

27. Lapidus CA: Kinesiology and mechanical anatomy of the tarsal joints. Clin Orth Rel Res 30:20, 1963

28. Hicks JH: The foot as a support. ACTA Anatomica 25:180, 1955
29. Jones RL: The human foot: an experimental study of its mechanics, and the role of its muscles and ligaments in the support of the arch. Am J Anatomy 68:1, 1941
30. McCarthy DJ, Gorecki GE: The anatomical basis of inferior calcaneal lesions. J Am Pod Assoc, 69:527, 1979
31. Gerster JC, Vischer TL, Bennani A, Fallet GH: The painful heel. Ann Rheum Dis 36:343, 1977
32. Furey JG: Plantar fascitis. JBJS 57A:672, 1975
33. Bordelon RL: Subcalcaneal pain. Clin Orth Rel Res 177:49, 1983
34. Perry J Anatomy and biomechanics of the hindfoot. Clin Orth Rel Res 177:9, 1983
35. Weiner BE, Ross AS, Bogdan RJ: Biomechanical heel pain: a case study. J Am Pod Assoc, 69:723, 1979
36. Neale D, Hooper G, Clowes CB: Adult foot disorders. p. 43. In Neale D (ed): Common Foot Disorders: Diagnosis and Management. Churchill Livingstone, Edinburgh, 1981
37. Mann R, Inman VT: Phasic activity of intrinsic muscles of the foot. JBJS 46A:469, 1964
38. Katoh Y, Chao EYS, Morrey BF, Laughman RK: Objective technique for evaluating painful heel syndrome and its treatment. Foot and Ankle 3:227, 1983
39. Graham CE: Painful heel syndrome: rationale of diagnosis and treatment. Foot and Ankle, 3:261, 1983
40. Tanz SS: Heel pain. Clin Orth Rel Res 28:169, 1963
41. Karr JP: A method to alleviate and cure the painful heel syndrome. J Am Pod Assoc 68:124, 1978
42. Marr SJ: The use of heel posting orthotic techniques for relief of heel pain. Arch Orth Trauma Surg 96:73, 1980
43. Leach RE, Dilorio E, Harney RA: Pathologic hindfoot conditions in the athlete. Clin Orth Rel Res 177:116, 1983
44. Frederick EC: Sport Shoes and Playing Surfaces. Human Kinetics Champaign, IL, 1984
45. Pavlov H, Heneghan MA, Hersh A, Goldman AB, et al: The Haglund syndrome: initial and differential diagnosis. Radiology 144:83, 1982
46. Helfet AJ: Developing conditions of the feet. p. 115. In Helfet AJ, Gruebel Lee DM (eds): Disorders of the Foot. JB Lippincott, Philadephia, 1980
47. Brody DM: Running injuries. Clinical Symposia 32:1, 1980
48. Johnson KA: Tibialis posterior tendon rupture. Clin Ortho Rel Res 177:140, 1983
49. Cowell HR: Talocalcaneal coalition and new causes of peroneal spastic flatfoot. Clin Orth Rel Res 85:16, 1972
50. Jayakumai S, Cowell HR: Rigid flatfoot. Clin Orth Rel Res 122:77, 1977
51. Frank SC: Management of limited subtalar motion. J Am Pod Assoc 50:390, 1960
52. Kyne PJ, Mankin HJ: Changes in intra-articular pressure with subtalar joint motion with special reference to the etiology of peroneal spastic flatfoot. Hosp Joint Dis 26:181, 1965
53. D'Amico JC, Shuster RO: Motion of the first ray. J Am Pod Assoc 69(1): 17, 1979
54. Hlavac HF: Compensated forefoot varus. J Am Pod Assoc 60(6): 229, 1970
55. Meyer JM, Tomeno B, Burdet A: Metatarsalgia due to insufficient support by the first ray. Int Orth 5:193, 1981
56. Shaw AH: The effects of a forefoot post on gait and function. J Am Pod Assoc 65(3):238, 1975
57. Bates BT, Ostering LR, Mason B, James LS: Foot orthotic devices to modify selected aspects of lower extremity mechanics. Am J Sports Med 7(6):338, 1979

58. Clarke TE, Frederick EC, Hamill C: The study of rearfoot movement in running. p. 166. In Frederick EC (ed): Sport Shoes and Playing Surfaces. Human Kinetics, Champaign, IL, 1984
59. Scheonhaus HD, Gold M, Hylinski J, Keating J: Computerized analysis of gait. J Am Pod Assoc 69(1):11, 1979
60. Walker DM: Mechanical therapy. p. 185. In Neale D (ed): Common Foot Disorders: Diagnosis and Management. Churchill Livingstone, Edinburgh, 1981
61. Price GFW: Metatarsus primus varus: including various clinicoradiologic features of the female foot. Clin Orth Rel Res 145:217, 1979
62. Bojsen-Moller F: Anatomy of the forefoot, normal and pathologic. Clin Orth Rel Res 142:10, 1979
63. Helfet AJ, Gruebel LD: Acquired deformities of the toes. p. 117. In Helfet AJ, Gruebel LD (eds): Disorders of the Foot. JB Lippincott, Philadelphia, 1980
64. Root ML, Orien WP, Weed JH: Clinical Biomechanics: Normal and Abnormal Function of the Foot. Vol. 2. Clin Biomech Corp, Los Angeles, 1977
65. Scheck M: Etiology of the acquired hammertoe deformity. Clin Orth Rel Res 123:63, 1977
66. Smith W: Evaluation of the adult forefoot. Clin Orth Rel Res 142:19, 1979
67. Morris MA: Morton's metatarsalgia. Clin Orth Rel Res 127:203, 1977
68. Oldenbrook LL, Smith CE: Metatarsal head motion secondary to rearfoot pronation and supination. J Am Pod Assoc 69(1): 24, 1979
69. Cawley MID, Smidt LA: Rheumatic disorders affecting the feet. p. 143. In Neale D (ed): Common Foot Disorders: Diagnosis and Management. Churchill Livingstone, Edinburgh, 1981
70. Helfet AJ, Gruebel Lee DM: The manifestations of rheumatoid disease in the foot. p. 159. In Helfet AJ, Gruebel Lee DM (eds): Disorders of the Foot. JB Lippincott, Philadelphia, 1980
71. D'Amico JC: The pathomechanics of adult rheumatoid arthritis affecting the foot. J Am Pod Assoc 66(4):227, 1976
72. Gilliland BC, Mannick M: Rheumatoid arthritis. p. 1987. In Wintrobe MM, Thorn GW, Adams RD, Braumwald E, Isselbacher KJ, Petersdorf RB (eds): Harrison's Principles of Internal Medicine. 7th Ed. McGraw-Hill, New York, 1974
73. Minaker K, Little H: Painful feet in rheumatoid arthritis. CMA 109:724, 1973
74. Vidigal E, Jacoby RK, Dixon StJA, et al: The foot in chronic rheumatoid arthritis. Ann Rheum Dis 34:292, 1975
75. Kirkup JR, Vidigal E, Jacoby R: The hallux and rheumatoid arthritis. ACTA Orth Scand 48:527, 1977
76. Simkin A: The dynamic vertical force distribution during level walking under normal and rheumatoid feet. Rheum Rehab 20:88, 1981
77. Grundy M, Blackburn, Tosh PA, et al: An investigation of the centers of pressure under the foot while walking. JBJS 57B:98, 1975
78. Gilliland BC, Mannik M: Reiter's syndrome, psoriatic arthritis, and arthritis associated with gastrointestinal diseases. p. 1998. In Wintrobe MM, Thorn GW, Adams RD, et al (eds): Harrison's Principles of Internal Medicine. 7th Ed. McGraw-Hill, New York, 1974
79. Chand Y, Johnson KA: Foot and ankle manifestations of Reiter's syndrome. Foot and Ankle 1:167, 1980
80. Wyngaarden JB: Gout and other disorders of uric acid metabolism. p. 607. In Wintrobe MM, Thorn GW, Adams RD, Braunwald E, et al. (eds): Harrison's Principles of Internal Medicine. 7th Ed. McGraw Hill, New York, 1974

81. Raymakers R: The painful foot. The Practitioner 215:61, 1975
82. Rask MR: Medial plantar neuropraxia (jogger's foot). Clin Orth Rel Res 134:193, 1978
83. Calvin WH, Devor M, Howe JF: Can neuralgias arise from minor demyelination?: spontaneous firing, mechanosensitivity, and after discharge from conducting axons. Exp Neurol 75:755, 1982.
84. Robson MC, Edstron LE: The diabetic foot: an alternative approach to major amputation. Surg Clinics N Am 57:1089, 1977
85. Helfet AJ: The swollen foot. p. 220. In Helfet AJ, Gruebel Lee DM (eds): Disorders of the Foot. JB Lippincott, Philadelphia, 1980
86. Dooley DM, Rasprak M: Modification of blood flow to the extremities by electrical stimulation of the nervous system. Southern Med J 69:1309, 1976
87. Huygens HJ: Unilateral painful vasospasm in the lower limbs of young women. Aust NZ, J Surg 45:147, 1975
88. Spillane JD, Nathan PW, Kelly RE, Marsden CD: Painful legs and moving toes. Brain 94:54, 1971

7 | Pain in Neuromuscular Disorders

L. Alan Stone

Pain, as traditionally viewed in neurophysiologic terms, is considered to be a medical problem with organic or physical characteristics. In the absence of physical findings, the pain is often considered to be nonorganic or psychogenic in origin and viewed as a behavior problem related to personality, motivation, or situation. This simplified, dichotomous interpretation of the pain experience suggests a complex physiologic process occurring within the sensory system involving receptors, transmitters, and integrative central mechanisms at the level of the cord, thalamus, and sensory cortex. Pain has not been viewed recently as a primary sensory modality received by specific nerve endings, conducted by special fibers, and pursuing selected pathways to the thalamus and cortex. There is no simple relationship between stimulus and subjective response as that relationship is affected by cognitive, motivational, and affective components leading to pain behavior.

The gate control theory of Melzack and Wall[1] first suggested the complex interrelationships of central nervous system influences on the reception, transmission, and perception of the pain experience. In their model, pain perception depends upon the relative intensity of discharge in larger and smaller sensory axons of peripheral nerves, the governing segmental influence of the internuncial neuronal pool of the dorsal horn of the spinal cord, and the modulating suprasegmental activity from cortical and subcortical regions. More recent understanding of pain has been advanced by the recognition of the existence of the opioid peptide enkelphalens and substance P in their possible roles as neurotransmittors in pain transmission.[2]

Pain in neuromuscular disorders, as in other disease processes, has been considered traditionally from one of two perspectives: acute and chronic pain states.

In the acute state, pain is defined as a reaction to an inflammatory process or to actual or impending tissue damage resulting from nociceptive input from the site of tissue insult. The stimulus for the acute pain experience may be mechanical, thermal, chemical, or electrical in nature, but the pain perception in this acute disease model depends upon the perception of a noxious stimulus in a normal sensory system.

Chronic pain states, which generally last longer than 6 months and which may start as an acute pain episode, require more than nociceptive input.[3] The origin of the pain is thought to be principally central and independent of peripheral nociceptive input. Chronic pain has a time dimension which makesit vulnerable to the effects of learning and conditioning and can be associated with the premorbid personality, motivational, and situational states. In learning theory, the central nervous system has the capability of storing memory information related to the pain experience. This pain experience may be triggered by afferent input, not necessarily nociceptive in nature. In chronic pain of central origin, normal afferent input may act on an altered sensory system resulting in abnormal processing of sensory information perceived as a pain experience. Chronic pain may also persist in an environment providing positive reinforcement for the pain behavior.

Benjamin Cruz has suggested a pain taxonomy to facilitate the understanding and management of pain syndromes.[3]

1.   Acute pain—arising from continued nociceptive input.

2.   Subacute pain—intermittent perception of nociceptive input (e.g., nocturnal paresthesia associated with carpal tunnel syndrome).

3.   Recurrent acute pain—intermittent nociceptive input with fluctuating disease states (e.g., migraine headaches).

4.   Progressive acute pain—nociceptive input associated with progressive disease states.

5.   Chronic constant pain—low level nociceptive input or no nociceptive input in patients who are copying with pain without seeking medical attention. These patients rely primarily on the over the counter pain medicine market, an industry which amounts to over one billion dollars a year in the United States.

6.   Chronic constant pain—without evidence of pathology or continued nociceptive input; patients who are not successfully coping with pain and are demanding of the medical system. This category is referred to as the chronic, intractable benign pain syndrome.

The success of medical management of the pain experience has varied with the pain classification. In the acute medical disease model, successful medical and/or surgical management of the cause of the disease has resulted in the relief from the pain symptoms. Analgesics, steroids, anti-inflammatory agents, local blocks, and other local or topical measures traditionally afford symptomatic relief. Surgical approaches, where indicated for pain relief, have been directed to various levels of the sensory system:

1. First sensory neuron—regions of the receptor area of the peripheral nerve, sensory root ganglion, and spinal nerve root (i.e., local blocks and rhizotomy).

2. Second sensory neuron—at the level of the spinal cord (i.e., cordotomies and tractotomies of the lateral spinothalamic tract).

3. Third sensory neuron—central synaptic connections of the thalamus to the cortex and hypothalamus (i.e., thalamotomies and cortectomies).

In the chronic pain states, medical and surgical management of pain has been less consistently successful. Pain may persist despite medical and surgical attempts to cure it and the persistence of pain suggests a behavioral cause rather than an organic one. The persistence of pain in the presence of medical and surgical therapies may be as disturbing to the practitioner as to the patient and contributes to the anxiety of the symptom complex and therapeutic relationship. Chronic pain, as a behavioral problem arising, perhaps, from a mix of antecedent nociceptive stimulation and contingent environmental consequences, suggests that a behavioral approach to treating the symptoms with techniques of behavior modification would be helpful.[4] The rationale for this approach is based upon the premise that chronic pain is a learned experience and that experience is sensitive or responsive to, and is partially controlled by, the immediate environment.[5]

An inclusive definition of pain is difficult to achieve given the complexity of the pain experience. Pain might be defined as an unpleasant experience associated with a number of adjective descriptions resulting from antecedent tissue insult of either historic or contemporary nature. More functionally, pain may be described as anything a patient says it is.[6]

The remainder of this chapter examines the more common pain syndromes associated with pathologic lesions at various tissue sites of the neuromuscular system. The discussion is not inclusive in breadth or depth of coverage, but will be hopefully representative of painful states associated with acute and chronic lesions of the neuromuscular system.

HEAD AND NECK

Thalamic (Central) Pain

Lesions producing central pain may involve the spinothalamic tract at any level from the spinal cord to the thalamus, as well as the central connections from the thalamus to the cortex, hypothalamus, cerebellum, and pallidum.

In cortical lesions, the mechanism of pain production is unknown, but alternate theories suggest either local irritation at the site of the lesion or release of cortical inhibitory influences on the thalamus as the probable casue for pain. The pain is spontaneous and occurs in the absence of usual extrinsic nociceptive stimuli and tends to be increased by certain stimuli such as anxiety and temperature changes. The severity of pain varies with time and is often described as an aching, burning, or cold, unpleasant sensation. The pain is often associated with signs of autonomic dysfunction such as cyanosis, decreased skin temperature, and increased sweating.

Brain stem lesions involving the thalamus are the most commonly recognized cause of central pain secondary to a variety of possible lesions: tumor, trauma, and inflammatory. The most common lesion is of vascular etiology involving occlusion of the arterial supply to the lateral nucleus of the thalamus.[7] Dejerine and Roussy first described the characteristics of the thalamic syndrome in 1906.[8] The symptom complex included (1) usually transient hemiparesis, (2) impairment of superficial and loss of deep sensation secondary to disruption of the medial lemniscus and spinothalamic tracts, (3) choreoathetoid movements, ataxia, and tremor secondary to the sensory deficit or involvement of the dentatorubrothalamic tracts, (4) spontaneous and intolerable, painful dysesthesias, (5) marked emotional lability, (6) diffuse vasomotor and other autonomic disturbances, and (7) occasional mental disturbance, dementia, and mutism.

Characteristically, thalamic pain appears after an interval of several weeks and varies in intensity from paresthesia to burning pain unaffected by analgesics. Hyperalgesia and hyperpathia are present with excessive reaction to stimulation of involved portions of the body. In extensive lesions, the entire contralateral half of the body may exhibit hyperpathic pain. Pain is increased with fatigue, apprehension, or other illness. The degree of sensory loss has little or no relationship to the intensity of the pain.

Treatment is a difficult therapeutic problem as traditional therapies offer little satisfaction;[7] sympathetic blocks and analgesics, including morphine, offer little relief. Tranquilizers may help with emotional lability. Rhizotomy of the trigeminal nerve may help the severe head pain, but high cordotomies and stereotactic surgical interruption of suprathalamic fibers offer mixed results. The only standard surgical procedure with a reasonable chance of success is a prefrontal lobotomy and then only for patients who are so incapacitated from the neurologic deficit that there is little hope for gainful function.

Other central nervous system lesions may mimic thalamic pain. Lesions within the midbrain, medulla, and spinal cord may present with a varying array of the thalamic pain symptom complex.

Cranial Neuralgias

A variety of cranial nerve lesions result in painful states of the head, face, and neck.

Trigeminal Neuralgia (Tic Douloureux)

Lesions of the 5th cranial, or trigeminal nerve may result in paroxysmal, unilateral facial pain associated with grimaces and contortions of the face. The pain is described as severe with a sensation of heat in one or more branches of the 5th cranial nerve. The painful attacks last only a few seconds to minutes with brief, relatively pain-free intervals between attacks. The attacks are often precipitated by normal sensory stimuli, particularly tactile or proprioceptive stimulation over trigger zones on the face. Recurrent attacks may last for a few days to months followed by periods of remission. There is no objective sensory loss or motor weakness.

The etiology is often unknown, but involvement may occur at any one of three levels:

1. Peripheral lesions secondary to a variety of traumatic, inflammatory, and neoplastic lesions of the head and face, paranasal sinus, and oral cavity. Local jawbone pathology and extraction of impacted wisdom teeth may precipitate the symptom complex.[9]

2. Trigeminal (gasserian) ganglion: lesions within the ganglion represent the most common pathology. Degenerative changes within the ganglion consisting of loss of cells, changes in the myelin sheaths, and axonal thickening have been described.[10] Trigeminal neuralgia has been associated with the herpesvirus.[11,12] The postherpetic pain and dysesthesias of herpes zoster more commonly affects the gasserian ganglion than any other sensory ganglion.[12]

3. Central lesions may occur secondary to vascular and neoplastic lesions of the pons, medulla, and upper cervical cord. Trigeminal neuralgia has been described as one of the first symptoms of multiple sclerosis, although the facial pain may be bilateral.[13]

Medical and pharmaceutical treatment is generally nonspecific and may include analgesics, anticonvulsants, nerve blocks, and alcohol injections. Neurosurgical methods are considered an essential element in the treatment, as reviewed by White and Sweet.[14]

Glossopharyngeal (Vagoglossopharyngeal) Neuralgia

The 9th cranial, or glossopharyngeal, nerve provides motor innervation to the posterior third of the tongue, tonsils, and nasopharynx. Symptoms consist of a paroxysmal, unilateral stabbing pain at the base of the tongue, behind the ear, and beneath the angle of the jaw. The pain is precipitated by proprioceptive trigger zones involving the functions of coughing, swallowing, and talking. Short bouts of pain may occur two to three times a year lasting for days to months with spontaneous remission.[15] The etiology is obscure and may be preceded by an upper respiratory infection and is sometimes associated with trigeminal neuralgia.

Geniculate Neuralgia

Geniculate neuralgia (Neuralgia of Hunt) is a rare symptom complex involving the geniculate ganglion, a vestigal sensory ganglion remnant with a variable sensory role in supplying the deep structures of the face, head, and portion of the ear. Clinical features consist of a paroxysmal, lancinating pain within the depths of the ear. Etiology is unknown except for those cases associated with herpes zoster infection (Ramsey-Hunt syndrome). In the latter case, the ear pain may be severe and continuous and associated with herpetic vesicular eruptions on the tympanum and in the external auditory canal. Occasionally, the pain may be associated with a 7th cranial palsy. Symptoms may improve spontaneously and intractable cases may require a surgical section of the nervus intermedius.

Tolosa-Hunt Syndrome

Tolosa-Hunt Syndrome consists of a painful ophthalmoplegia characteristized by periorbital pain with involvement of the cranial nerves (III, IV, V, and VI) passing through the cavernous sinus.[16] Partial or total paralysis of the extraocular muscles may occur. The syndrome is characterized by exacerbations and remissions with occasional residual neurologic deficits. The etiology is generally secondary to an indolent, nonspecific inflammation or granuloma at the level of the anterior cavernous sinus and superior orbital fissure. The pathologic process is highly sensitive to high dose steroid therapy.

Spenopalatine Neuralgia

Spenopalatine neuralgia is an idiopathic symptom complex with continuous, unilateral pain of the lower portion of the face with the maximal site of pain at the base of the nose and extending back to the ear. The pain may radiate to the neck and arm and may be accompanied by rhinorrhea, nasal congestion, and tinnitus. The symptom complex is more common in females and may be associated with a migraine variant due to vasodilation of the internal medullary artery.

Raeders Paratrigeminal Syndrome

Raeders paratrigeminal syndrome results in oculosympathetic nerve involvement with trigeminal symptoms produced by a lesion in the region of the trigeminal ganglion. Clinical features consist of periorbital pain in the opththalmic division of the trigeminal nerve, occasional anhidrosis, ptosis, and miosis. The pain is unilateral and of a deep and persistent quality characterized by periodic exacerbations. Two subgroups of patients exist with this symptom complex:[17] (1) a subgroup without associated middle cranial nerve involvement, and (2) a subgroup with associated involvement of cranial nerves II, III, IV, and VI.

In the former group, the process tends to be benign and self-limiting without definite etiology, although vascular and inflammatory lesions of the region of the trigeminal ganglion are suspect. With additional cranial nerve involvement, aggressive evaluation and etiologic treatment is required to manage a pathologic process in the middle cranial fossa. Tumors, vascular lesions, infections of the sinus, ear, and teeth, and pneumonia have been associated with the group with middle cranial nerve involvement.

Atypical Facial Pain

A number of patients present with facial pain of no demonstrable cause; the pain tends to be of long duration and unresponsive to analgesic therapy. The character, location, and duration of pain varies among patients, but is rarely limited to the areas supplied by the various cranial nerves. There is no accepted etiology for the pain, but in some cases, there is an autonomic phenomena consisting of lacrimation and rhinorrhea, which suggests a neurovascular disorder related to migraine. A possible psychologic etiology is suggested by Dalessio based upon the association of the symptoms with depression, neurotic traits, gastro-intestinal complaints, and hysterical motorsensory deficits.[18] Glazer also recognized these traits and thought them to be the result of chronic pain.[19]

SPINE

Spinal cord lesions may manifest by weakness, spasticity, incontinence, pain, paresthesia, and numbness depending upon the site and type of lesion. Pain may be of three types:[20]

1. Radicular pain in the affected dermatone: the pain has been described as dull, boring, or, more characteristically, lancinating with exacerbation by increased thoracic—abdominal pressure.
2. Tract pain secondary to irritation or anatomic disruption of the internuncial neuronal pool and/or the ascending spinothalamic tracts: a diffuse pain which is usually referred to areas below the level of the lesion and fails to conform to a dermatomal or peripheral nerve distribution.
3. Vertebral pain secondary to a destructive lesion of bone: the pain is felt as a deep ache. In metastatic vertebral lesions, pain may be felt in the vertebrae before radiographic changes or other features of the disease become evident.

Any lesion that constricts the spinal canal may cause neurologic symptoms; the lesion may be a result of direct compression of the spinal cord and accompanying roots or interference with their blood supply. The severity of neurologic symptoms depends upon the degree of compression and the rapidity with which it develops. Sudden, rapid compression results in more severe symptoms, while gradual compression results in an insidious onset of symptoms. Most spinal constrictive lesions are benign and cause neurologic changes by direct compression, rather than by invasion and destruction.[21] The spinal cord can be constricted by a wide variety of lesions: (1) Intraspinal: tumors, Pagets disease, rheumatoid arthritis, etc., and (2) Extraspinal: degenerative disc disease, narrowing of spinal canal, metastases, infections, vascular lesions, trauma, etc.

Syringomyelia

Syringomyelia is a chronic symptom complex involving the spinal cord and/or the medulla characterized by the development of cavitation and gliosis within the substance of these structures.[22] Cavity formation occurs more commonly at certain levels: (1) brain stem (syringobulbar): bulb and upper cervical cord with cranial nerve involvement, (2) cervicordorsal cord: the most common location, and (3) lumbosacral.

The symptoms will vary with the site of involvement, but typically consist of sensory dissociation with loss of pain and temperature, but retention of touch, lower motor neuron involvement, impairment of long tract function, and trophic disorders. In the later stages of the disease with extension of the gliosis, pyramidal, and extrapyramidal involvement may result in spastic paralysis below the level of the lesion, while disturbances in touch and proprioception occur from dorsal column involvement.

Classically, the cavitation affects the decussating nociceptive and thermoceptive fibers initially with resultant hypalgesia, analgesia, and thermoanesthesia. However, Spiller has noted, in some cases, pain of a boring, lancinating nature in affected areas.[23] He believed this pain to be of central origin related to involvement of internuncial neuronal cells and spinothalamic tract fibers.

The disease commonly occurs between the ages of 25 to 40 with a higher incidence in males.[24] There is no single cause for the progressive, degenerative disorder, but the symptom complex may arise from a variety of causes:

1. *Congenital*: embryonic deficit resulting from incomplete or imperfect closure of the neural tube during the third to fourth week of intrauterine life or from intramedullary vascular anomaly

2. *Acquired*: deficit may arise from spinal cord tumor, hemorrhage, deficient blood supply, and arachnoiditis secondary to trauma.

Fredrichs Ataxia

Fredrichs ataxia is an autosomal recessive inherited ataxia characterized by pathologic degeneration of the posterior columns of the spinal cord and the dorsal roots with sparing of the anterior horn cells and ventral roots. Pain and temperature perception are normal with alteration in position and vibration senses in the early stages with symptoms of unsteady gait in the absence of muscle weakness or wasting. In the later stages, severe ataxia may be present with dysarthria. Occasionally, patients will describe a stabbing pain in the legs relieved by movement.

Tabes Dorsalis

Tabes dorsalis is a clinical syndrome resulting in loss of joint position and deep pain sensation with preservation of superficial pain and temperature from syphilis. Neurologic involvement of the spinal cord region may result in (1) chronic inflammatory meningitis with endarteritis and thrombosis of small arteries, (2) posterior column degeneration, and (3) degeneration of posterior roots. Occasionally, the lateral pyramidal tracts and cranial sensory nerves are involved. The degeneration and fibrosis of the posterior column and roots occurs as a result of the syphilitic inflammation, while injury to nerve fiber may result from meningitis, direct inflammation, or presence of the spirochete. Pathologic changes are more pronounced in the lumbar portion of the cord and severe aching and lancinating pains in the legs may be present.

Herpes Zoster

Herpes zoster, or postHerpetic neuralgia, results from the varicella virus infection of the posterior root ganglia. The acute, self-limiting viral infection produces inflammatory lesions in the posterior root ganglia characterized by round cell infiltration, hemorrhage, and axon degeneration.[25] The lesions may spread to the same segment of the spinal cord with inflammation of posterior and anterior horns with destruction of anterior horn cells and occasionally, long-tract involvement.[26] The disease is characterized by pain and vesicular eruptions in the dermatomal distributions of the involved ganglia. The pain may be present for up to 3 weeks prior to the vesicular eruptions and in 10 to 20 percent of the cases, a severe and persistent, intractable pain may occur within the area of the original cutaneous eruptions.[27] The disease is thought to be a reactivation of the varicella virus which has lain dormant in the dorsal root ganglion since a childhood infection with chicken pox. The disease is especially common in older people and in those with debilitating conditions like Hodgkin's disease and the lymphomas. The infection is generally unilateral and most commonly affects single dermatomes of the thoracic spine.

Vascular Lesions

Vascular lesions of the spinal cord occur from a variety of causes secondary to occlusion, infarction, or hemorrhage within the vascular network of the spinal and radicular arteries to the cord.[28] Atherosclerosis of the spinal arteries is the most common cause of a vascular myelopathy. The disease may present as an abrupt onset with an established defect or develop progressively. The insidious onset form is generally heralded by pain and dysesthesia at the level of the infarct. The anterior spinal artery is the most common site of involvement at the level of the thoracic spine. Signs include loss of spinothalamic sensation and an upper motor neuron lesion below the level of involvement. Transient ischemic attacks may occur with restricted spinal cord arterial supply. Symptoms may mimic those of intermittent claudication of the legs with progressive pain in the legs with activity. The pain may last for 10 minutes or more after walking in contrast to typical intermittent claudication, which is generally relieved by rest. Additionally, transient ischemia of the spinal cord may be accompanied by neurologic symptoms of weakness, numbness, and sphincter disturbances with walking.

Hemorrhage or infarction of the spinal cord appears as an abrupt onset of neurologic symptoms and signs referable to the spinal cord with a full range of motor, sensory, and autonomic involvement. Infarction of the anterior spinal artery secondary to emboli formation from trauma or a mural thromboemboli detached from the aorta may result in neurologic deficit. Sensory symptoms may be minimal or severe at onset with radicular, diffuse, or poorly defined pain and paresthesia. Hemorrhage secondary to rupture of a vascular malformation, anticoagulation therapy, or blood dyscrasias may result in bleeding into the epidural space with a resultant compressive hemotoma producing rapid damage to the spinal cord. The clinical picture is one of severe back pain at the level of the lesion, followed swiftly by paraparesis and then paraplegia.

Degenerative Disc Disease and Spinal Spondylosis

Degenerative disc disease with either foraminal encroachment from osteophyte formation and/or frank herniation of the intervertebral disc occurs less frequently in the cervical spine than in the lumboscral spine. Because the posterior longitudinal ligament is weaker in its central portion, herniations are likely to be either midline with compression of the spinal cord or posterolateral with encroachment upon the nerve root in proximity to the intervertebral foramen. Overt trauma may result in posterior herniation with anterior cord compression. More commonly, there is no clear history of trauma, and neurologic symptoms arise from progressive degenerative changes resulting in nerve root compression or spinal canal encroachment. Degenerative changes include loss of water content with fragmentation, narrowing, and ossification of the disc; these changes stimulate a sclerotic reaction in adjacent vertebrae so that osteophyte formation proliferates and protrudes into the spinal canal and adjacent intervertebral foramen.[29] The dura and root sleeves fibrose and thicken with resultant decrease in mobility of the cord and roots because of adhesions. Vertebral subluxations and a thickened ligamentum flavum accentuate the risk of cord compression particularly during neck extension.[30]

Typical symptoms in nerve root compression include cervical pain radiating into the shoulder girdle and upper extremity in a dermatomal distribution. Most common sites of involvement are at the C5-6 and C6-7 interspaces. Pain is frequently most prominent in the scapular region[31] and is aggravated by head and neck motions. Associated with the radicular pain are sensory dysesthesias, motor weakness, and reflex changes.

With spinal cord involvement, the typical motor and sensory radicular signs and symptoms may be seen at the level of the lesion with superimposed signs and symptoms of long tract involvement distal to the level of the lesion. Paraparesis with sensory involvement and bowel and bladder dysfunction may occur to a varying degree in the lower extremities. Trauma involving hyperextension of the head and neck can precipitate immediate and persistent symptoms. More commonly, the natural history is one of insidious onset and slow progression with long periods of neurologic stability. Symptoms begin in the fifth or sixth decade and involve the lower extremities. Stiffness and fatigue develop with hyperreflexia, extensor plantar response, spasticity, and motor weakness. A loss of vibration sense occurs and pain is generally not a prominent feature, although a number of patients may complain of a burning sensation in the soles of the feet.

Thoracic spondylosis with disc herniation is uncommon.[31] Motions of the thoracic spine are limited by the ribs and intercostal muscles protecting the thoracic discs from the stresses and strains seen in the cervical and lumbar spine. When disc protrusions occur, they are more common in the lower four thoracic vertebrae with T11 being the most commonly affected level.[32] Disc protrusion will result in radicular pain with lateral encroachment into the foramen. The pain may mimic that of intercostal neuralgia, pleuritis, heart disease, gallbladder, and other abdominal complaints. With a midline compression, spinal cord compression will occur with motor and sensory impairment below the level of the lesion with bowel and bladder dysfunction.

Spinal Cord Trauma

Trauma to the spinal cord can occur as a result of four types of injuries:[33]

1. Skeletal lesions: compressed vertebrae, comminuted fracture, facet dislocation.

2. Impact injuries with hemorrhage and edema resulting in decreased perfusion and ischemia.

3. Closed spinal injury: flexion extension injury, vertical compression trauma, rotational injury.

4. Penetrating injuries.

Following injury to the spinal cord with interruption of the ascending sensory tracts, sensory deficits of varying degrees may ensue. Pain associated with neurologic deficit is of various types:

1. Root: radicular pain.

2. Hyperpathic pain: a zone of hyperpathia develops at the level of the lesion which may involve one or more dermatomes and result in a bandlike

tightness and burning pain; this area may become a hypersensitive trigger point which will precipitate local or more diffuse spasms below the level of the lesion and cause hyperactivity of the autonomic nervous system.

3. Central pain secondary to interruption and irritation of the internuncial pool and spinothalamic tract.

4. Phantom sensation: similar to that experienced by amputees.

The central pain associated with spinal cord injury occurs below the level of the lesion and is often an intense tingling, burning pain which cannot be localized.[34] Almost all paraplegics have this pain, which is resistant to analgesics. The pain is not intrinsic to the isolated cord segment, and alcohol injection of this area will not relieve the pain; but if the distal portion of the proximal segment of the intact cord above the lesion is injected with Novocain, the burning pain disappears.[35]

Brown-Sequard Syndrome

The Brown-Sequard syndrome follows lateral hemisection of the spinal cord and is characterized by the following features:

1. Ipsilateral upper motor neuron paralysis and loss of tactile discrimination, position, and vibration distal to the lesion.

2. Contralateral loss of pain and temperature distal to the level of the lesion because of the crossing over of the spinothalamic tracts; usually, the level of pain and temperature loss is one to several segments below the level of the lesion.

Myelitis

Myelitis is a nonspecific term indicating inflammation of the spinal cord secondary to a variety of possible etiologic factors:

1. Viral: poliomyelitis, rabies, type E encephalitis.
2. Bacterial.
3. Rickettsial, fungous, and parasitic infections.
4. Acute spontaneous inflammation: a postinfectious or postvaccination myelitis based upon an abnormal or excessive host immune response is the most common cause of an acute transverse and ascending myelitis.[36] However, in more than half of the patients with acute transverse myelitis, no clear history of an antecedent event, such as a respiratory infection, trauma, and injection, can be determined.[37]

The mid- to high thoracic segments are most commonly involved with an acute onset and two thirds of the patients reaching maximal neurologic involvement within 24 hours of onset. Initial symptoms consist of diffuse paresthesia in the lower extremities with occasional, severe back pain. A rapid, but incomplete sensory loss involving pain and temperature primarily develops within a short period. Frequently, there is a dermatomal band of hyperalgesia at the margin between normal sensation above the lesion and the severe sensory loss below the level of the lesion. Autonomic and motor symptoms and signs complete the clinical picture. With ascending lesions, the symptoms start in the legs with progressive ascent of motor and sensory loss on a segment by segment basis.

Myelopathy

Myelopathy occurs in a variety of diseases in which noninflammatory responses dominate the clinical picture. The myelopathy may develop as a consequence of toxic, nutritional, metabolic, and necrotizing spinal diseases. Toxic myelopathy may be secondary to arsenic exposure, injection of contrast media with the radiopaque iodides, and spinal anesthesia. Physical agents such as radiation therapy and electrical injury may also precipitate myelopathy. Peripheral nerves and nerve roots are more resistant than the central nervous system to radiation damage, but may degenerate following deep radiation therapy.[38] Usually, signs and symptoms of myelopathy dominate with an occasional sudden onset indicating infarction due to radiation-induced endarteritis.

Extradural and intradural compression syndromes may result in myelopathy. A common cause of extradural compression is metastatic carcinoma with changes in the spinal cord relating to both mechanical displacement and ischemia.[39] Intrinsic tumors are usually primary and of glial origin with ependymomas being twice as common as astrocytomas.[40] Pain may result from radicular or vertebral compression, as well as damage to the internuncial cells and spinothalamic tract.

EXTREMITIES

Extremity pain secondary to a pathologic lesion of the neuromuscular system may result from either a neuropathic or myopathic disease process.

Peripheral Neuropathy

Lesions of the peripheral nervous system may occur at a variety of tissue site levels of the lower motor neuron and first sensory neuron. Lesions of the anterior horn cell and dorsal root ganglion are discussed in the preceeding sections. The relative exposure of the plexus and peripheral nerve make them particularly vulnerable to trauma and damage by a variety of physical agents.

Peripheral neuropathies may be divided into two broad categories of pathology with common characteristics unique to each. Polyneuropathies are characterized by a diffuse, symmetrical sensorimotor disturbance affecting multiple nerve distributions and are associated with agents that act diffusely on the peripheral nervous system such as toxic disorders, deficiency states, immune reactions, infectious agents, and genetic disorders. Isolated nerve lesions (mononeuropathies) or multiple isolated nerve lesions (mononeuritis multiplex) result from processes that produce local damage to nerves. Mechanical injuries involving compression, traction, or penetrating wounds, and thermal, electrical, vascular, and neoplastic are common precursors to local nerve damage. Commonly, an isolated nerve lesion may be superimposed upon a systemic polyneuropathy as may occur with diabetic polyneuropathy.

A variety of classification schemes exist to describe the nature and degree of nerve insult. Seddon has proposed the following functional classification of nerve injury:[41]

1. Neuropraxia: an anatomic or biochemical disruption in the myelin sheath with the anatomic continuity of the axon remaining intact.
2. Axonotmesis: anatomic interruption of the axon resulting in Wallerian degeneration with preservation of the connective tissue framework of the nerve.
3. Neurotmesis: anatomic interruption of the axon and disruption of the connective tissue framework.

The process of Wallerian degeneration involves the dissolution of the axon and its myelin sheath and occurs throughout the nerve at and distal to the site of the lesion within a given time frame of 2 to 3 weeks. Retrograde changes in nerve may also occur as a result of axonal disruption and may progress to include the parent anterior horn cell and first sensory ganglion, a process referred to as chromatolysis. Retrograde changes affect sensory fibers more than motor fibers and depend upon the severity of tissue insult and the proximity of the lesion to the parent cell. The greater the degree of tissue insult and the more proximal the level of the lesion, the greater is the likelihood of developing retrograde changes in the peripheral nerve and its parent cell. Retrograde disturbances may extend beyond the parent cell originally involved by inducing trans-synaptic effects in related axons. Depression and failure of synaptic transmission, abnormalities in the pattern of synaptic activity, and unfavorable effects of integrative functions have been described for neurons during the period of chromatolysis.[42]

Many peripheral nerve lesions present as a mixed involvement of demyelination, axonal degeneration, and connective tissue framework disruption variously affecting individual axons within the nerve trunk. Lesions initially presenting as a locally demyelinating event may evolve into one characteristized by axonal degeneration. The consequences of the nerve injury will depend upon the type and degree of tissue insult. Local neuropraxic lesions will present with weakness or paralysis, sensory loss, and dysesthesias in the given nerve distribution with spontaneous return of function within weeks to months.

Diffuse demyelinating neuropathy seen in some forms of hereditary and infectious polyneuropathies may have a more protracted time course with progressive involvement in the former and variable degree of return of function in the latter.

Peripheral nerve lesions resulting in axonal degeneration will result in a variety of symptoms and signs depending upon the severity and extent of the lesion.

1. Paresis or paralysis of voluntary movement will occur in the affected distribution with subsequent development of atrophy and trophic changes.

2. Sensory loss: patterns of sensory loss may vary from hypesthesia to anesthesia variously affecting the sensory modalities depending upon the lesion.[43] In some forms of hereditary sensory neuropathy there may be loss of small diameter myelinated and unmyelinated axons subserving pain and temperature sensibility. Selective loss of larger myelinated sensory axons occurs in Fredrich's ataxia with loss of touch, pressure, joint position, and two point discrimination. More commonly, there is simultaneous loss of all sensory modalities.

3. Sensory dysesthesias: a variety of sensory disturbances may occur in peripheral nerve lesions:

    (A) Paresthesia is usually described as a tingling sensation or as thermal in nature.

    (B) Hyperesthesia or hyperpathia is described as an unpleasant quality added to cutaneous sensation and is associated with an altered sensory threshold. Stimuli that are normally neutral or even pleasant in affective tone may be uncomfortable or sometimes excruciatingly unpleasant.[44] Such sensations are usually precipitated by light moving stimuli rather than firm pressure and are usually found following partial nerve injuries or during recovery from nerve injuries. The hyperesthetic feet of a patient with alcoholic neuropathy and the affected skin areas of postherpetic neuralgia are examples.

4. Pain may be a troublesome symptom in a variety of peripheral nerve lesions. Certain localized nerve lesions may be associated with pain in the distribution of the nerve, locally within the nerve at one site, or a diffusely radiating pain. Some generalized neuropathies are uniformly painless while others are attended by pain of various types;

    (A) General deep seated aching sensation typified by the nocturnal pains in the lower legs in diabetic neuropathy.

    (B) Severe, lancinating pains in some forms of hereditary sensory neuropathy.

    (C) Severe, intractable pain of causalgia associated with high velocity injury to peripheral nerve.

5. Ataxia: sensory ataxia may result from disruption in proprioceptive fibers leading to incoordination and tremor.

6. Autonomic involvement: disturbances in autonomic nervous system

function may occur as a result of a peripheral nerve injury. Localized lesions of T1 or of the cervical sympathetic chain may result in Horner's syndrome. Orthostatic hypotension can occur secondary to the defects in vasomotor function. Anhidrosis will result from deficient sudomotor function in the cutaneous distribution of the involved peripheral nerve. Disturbances in genitourinary function may result in an atonic bladder.

Causalgia

Causalgia represents an occasional, severe, spontaneous, and persistent pain syndrome following peripheral nerve injury. The pain has been described as an intense burning sensation which may spread beyond the territory of the involved nerve and which may be associated with vasomotor and dystrophic changes. The occurrence of causalgia is most frequently related to incomplete or partial injuries to the median and posterior tibial nerves and to the medial cord of the brachial plexus. These nerve distributions contain the bulk of the sensory fibers to the skin and the greater number of sympathetic fibers and have the greater representation in the spinal ganglia and central nervous system. The lesions are often proximal in origin with 90 percent of them occurring above the elbow and above the knee.[45] Multiple involvement of nerves is frequent and onset usually occurs within 24 hours of the injury, but may be delayed for several weeks. According to Sunderland, causalgia usually follows high velocity missile wounds, less commonly, traction injuries, and rarely, other forms of nerve damage such as arterial and venous occlusions.[46] There is no good correlation between the severity of pain and the anatomic lesion or the degree of damage to non-neural tissue. The pain tends to be more severe in the hand and foot and is aggravated by emotional and environmental factors and tends to persist for longer than 5 weeks. There are variable sympathetic effects noted with causalgia. Increased sweating is noted in some cases with absence of sweating noted in other cases. Peripheral blood flow may be increased or decreased, which suggests that disturbances of vasomotor function are not responsible for the pain.

Sympathetic block often abates the pain temporarily and, in some cases, can give permanent and complete relief from the symptoms.[45] Sympathectomy at the preganglionic level can relieve the symptoms in 70 to 80 percent of the cases. Other surgical procedures for pain relief have been performed at multiple tissue sites in the sensory pathway from receptor to cortex with some success, but with a tendency for symptoms to recur.

The etiology of causalgia is obscure with a number of theories postulated over the years as reviewed by Sunderland.[46] Lewis and Davis and Pollock, in separate studies as reported in Sunderland, suggested a peripheral factor related to the release of a pain producing substance at the site of injury. Nathan suggested that the pain impulses originated at the site of nerve trunk damage and not at the peripheral terminations of the involved nerve.[47] Doupe et al suggested that damaged segments in mixed nerve at the site of insult might form artificial synapses through which impulses in efferent sympathetic fibers might excite adjacent sensory fibers leading to widespread peripheral and central effects.[48] Livingston, as reported in Sunderland, suggests that causalgic pain is central, rather than peripheral in origin and results from retrograde changes in the cord. A disorganized cord activity ensues and results in abnormal function in the presence of altered or absent peripheral sensory input. An abnormal state of activity develops in the internuncial neuron pool in the posterior horn of the spinal cord, which is believed to originate initially from impulses discharged centrally from the injured segment. The altered peripheral sensory input combined with the afferent input from the proximal segment of the injured tissue combine to convert the cord neurons into a hypersensitive foci, which continues to operate, becomes self-sustaining, and spreads to involve higher centers.

Phantom Limb Sensation

Phantom limb sensation occurs after most traumatic and surgical amputations of the arm and leg. Phantom limb sensations are not present in congenital amputations and tend to be absent in younger patients with noncongenital amputation before the development of body image at approximately 8 years of age.[49] Phantom limb sensation may, in fact, occur with any interruption of the sensory pathway between the periphery and the sensory cortex and commonly occurs in spinal cord injury and brachial plexus lesions.

A variety of sensations may be associated with the phantom limb. The phantom describes a positive sensation of numbness or tingling associated with an appreciation of the peripheral parts of the limb. More pronounced paresthesias of a thermal quality may occur with sudden lancinating or cramplike pains. The phantom sensation usually subsides within a few months, but may persist as either an intermittent or continuous sensory experience.

The etiology of phantom limb sensation and pain is obscure and may partially relate to the emotive aspect of limb amputation.

Local factors related to surgical trauma contribute to the early perception of phantom limb sensation from the volley of afferent impulses at the site of amputation. Persistent phantom sensations may also relate to neuroma formation, adhesions at the site of amputation, and influences associated with blood supply and tissue nutrition.

Retrograde changes following nerve trunk section may affect the proximal nerve trunk, posterior root ganglia, spinal cord, and cortex. These neuronal and transsynaptic changes contribute to an altered state of central processing of sensory information.

Elimination of normal sensory inflow from the limb further imbalances the established pattern of neuronal activity and contributes to altered central processing of sensory information.

The combination of retrograde neuronal changes and altered peripheral sensory inflow may combine, as was discussed for causalgia, to disorganize sensory circuits so that they discharge independently of peripheral foci for irritation. Hyperexcitable pools of neurons become foci of abnormal sensations initiating new central pathways which become so conditioned that the individual experiences continuous pain. The consolidation of central irritable foci makes difficult any attempt to control, relieve, or cure pain by procedures directed at the periphery.[50] In most cases, disorganized central circuits gradually diminish with establishment of a new equilibrium. At the same time, hyperexcitable and unstable neuronal systems may continue to respond to stimuli from stump tissues, environmental stimuli, and activity elsewhere in the central nervous system and precipitate intermittent periods of pain and phantom sensation. In other cases, abnormal activity originating in a disorganized neuronal pool may persist to maintain and intensify the phantom state leading to a continuation of unpleasant sensory phenomena.

Shoulder Hand Syndrome (Sudecks Atrophy)

The shoulder hand syndrome is one of a number of variously caused disorders with a similar clinical presentation of pain, numbness, and motor disability produced by circulatory and neural disturbances.[51] Three stages of the syndrome exist: (1) painful disability of the shoulder with swelling and stiffness of the hand and fingers with either an acute painful onset or insidious development over a period of 3 to 6 months, (2) gradual relief of pain and dysfunction at the shoulder with decreased swelling of the hand, but with increasing stiffness and deformity of the fingers and developing osteoporosis, and (3) trophic changes in the hand with persistent stiffness and deformity.

Many conditions may precipitate the syndrome. The syndrome has been associated with myocardial infarction, angina, cervical osteoarthritis, cerebral vascular disease, and peripheral nerve trauma among a variety of other causes. The pathophysiology is not clear, but nociceptive stimuli from the site of tissue insult is thought to initiate autonomic reflex activity with vasodilation and to stimulate reflex activity within the internuncial neuronal pool of the spinal cord to initiate the painful state.[51]

Treatment has been directed to management of the underlying pathology, blocking the effect of the nociceptive stimuli with stellate ganglion injections, steroids, and analgesics and utilizing the modalities of physical therapy for the musculoskeletal dysfunction.

Mononeuropathies

Entrapment Neuropathies. Local injury to peripheral nerve may occur as a result of mechanical compression, or ischemia, at points where the nerve may pass through rigid anatomic canals or beneath tight ligamentous or fascial bands. Entrapment may occur more readily when inflammation or degeneration is present in adjacent joints and tendons or where the nerve travels a superficial course exposing it to repeated environmental trauma. Any space-occupying lesion, adjacent tissue hyperplasia, or edematous anatomic region may also compress nerve trunk.

Phrenic Nerve. The phrenic nerve originates from the anterior primary division of C3–C5, and descends in front of the scalenus anticus muscle to pass behind the subclavian vessels to enter the mediastinum. In the mediastinum, the nerve lies between the pericardium and the pleura where it divides into multiple branches to innervate the diaphragm. In its course from the cervical spine to the diaphragm, the nerve may be surrounded by neoplasm, and compressed by enlarged lymph nodes and inflammatory tissue. Sensory symptoms consisting of persistent pain in the C5 dermatome of the shoulder and arm may herald the onset of motor paralysis.[52] Diaphragmatic tics may also be present.

Median Nerve. One of the most common sites of entrapment in man occurs with the median nerve at the wrist, as it passes with the long flexor tendons through the carpal tunnel under the cover of the transverse carpal ligament. Any condition that increases the volume of the structures within the canal or any pathologic distortion of the walls of the canal may produce a compressive lesion of the nerve.[53]

Main clinical features include pain and paresthesia in the median nerve distribution of the hand with occasional retrograde pain radiation to the arm and shoulder. Symptoms tend to be worse at night and increased upon repetitive hand activities and certain posturing of the hand. Thenar intrinsic musculature weakness and wasting may be present in chronic lesions and Raynaud's phenomenon may be a variable occurrence. The syndrome is most common in postmenopausal females and in individuals with occupational or recreational activities requiring repetitive hand function.

A less common site of median nerve entrapment occurs at the elbow when the nerve enters the forearm between the two heads of the pronator teres. *Pronator syndrome* is characterized by pain, hypesthesia, paresthesia, and weakness in the median nerve distribution below the elbow.

Ulnar Nerve. The ulnar nerve may be subject to entrapment at a variety of sites in the neck and arm. Compressive lesions may occur at the level of the wrist and hand and the nature of the symptoms and signs will vary with the exact anatomic site of involvement, as described by Ebeling et al.[54] The ulnar nerve runs a superficial course as it passes behind the medial epicondyle of the humerus to enter the forearm under the cover of the flexor carpi ulnaris muscle. At this level in the cubital tunnel, the nerve is subjected to environmental trauma relating to postural habitus, as well as to underlying arthritic changes and structural deformities of the elbow. In the upper arm segment, the nerve in its superficial course may also be subjected to external pressure on the outstretched upper arm.

Compression of the ulnar nerve may occur as part of the symptom complex of the thoracic outlet syndrome. Compression of the lower trunk of the brachial plexus and/or subclavian vessels may occur at a variety of tissue sites within the thoracic outlet.[55] Symptoms will depend upon whether nerve or vascular structures or both are involved. According to Reuss, 97 percent of the patients with thoracic outlet syndrome have neurologic, rather than vascular symptoms.[56] The majority of cases have intermittent pain of insidious onset with a burning dysesthesia aggravated by exercise and elevation of the arm. Raynaud's phenomenon and signs of venous compression may also be present. Pain and paresthesia occur primarily in the C8–T1 distribution, but pain may also be referred to the neck, scapula, and pectoral region.

The subclavian steal syndrome represents a symptom complex often confused with thoracic outlet syndrome.[7] The former is characterized by a reversed retrograde flow in the vertebral artery secondary to an atherosclerotic lesion of the subclavian artery which results in a siphoning effect on vertebrobasilar circulation. Symptoms of cerebral ischemia occur with arm pain, paresthesia, and weakness and are aggravated by exercise and activity.

Radial Nerve. The radial nerve is subjected to compression at four potential sites along its pathway. In the axilla, the nerve is subjected to environmental trauma from an improperly used crutch or other local deforming force in the axilla. At the level of the spiral groove, the radial nerve passes from the medial to the lateral side of the upper arm in a relatively superficial course around the humerus. Trauma to the nerve at this level can occur from an improperly placed needle injection or from resting on the arm as may occur during sleep in Saturday night palsy. Entrapment of the deep motor branch (posterior interosseous) of the radial nerve may occur at the elbow where the motor branch passes under a fibrous arch formed by the suppinator and the extensor carpi radialis longus muscles (arcade of Froshe). Symptoms are often associated with activities involving repeated forceful suppination of the forearm and extension of the wrist: a condition often associated with lateral epicondylitis.[57] Patients complain of proximal forearm pain often at night or after use of the arm. Muscle weakness and wasting may occur in the absence of a sensory deficit. Entrapment of the sensory branch of the radial nerve (superficial radial nerve) may occur in the forearm after the nerve emerges from under the cover of the brachioradialis. Entrapment can be secondary to an aberrant course through the extensor carpi radialis brevis or from pressure secondary to a tight watch band or handcuffs. Painful dysesthesias occur in the distal radial aspect of the forearm.

Lateral Femoral Cutaneous Nerve. Meralgia paresthetica is a common, annoying, benign entrapment of the lateral femoral cutaneous nerve of the thigh. The nerve originates from L2 and L3 and runs across the ileum to enter the thigh through an opening formed by the attachment of the inguinal ligament to the anterior superior iliac spine. The nerve may be compressed at the point of entrance to the thigh and will precipitate the characteristic burning pain and hypersensitivity of the anterolateral thigh. The symptoms are often related to wearing corsets, belts, and trusses or tight fitting jeans.[58]

Femoral Nerve. The femoral nerve arises from the lumbar plexus and runs along the lateral border of the psoas before entering the thigh deep to the inguinal ligament. Compression of the femoral nerve often induces spontaneous pain in the groin and thigh along with a variable amount of motor weakness and sensory deficit in the anterior medial thigh. Entrapment of the femoral nerve in the inguinal region is uncommon, but may be associated with inguinal hernia or scarring in the area. More proximal lesions may occur from the use of retractors during abdominal surgery or from a retroperitoneal hematoma developing as a complication of hemophilia or in patients receiving anticoagulation therapy.[59]

Following vascular reconstructive surgery in the legs, a transient dysesthetic pain and paresthesia of the medial knee and leg may result from involvement of the sensory termination of the femoral nerve (saphenous neuralgia).

Obturator Nerve. The obturator nerve originates from the ventral divisions of L2–L4, pierces the iliopsoas, and descends across the pelvis to enter the thigh through the obturator canal. Compression may occur anywhere along its course as a result of tumor, inflammation, pelvic fractures, or positioning in the lithotomy posture. Compression of the nerve results in hip, thigh, and knee pain with sensory impairment of the medial thigh and motor weakness in the adductor muscle group. The knee pain with obturator neuropathy can be confused with intrinsic knee joint pathology.

Sciatic Nerve. The sciatic nerve is the largest nerve in the body and arises from multiple levels of the lumbosacral spine. The nerve leaves the pelvis through the sciatic notch after passing through or below the pyriformis and lies under the cover of the gluteus maximus to reach the posterior thigh. At a variable distance along the posterior thigh, the nerve divides into its terminal divisions: common peroneal and posterior tibial nerves. Prior to that division, the nerve may be compressed at several levels: (1) level of the nerve root, (2) sciatic notch secondary to external trauma from prolonged sitting or a fall, or as a consequence of anomalies of the pyriformis, and (3) level of the hip joint consequent to joint replacement and other operative hip procedures. Lesions may present with pain and other signs in the sciatic nerve distribution.

Common peroneal nerve compression occurs primarily at the fibular head where the nerve is superficial, fixed, and angulated as it wraps around the neck of the fibula. The limited mobility of the nerve at this level makes it vulnerable to traction injuries as may occur with inversion ankle sprains. Compression may occur from a tight fitting cast, postural habits of crossing one leg over the other, and in occupations requiring prolonged kneeling or squatting. Compression at this site involves the deep peroneal branch more than the superficial peroneal branch and symptoms may include pain and paresthesia over the anterolateral leg with a variable amount of motor weakness.

Entrapment of the deep peroneal branch at the ankle under the inferior extensor retinaculum may occur as a result of repetitive microtrauma from shoe wear or from ankle sprain (anterior tarsal tunnel syndrome).

Entrapment of the superficial peroneal branch may occur at the site it pierces the deep fascia of the lower one third of the leg and divides into its terminal branches. The opening in the fascia provides a site for entrapment secondary to an inversion ankle injury or as a result of a fascial defect with muscle herniation at the point of nerve exit. Pain and numbness occur in the lateral third of the leg and dorsum of the foot and tend to be aggravated by exercise and walking.

Proximal compression of the posterior tibial branch of the sciatic nerve is uncommon, but may occur in the popliteal fossa secondary to vascular malformations, cysts, and hematomas. Compression of the nerve may occur at the ankle where it passes behind the medial malleolus and under the flexor retinaculum (tarsal tunnel) with the posterior tibial vessels. The most common complaints of patients with tarsal tunnel syndrome are pain and burning dysesthesia confined to the sole of the foot; rarely is there a motor deficit.[60] The symptoms are aggravated by prolonged standing and walking. Compression may occur as a result of osteoarthritis and post-traumatic deformities, chronic swelling and tenosynovitis, and hyperpronation of the subtalar joint.

Direct compression of the plantar nerves may occur in the foot from prolonged standing, hyperpronation, and tenosynovitis of the plantar tendon sheaths. The interdigital nerves may be compressed in inflammatory processes such as rheumatoid arthritis or from excessive hyperextension of the metatarsal phalangeal joints, as occurs with deep squatting. Morton's neuroma results from recurrent compression of the interdigital nerves to the third and fourth toes from a variety of causes including ill fitting shoe wear.

Pudendal Nerve. The pudendal nerve is formed from the S2–S4 nerve roots and passes between the coccygeus and pyriformis muscles to exit from the pelvis through the lesser sciatic foramen. The nerve divides into terminal motor and sensory branches to the anal and perineal regions and to the mucous membranes of the urethra and to the penis and clitoris. Clinical features of involvement include pain referred to the perineum and genital region with spread to the groin, leg, and abdomen. The pain is often severe and paroxysmal and is associated with a hyperesthesia. Symptoms may arise from compressive or irritative lesions at any point along the course of the nerve and can occur as pressure neuralgias in cyclists and horsemen. Lower pelvic tumors and herpes zoster are other primary etiologic agents.

Polyneuropathy

Pathologic processes that result in a bilaterally symmetrical disturbance of function tend to be associated with agents that act diffusely on the peripheral nervous system. A progressive mixed sensory-motor polyneuropathy generally appears initially in a distal distribution in the lower extremities with motor weakness and wasting with a glove and stocking sensory deficit, pain, and autonomic involvement. Symptoms and signs of the polyneuropathy will ascend the lower extremities and will involve upper extremity nerve distributions at a later stage. Symptoms of sensory nerve involvement will depend on whether there is large or small fiber involvement, the rate of degeneration, the type of nerve injury, and whether all or just the distal part of the axon is affected. Negative symptoms with loss of sensory units may include loss of sensation and deficits in motor activities requiring afferent input. Positive symptoms represent excessive neural activity related to injured axons or regenerated axonal sprouts and may include varying degrees of paresthesia, dysesthesia, hyperalgesia, and pain of an aching or burning quality.

Uremia. The neuropathy associated with uremia is seen only in end stage renal disease and is not part of the symptom complex in acute renal failure.[61] Decreasing renal function is associated with the development of the neuropathy and the latter is presumably related to the accumulation of toxic metabolites. The etiology of the neuropathy is unclear as hemodialysis does not appear to improve peripheral nerve function, but successful kidney transplant does. Typically, uremic neuropathy is a progressive symmetric, predominantly sensory neuropathy. Symptoms may include paresthesia, burning pain, and other hyperalgesic phenomena and will be followed subsequently by motor involvement.

Malignant Disease. Multiple neurologic syndromes have been described in malignancy affecting both central and peripheral nervous systems, including the neuromuscular junction, as well as primary muscle disorders. These syndromes may present in combination and are often associated with carcinoma of the lung.

Peripheral nerve involvement associated with malignancy may occur secondary to (1) direct compression by tumor or hemorrhage or (2) remote effects of tumor. In the latter instance, the incidence of neuropathy varies with the type of carcinoma and the criteria used to diagnose the neuropathy. When pathologic or electrophysiologic criteria are used, the incidence of neuropathy approaches 50 percent.[62] Many possible mechanisms for the production of polyneuropathy have been suggested, but the etiology remains obscure. McLeod has identified the following as possible agents: direct infiltration, toxic factors released by the tumor, alterations in enzyme activity and metabolism, nutritional deficiencies, vascular lesions, viral infections, and immunologic responses.[62]

The symptoms of neuropathy may precede the diagnosis of tumor by a variable period of up to 6 months. Sensory symptoms predominate and include numbness, paresthesia, and aching limb pains. Motor weakness and wasting usually occur later in the illness. The course of the neuropathy is generally one of an insidious onset with slow progression unaffected by the removal of the tumor.[63]

Nutritional Deficiency and Chronic Alcoholism. The mechanism of nutritional neuropathies may result from chronic alcoholism, food faddism, malabsorption, and drugs and is generally a result of dietary imbalance rather than starvation. Vitamins are essential for normal cell metabolism as important components of enzyme systems. The vitamin B complexes are important to catabolic reactions in the metabolism of carbohydrates required as an energy source in the function of both the central and peripheral nervous systems.

The neuropathy of vitamin B_1 (thiamine) deficiency (beriberi) is often associated with chronic alcoholism as a result of substituting alcohol for food in diets containing thiamine or as a result of inadequate absorption resulting from chronic gastritis seen in alcoholism.[64] Nonalcohol-related thiamine deficiency is seen in some cultures with inadequate dietary intake of thiamine.

The typical neuropathy is one of insidious onset with a symmetrical, ascending polyneuritis characterized by pain and paresthesia in the lower extremities initially. Distal vasomotor and sudomotor abnormalities are consistently present with later development of motor weakness and wasting. The disturbance in autonomic function gives rise to the burning feet syndrome characterized by severe burning pain and hyperesthesia in the feet and legs associated with hyperhydrosis of the feet and occasionally the hands. Pain may become the dominant symptom in the nutritional-alcoholic neuropathies and the pain may become so severe as to preclude walking and manipulating objects with the hands.

A subgroup of alcoholics exist who develop a rapid onset neuropathy with rapid progression of symptoms. The onset is related to bouts of heavy drinking on a background of severe nutritional deficiency.

Vitamin B_{12} deficiency states resulting in pernicious anemia are characterized by macrocytic anemia, bone marrow hyperplasia, and subacute combined degeneration of the spinal cord. Deficiency usually occurs as a result of the inability to absorb the vitamin from the gastronintestinal tract. The nerve pathology is one of degenerative and demyelinating lesions of the dorsal lateral columns of the spinal cord and peripheral nerves. Anterior horn cells may show chromatolysis. The disease is one of late adult life with insidious onset of gradually increasing weakness, anorexia, diarrhea, and abdominal pain. Neurologic symptoms develop in 80 to 95 percent of the patients with the initial appearance of symmetrical numbness and paresthesia with shooting pains in the extremities.[64]

Fabry's Disease.   Fabry's disease is a sex-linked recessive genetic disorder of lipid metabolism characterized by intense sensations of burning pain in the feet and lower legs. The severe pains often preclude walking. Typically, the disease occurs in young males and results in organ system involvement secondary to lipid deposition in the vasculature.[65] There is variable involvement of the central, peripheral, and autonomic nervous systems with fiber loss and degenerative changes in unmyelinated nerve fibers.[66] A reddish purple maculopapular rash of the inguinal, perineal, and gluteal regions accompany the neurologic disorder. Progressive uremia and renal failure are a frequent cause of death.

Inherited Disorders of Motor, Sensory, and Autonomic Neurons.   The hereditary neuropathies refer to a group of disorders referred to in the past by a variety of terms such as Charcot-Marie-Tooth disease, Roussy-Levy syndrome, and Refsum's disease. Many of these syndromes show predominant involvement of peripheral motor neurons, but a variety show preferential involvement of peripheral sensory neurons. As a group, the latter category demonstrates a slowly progressive, symmetrical, and diffuse neuropathic deficit characterized by degeneration of unmyelinated and myelinated small diameter axons. Degeneration of spinal ganglion neurons has also been noted to occur.[43] Symptoms may include hypesthesia, frank sensory loss with insensitivity to pain, ulcer formation, and severe, intermittent, lancinating pain. Sensory loss occurs predominantly in the legs and feet and is characterized more by loss of pain and temperature, and anhidrosis with slight to moderate motor weakness. Symptoms in some cases are often confused with syringomyelia. In some cases, there may be severe recurring pains in the shoulders, as well as the legs and feet. These attacks may be related to the rapidity of progression of the disease and to the degree of involvement of pain fibers. The attacks may last for hours, days, or weeks and are followed by a variable period of remission. The primary site of pathologic insult is controversial with variable lesions noted in the posterior columns of the spinal cord, posterior roots, spinal ganglia, and peripheral nerves.

Toxic Neuropathy. A variety of toxic agents including metals, industrial agents, and drugs may result in neuropathy. With the exception of lead, which produces a motor neuropathy, most other toxic agents produce a characteristic pattern of polyneuropathy. A mixed sensorimotor involvement of symmetrical, distal distribution affects the lower limbs more than the upper limbs. Sensory symptoms predominate and consist of paresthesia, burning dysesthesias, pain, and hypersensitivity. The autonomic nervous system is involved in the more severe forms of polyneuropathy. Primary pathologic changes are secondary to axonal degeneration.

Acute Inflammatory Demyelinating Polyneuropathy. Several types of postinfectious polyneuritis occur as a consequence of an antecedent illness, generally an upper respiratory infection. Other illnesses associated with this type of neuropathy include bacterial infection, recent immunization, and animal and insect bites. Viral or bacterial invasion of neural structure has not been demonstrated and the lesion is thought to be an immunologic response with lymphoid cell infiltration resulting in demyelination and occasional axonal degeneration of neural structure.[67]

The symptom complex may be predominantly motor as occurs in the Landry-Guillain-Barré-Strohl syndrome. A mixed motor-sensory neuropathy and a predominantly sensory neuropathy may also occur. The symptoms begin with an insidious onset of motor and/or sensory symptoms in the lower limbs with progression to the upper limbs and occasionally the cranial nerves within days. The lesions may affect spinal roots, ganglia, and the central nervous system, as well as peripheral nerves. In the sensory form of involvement, severe lancinating pains of the shoulder and pelvic girdles may develop over a period of hours or days. The pain may be associated with sensory loss resulting in ataxia and incoordination. The disease tends to crest within a few days, but recovery tends to be less complete than in patients with the predominantly motor form. Many patients are left with a residual sensory deficit with persistent pain.

Diabetic Neuropathy. Peripheral neuropathy is seen as a complication of early onset insulin-dependent diabetes and in adult onset diabetes. The neuropathy associated with diabetes may take a variety of forms. Attempts to classify the forms of diabetic neuropathy have been complicated by the tendency for mixed syndromes to occur in any one patient. Thomas has suggested the following functional classification:[68] (1) sensory polyneuropathy, (2) mononeuropathy, and (3) multiple mononeuropathy.

The predominantly sensory, symmetrical polyneuropathy of gradual onset is the most frequent form of neuropathic deficit in diabetic subjects. In some cases, the occurrence of neuropathy may precede the diagnosis of adult onset diabetes. An uncertain relationship exists between the adequacy of diabetic control of carbohydrate metabolism and the development of the neuropathy, but in general, the more severe degrees of nerve damage occur in individuals with inadequate diabetic control.[69] An acute onset of a symmetrical polyneuropathy may follow a history of emotional stress, intercurrent infection, surgery, or even initiation of diabetic treatment.[70] Other possible etiologic factors in the neuropathy include toxic metabolites and the microangiopathy associated with atherosclerosis of the small nutrient arteries to nerve.

In many cases, clinical examination may reveal abnormalities in the absence of symptoms. In the symptomatic patient, numbness and a burning paresthesia may occur in the feet and legs with an aching pain that tends to be worse at night. Occasionally, a severe sensory neuropathy develops with distal loss of cutaneous sensibility, deep pain, joint position, and vibration in all four limbs. A sensory ataxia will develop and the loss of pain sensibility contributes to the development of plantar ulcers and neuropathic arthropathy. This syndrome of diabetic pseudotabes can be accompanied by the presence of lancinating leg pains and autonomic changes.

Isolated or multiple isolated nerve lesions may also be associated with diabetes. Isolated lesions of the 3rd, 4th, 6th, and 7th cranial nerves may occur alone or in varying combinations. Isolated lesions of the femoral nerve occur as well as compression of individual nerves at the common sites for the peripheral entrapment neuropathies.

Demyelination of peripheral nerve has been identified as an important component of the peripheral nerve changes based upon nerve conduction studies.[71] The peripheral demyelination may be either primary relating to a disturbance in Schwann cell function or secondary to primary axonal involvement. Neuropathic lesions have been identified not only in peripheral nerve trunk, but also in spinal roots, dorsal root ganglion cells, and anterior horn cells.[72]

A third form of diabetic neuropathy manifests as an upper lumbar plexus neuropathy referred to as diabetic amyotrophy.[73] The syndrome presents in one of two forms. The first type occurs in the middle-aged adult onset diabetic with an abrupt onset of severe pain in the hip and anterior thigh associated with weakness of the quadriceps, iliopsoas, and adductors. The pain gradually resolves over several weeks. The pathogenesis is thought to be an acute impairment of blood supply to the superior portion of the lumbar plexus.

The second type begins in the middle-aged or elderly patients with mild, recently discovered diabetes. The syndrome is characterized by a progressive, debilitating disorder, which starts insidiously with a deep aching and burning pain in the hips and thighs. A steadily progressive weakness of proximal and distal muscles ensues and patients frequently become bedfast with cachexia, pain, and diffuse weakness. The pain worsens for weeks and months before gradually decreasing. The pathogenesis is thought to be an acute infarction of small vessels resulting in ischemic mononeuropathy multiplex.[74]

Multiple Mononeuropathy (Mononeuropathy Multiplex)

Single peripheral nerves may become involved sequentially in both time and space in a distribution dissimilar to the distal symmetrical distribution associated with polyneuropathy. Typically, the patient develops weakness, paresthesia, and dysesthetic pain in the distributions of the involved nerves. This syndrome may be seen in a variety of conditions: necrotizing angiitis, vasculopathies, and in inflammatory disorders.

Brachial Neuralgia. Brachial neuralgia, an acutely painful syndrome, is known by a variety of names—brachial amyotrophy, Parsonage-Turner syndrome—and is characterized by a sudden onset of continuous pain in the shoulders with radiation to the neck and arm. Weakness with wasting rapidly develops in the shoulder girdle and upper arm musculature. The lesions may involve one or more single peripheral nerves at the root or plexus levels and typically involves the distribution of the upper trunk.[75] Occasionally, other nerve distributions in the upper and lower extremity are involved. The syndrome is more common in males with 90 percent of the patients recovering within 3 years. The etiology is uncertain with 50 percent of the patients having an antecedent history of a viral infection, recent vaccination, surgery, or unrelated trauma. On that basis, an immunologic response mechanism based upon an allergic vascular disturbance with edema of neural structures has been postulated as the pathologic lesion. In the remaining cases, there is no clear history of an antecedent event likely to precipitate an immune response.

Heredofamilial Brachial Plexus Neuropathy. This genetic syndrome of autosomal dominance inheritance is also characterized by excruciating shoulder pain with severe weakness and wasting in the shoulder girdle musculature. In contrast to brachial neuralgia, lower cranial nerve involvement and isolated mononeuropathies in other extremities may be seen in this genetic disorder.[76] The clinical course is benign and self limiting with full recovery after several months.

Porphyric Neuropathy. Porphyric neuropathy is a genetically determined metabolic disorder characterized by an overproduction and excretion of porphrin and porphyrin precursors.[77] Clinical features include:

1. Abdominal pain suggestive of an acute surgical emergency
2. Psychological disturbances consisting of a feeling of restlessness associated with insomnia, crying, and neurotic hysterical behavior
3. Neurologic symptoms beginning with back and upper extremity pain with paresthesia with later development of proximal upper extremity motor weakness. The neuropathy progresses to include cranial nerves and central nervous system involvement with mental disturbance and seizure; the neuropathy is often precipitated in response to barbituate medication given to treat the psychologic manifestations.

The etiology is thought to be a primary disturbance in neuronal metabolism with resultant patchy destruction of axons and myelin sheaths with chromatolysis of anterior horn cells, dorsal root ganglia, autonomic cells in the spinal cord, bulbar region, cerebellum, and cortex. The neuropathy is the frequent cause of death, but if patients survive, most will recover from the neuropathy, although relapses may occur.

Multiple Myeloma. Multiple myeloma is a malignant disorder of uncontrolled proliferation of the plasma cell system with infiltration of these cells into bone and other tissues. Anemia, renal failure, and pathologic fracture are common consequences. Neurologic complications include (1) compression of the spinal cord and roots by collapsed vertebrae or by extradural deposits of myeloma, (2) cranial nerve palsies, (3) mononeuropathies secondary to compression by a myelomatous mass, and (4) polyneuropathy. The symptoms of neuropathy may precede the diagnosis of multiple myeloma by months. Pain in the arms and legs is a significant component of the disease in addition to the characteristic bone pain. The neuropathic changes are secondary to direct infiltration of myeloma into neural structures. Degeneration of myelin sheath and axon cylinders occurs with chromatolysis in the anterior horn cells.[79]

Collagen Disease and Necrotizing Angiopathy. Disorders of diffuse connective tissue involvement may give rise to a variety of neurologic manifestations. These neurologic changes are generally secondary to immunologically induced inflammatory changes in the walls of the arterioles and capillaries with resultant occlusion and local ischemia of the epineural vasculature. Patients may develop an abrupt onset neuropathy with subsequent involvement of other nerve distributions. A diffuse array of symptoms will be associated with the multiple sites of ischemic occlusion superimposed upon connective tissue disorder. Fever, arthralgia, weight loss, and other systemic symptoms will be associated with focal or diffuse motor and sensory involvement of both the central and peripheral nervous systems. Burning pain is a frequent complication of the vascular lesions.

In periarteritis nodosa, peripheral nerves are involved in 50 percent of the cases with either a polyneuritis, mononeuritis multiplex or, occasionally, as ascending paralysis of the Landry-Guillain-Barré-Strohl type.[80] Similar changes have been described in scleroderma, rheumatoid arthritis, Wegener's granulomatosis, and Sjögren's syndrome. In rheumatoid arthritis, the neuropathy may also take the form of a focal compression neuropathy associated with periarticular inflammatory changes.[81] Carpal tunnel syndrome is a common occurrence in rheumatoid arthritis.

Restless Leg Syndrome

The symptom complex of restless leg syndrome was described by Ekbom as an ill-defined discomfort in the legs at rest.[82] Clinical features include pain and paresthesia in the lower limbs at rest with an irresistible tendency to move the limbs or to get up and walk for symptomatic relief. The symptoms are generally symmetrical and may occasionally involve the thighs and upper extremities. The pain may last for 10 minutes up to several hours and may run a course over several years with spontaneous remissions and exacerbations. Objective findings are minimal, although the syndrome is commonly associated with anxiety, tension, and mild depression. No definite etiology has been defined, although Ekbom showed that 50 percent of patients had decreased serum iron. The symptoms may be induced by pregnancy and have been associated with a variety of neuropathic conditions related to diabetes, uremia, and malignancy, among other conditions.

Muscle Disorders

Muscle is subject to a variety of inflammatory processes of which pain may be a significant component. Bacterial, viral, parasitic, and granulomatous conditions may precipitate an inflammatory process in muscle. More commonly, the myopathy is secondary to an idiopathic inflammation which is often associated with disturbances in the immune system.[83]

Polymyositis and Dermatomyositis

Polymyositis and dermatomyositis represent another manifestation of collagen disorders affecting skeletal muscle and/or skin. The two conditions are similar except that in dermatomyositis, skin lesions are a characteristic feature of the disease. Bohan and Peters have classified this connective tissue disorder into the following groups.[84]

1. Primary idiopathic polymyositis
2. Primary idiopathic dermatomyositis
3. Dermatomyositis/polymyositis associated with neoplasia
4. Childhood dermatomyositis/polymyositis associated with vasculitis
5. Dermatomyositis/polymyositis associated with collagen vascular disease

The pathologic lesion in muscle is one of mixed degenerative and regenerative changes with necrosis, fibrosis, and atrophy of muscle fibers with interstitial infiltrations. The etiology is unknown in many cases, but in others, the lesions in muscle fibers can be related to vascular insufficiency. There is thickening of small vessel walls with infiltration and degeneration of capillary beds.[85]

The disease is more common in childhood and in the fifth and sixth decades of life with males more affected than females. Onset of symptoms may begin with a variety of systemic signs: fever, malaise, myalgia, and gastrointestinal distress. Skeletal muscle involvement, with or without cutaneous skin lesions, appears as a symmetrical proximal weakness affecting pelvic and shoulder girdle musculature. Weakness of anterior neck muscles is also prominent. Bulbar weakness is unusual, but distal extremity muscles become involved as the disease progresses. When pain is present, it is described as a deep aching within muscle associated with muscle swelling and induration with local tenderness.

The disease runs a variable course with three predominant outcomes: (1) single acute attack with recovery, (2) remitting, relapsing illness with imperfect recovery, (3) chronic, indolent form with progressive involvement. Treatment is with steroids and immunosuppressive agents.

Polymyalgia Rheumatica

There are many illnesses in which muscle pain is a prominent symptom; some are nebulous and difficult to diagnose. In polymyalgia, muscle pain and stiffness occur after a period of rest and are relieved by exercise and activity. The etiology is unknown, although some patients present with a low grade fever. A good response is often noted to prednisone.[83]

Myoglobinuria

With acute insult to muscle tissue, myoglobin may be released into the serum and thence into the urine. This release may occur in normal muscle under the stress of excessive exercise or may occur as a result of a crush injury or metabolic anomaly.[86]

Hereditary myoglobinuria represents a genetic metabolic disorder of phosphorylase deficiency and can give rise to fatigue, pain, and myoglobinuria with exercise.[87] These symptoms may be associated with weakness, headaches, nausea, and vomiting. The large muscle groups of the arms and legs are most often affected. After an acute attack, muscle function returns to normal within 1 to 3 weeks. Renal failure is the most serious complication of myoglobinuria.

Nutritional Myopathy

Nutritional myopathies, as was true for some forms of nutritional neuropathies, are a well recognized complication of chronic alcoholism.[88] The typical illness takes two forms: (1) acute attack of muscle pain, swelling, and weakness primarily in the thigh muscles with associated myoglobinuria and (2) chronic progressive proximal weakness of shoulder and pelvic girdle musculature.

Abnormal Muscle Activity

Abnormal and repetitive muscle activity occurs as a part of many different disorders as seen in myokymia, muscle spasms related to calcium deficiency, and myotonia. In the stiff man syndrome, there is a painful, sustained repetitive activity of muscle fibers. The disease is one of adult life and is characterized by painful and uncontrollable contractions of muscles, particularly in the hips, thighs, and shoulders.[89] The limbs are held rigid and immobile and voluntary movements may not be possible. The sustained contractions or spasms disappear during sleep or anesthesia only to return upon awakening. The spasms may also be relieved by peripheral nerve block and curarization.

The physical examination reveals no definitive neurologic abnormality other than the sustained muscle contractions. The origin of the disease is not clear, but may be related to overactivity of the gamma efferent system from suprasegmental influences. High doses of diazepam (Valium) have afforded effective symptomatic relief.

REFERENCES

1. Melzack R, Wall P: Pain mechanisms: a new theory. Science 150:971, 1965
2. Snyder S: Brain peptides as neurotransmittors. Science 209:976, 1980
3. Cruz B: Pain taxonomy and physiology. Fifth Annual Colorado Pain Symposium: The Surgical Management of Pain. Pain Control Center of Boulder Memorial Hospital and the University of Colorado School of Medicine. Jan 8–15, 1983, Aspen, Colorado
4. Fordyce W, et al: Operant conditioning in the treatment of chronic clinical pain. Arch Phys Med Rehab 54:399, 1973
5. Fordyce W: Behavioral Models for Chronic Pain and Illness. CV Mosby, St. Louis, 1976
6. Marskey H, Spear F: The concept of pain. J Psycho Som Res 11:59, 1976
7. Mircea A, Morariu M: Major Neurological Syndromes. Charles C Thomas, Springfield, IL, 1979
8. Dejerine J, Roussy G: Le syndrome thalamique. Rev Neurol 14:521, 1906
9. Ross G, Wolf J, Chipman M: The Neuralgias. In Baker A (ed): Clinical Neurology. Harper & Row, Philadelphia, 1983
10. Beaver D, Moses H, Ganote C: Electron microscopy of trigeminal ganglion III: trigeminal neuralgia. Arch Pathol 79:571, 1969
11. Behrman S, Knight G: Herpes simplex associated with trigeminal neuralgia. Neurology 4:525, 1954
12. Hope-Simpson R: The nature of herpes zoster: a long term study and a new hypothesis. Proc Roy Soc Med 58:9, 1965
13. Chakravorty B: Association of trigeminal neuralgia with multiple sclerosis. Arch Neurol 14:95, 1966
14. White J, Sweet W: Pain and the neurosurgeon: a forty year experience. Charles C Thomas, Springfield, IL, 1969
15. Chawla J, Falconer M: Glossopharyngeal and vagal neuralgia. Br Med J 3:529, 1967
16. Smith J, Taxdal D: Painful ophthalmoplegia—the Talosa-Hunt syndrome. Ophthalmologica 61:1466, 1966
17. Boniuk M, Schlezinger N: Raeders syndrome. Am J Ophthalmot 54:1074, 1962
18. Dalessis D: Some reflections on the etiologic role of depression in head pain. Headache 8:28, 1968
19. Glazer M: Atypical facial neuralgia: diagnosis, cause, and treatment. Arch Intern Med 65:340, 1940
20. De Meyer W: Anatomy and clinical neurology of the spinal cord. In Baker A (ed): Clinical Neurology. Harper & Row, Philadelphia, 1983
21. Mulder D, Dale A: Spinal cord tumors and discs. In Baker A (ed): Clinical Neurology. Harper & Row, Philadelphia, 1983
22. Finlayson A: Syringomyelia and related conditions. In Baker A (ed): Clinical Neurology. Harper & Row, Philadelphia, 1983
23. Spiller W: Central pain in syringomyelia and dysesthesia and overreaction to sensory stimuli in lesions below the optic thalamus. Arch Neurol Psychiat 10:491, 1923
24. McIlroy W, Richardson J: Syringomyelia: a clinical review of 75 cases. Can Med Assoc J 593:731, 1965

25. Finneson B: Diagnosis and Management of Pain Syndromes. 2nd Ed. WB Saunders, Philadelphia, 1969
26. Baringer J, Townsend J: Herpes virus infection in the peripheral nervous system. In Dyck P, Thomas P, Lambert E (eds): Peripheral Neurology, Vol. 3. WB Saunders, Philadelphia, 1975
27. Burgoon C, Burgoon J, Baldridge G: The natural history of herpes zoster. JAMA 164:265, 1957
28. Moosy J: Vascular disease of the spinal cord. In Baker A (ed): Clinical Neurology. Harper & Row, Philadelphia, 1983
29. Brain W, Wilkenson M: Cervical Spondylosis and other Diseases of the Cervical Spine. WB Saunders, Philadelphia, 1967
30. Stoltman H, Blackwood W: The role of the ligamentum flava in the pathogenesis of myelopathy in cervical spondylosis. Brain 87:45, 1964
31. Carson J, Gumpert J, Jefferson A: Diagnosis and treatment of thoracic intervertebral disk protrusion. J Neurol Neurosurg Psychiat 34:68, 1971
32. Love J, Schorn V: Thoracic disk protrusion. JAMA 191:627, 1965
33. Boshes B: Trauma to the spinal cord. In Baker A (ed): Clinical Neurology. Harper & Row, Philadelphia, 1983
34. Pollock L, et al: Management of residuals of injuries to the spinal cord and cauda equina. JAMA 146:1551, 1951
35. Druchman R: Central pain of spinal cord origin. Neurology 15:518, 1965
36. Plum F, Olson M: Myelitis and myelopathy. In Baker A (ed): Clinical Neurology. Harper & Row, Philadelphia, 1983
37. Altrocchi P: Acute transverse myelopathy. Arch Neurol 9:111, 1963
38. Stoll B, Andrew J: Radiation induced peripheral neuropathy. Br Med J 2:834, 1966
39. Brice J, McKissock: Surgical treatment of malignant extradural spinal tumors. Br Med J 1:1341, 1965
40. Slooff J, Kernohan J, McCarty C: Primary Intramedullary Tumors of the Spinal Cord and Filum Terminale. WB Saunders, Philadelphia, 1964
41. Seddon H: Three types of nerve injury. Brain 66:237, 1943
42. Sunderland S: Degeneration of the axon and associated changes. In Nerves and Nerve Injuries. E & S Livingstone, London, 1968
43. Dyck P, Ohta M: Neuronal atrophy and degeneration predominantly affecting peripheral sensory neurons. In Dyck P, Thomas P, Lambert E (eds): WB Saunders, Philadelphia, 1975
44. Walters A: The differentiation of causalgia and hyperpathia. Can Med Assoc J 80:105, 1969
45. Richards R: Causalgia: a centennial review. Arch Neurol 16:339, 1967
46. Sunderland S: The painful sequelae of injuries to peripheral nerve: causalgia. In Nerves and Nerve Injuries. E & S Livingstone, London, 1968
47. Nathan P: On the pathogenesis of causalgia in peripheral nerve injuries. Brain 70:145, 1947
48. Doupe J, Cullen C, Chance G: Post traumatic pain and causalgia syndrome. J Neurol Neurosurg Psychiat 7:33, 1944
49. Sunderland S: Disturbances of sensation associated with amputation stumps: general considerations. In Nerves and Nerve Injuries. E & S Livingstone, London, 1968
50. Sunderland S: Stump pain and abnormal sensory phenomena superimposed on the phantom state. In Nerves and Nerve Injuries. E & S Livingstone, London, 1968

51. Steinbrocher O, Argyros T: Shoulder hand syndrome. Med Clin North Am 42:1533, 1958

52. Wilson S: Phrenic neuralgia. In Bruce A (ed): Neurology. 2nd Ed. Williams & Wilkins 1:292 Baltimore, 1955

53. Taylor N: Carpal tunnel syndrome. Am J Phys Med 50 No. 4:792, 1971

54. Ebeling P, Gilliatt P, Thomas P: A clinical and electrical study of ulnar nerve lesions in the hand. J Neurol Neurosurg Psychiat 23:1, 1960

55. Roos D, Owens, J: Thoracic outlet syndrome. Arch Surg 93:71, 1966

56. Reuss D: Thoracic outlet syndrome. Fifth Annual Colorado Pain Symposium: The Surgical Management of Pain. Pain Control Center of Boulder Memorial Hospital and University of Colorado School of Medicine. Jan 8–15, 1983, Aspen, Colorado, 1983

57. Roles N, Maudsley R: Radial tunnel syndrome. J Bone Joint Surg 54B:499, 1972

58. Kitchen C, Simpson J: Meralgia paresthetica: a review of 67 patients. Acta Neurol Scand 48:547, 1972

59. Young M, Norris J: Femoral neuropathy during anticoagulation therapy. Neurology 26:1173, 1976

60. DiStefano V, Sack JT, Whittaker R, et al: Tarsal tunnel syndrome: a review of the literature and two case reports. Clin Orthop 88:76, 1972

61. Asbury K: Uremic Neuropathy. In Dyck P, Thomas P, Lambert E (eds): Peripheral Neuropathy. Vol. 2. WB Saunders, Philadelphia, 1975

62. McLeod J: Carcinomatous neuropathy. In Dyck P, Thomas P, Lambert E (eds): Peripheral Neuropathy. Vol. 2. WB Saunders, Philadelphia, 1975

63. Croft P, Wilkinson M: The course and prognosis in some types of carcinomatous neuromyopathy. Brain 92:1, 1969

64. Victor M: Polyneuropathy due to nutritional deficiency and alcoholism. In Dyck P, Thomas P, Lambert E (eds): Peripheral Neuropathy. Vol. 2. WB Saunders, Philadelphia, 1975

65. O'Brady R, King F: Fabry's disease. In Dyck P, Thomas P, Lambert E (eds): Peripheral Neuropathy. Vol. 2. WB Saunders, Philadelphia, 1975

66. Ohnishi A, Dyck P: Loss of small peripheral sensory neurons in Fabry's Disease. Arch Neurol 31:120, 1974

67. Arnason B: Inflammatory polyradiculoneuropathies. In Dyck P, Thomas P, Lambert E (eds): Peripheral Neuropathy. Vol. 2. WB Saunders, Philadelphia, 1975

68. Thomas P: Metabolic neuropathy. J Coll Phys Lond 7:154, 1973

69. Fry I, Hardwick C, Scott G: Diabetic neuropathy: a survey and follow up of 66 cases. Guys Hosp Rep 111:113, 1962

70. Thomas P, Eliasson S: Diabetic neuropathy. In Dych P, Thomas P, Lambert E (eds): Peripheral Neuropathv. Vol. 2. WB Saunders, Philadelphia, 1975

71. Gilliatt R, Willison R: Peripheral nerve conduction in diabetic neuropathy. J Neurol Neurosurg Psychiat 25:11, 1962

72. Greenbaum D: Observations on the homogenous nature and pathogenesis of diabetic neuropatɪy. Brain 87:215, 1964

73. Garland, H: Diabetic amyotrophy. Br J Clin Prac 15:9, 1961

74. Raff M, Sangalang V, Asbury A: Ischemic mononeuropathy multiplex associated with diabetes mellitus. Arch Neurol 18:487, 1968

75. Tsairis P, Dyck P, Mulder D: Natural history of brachial plexus neuropathy: report of 99 cases. Arch Neurol 27:109, 1972

76. Smith B, Ramakris T, Schlagen R: Familial brachial neuropathy: two case reports with discussion. Neurology 21:941, 1971

77. Ridley A: Porphyric neuropathy. In Dyck P, Thomas P, Lambert E (eds): Peripheral Neuropathy. Vol. 2. WB Saunders, Philadelphia, 1975

78. Collins R, et al: Neurologic manifestations of intramuscular coagulation in patients with cancer. Neurology 25:795, 1975

79. Davis L, Drachman D: Myeloma neuropathy: successful treatment of two cases and review of cases. Arch Neurol 27:507, 1972

80. Conn D, Dych P: Angiopathic neuropathy in connective tissue disease. In Dyck P, Thomas P, Lambert E (eds): Peripheral Neuropathy. Vol. 2. WB Saunders, Philadelphia, 1975

81. Pallis C, Scott J: Peripheral neuropathy in rheumatoid arthritis. Brit Med J 1:1141, 1965

82. Ekbom K: Restless leg syndrome. Neurology 10:868, 1968

83. Brooke M: A Clinician's View of Neuromuscular Diseases. Williams & Wilkins, Baltimore, 1977

84. Bohan A, Peters J: Polymyositis and dermatomyositis. N Engl J Med 292:344, 1975

85. Jerusalem F, et al: Morphometric analysis of skeletal muscle capillary ultrastructure in inflammatory myopathies. J Neurol Sci 23:391, 1974

86. Olerud J, Homer L, Carroll H: Serum myoglobin levels predicted from serum enzyme values. N Engl J Med 243:483, 1975

87. Larsson L, et al: Hereditary metabolic myopathy with paroxysmal myoglobinuria due to abnormal glycolysis. J Neurol Neurosurg Psychiat 27:361, 1964

88. Ekbom K, et al: Muscular affections in chronic alcoholism. Arch Neurol 10:449, 1964

89. Gordon E, Januszko D, Kaufman L: A critical survey of the stiff man syndrome. Am J Med 42:582, 1967

8 Transcutaneous Electrical Nerve Stimulation: Its Uses and Effectiveness with Patients in Pain

Jeffrey S. Mannheimer

Transcutaneous electrical nerve stimulation (TENS) is the transmission of electrical energy across the surface of the skin to the nervous system. Electricity is a natural phenomenon within all types of living tissue. The brain constantly receives and intergrates electrical signals indicative of all environmental (external) and bodily (internal) events including that of pain.

One type of electrical impulse that can signal impending damage, merely annoy, partially hinder, or totally incapacitate is the impulse of nociception. The nociceptive impulse mediating the sensation of pain is also a prime impetus that brings the patient to a health practitioner.

Throughout history relief from pain has been sought by various means. Historical references to pain relieving modalities include herbs, potions, heat and cold applications, acupuncture techniques, drugs, surgery, meditation, hypnosis, and electricity. TENS incorporates an early method of pain relief that has now been refined and simplified for ease of application via the use of new scientific and technologic advances.

Historical references to the use of electricity to decrease or control pain begin in the year 46 A.D. when a Roman physician, Scribonius Largus, described how the electric stimulus for a torpedo fish (electric eel) was able to provide pain relief for headache and gout.[1,2] One of the first commercially available TENS devices that was battery powered and touted for pain control, among many other indications, appeared in 1919 and was known as the *electreat*.[3] In its original design the electreat had only one adjustable parameter, amplitude, with pulse rate and width being fixed. The device produces a strong electrical paresthesia and is still in use in its original form.

Publication of Melzack and Wall's gate control theory[4] in 1965 produced a reawakening of scientists and clinicians involved in pain research and management. Based upon the original tenets of this theory, that has since been reviewed and analyzed by many,[5] Shealy and Mortimer, in 1967, developed a stimulator that transmitted electrical impulses to surgically implanted electrodes over the dorsal columns of the spinal cord.[6,7] This device became known as the dorsal column stimulator (DCS) and was used exclusively for patients with chronic intractable pain.

DCS usage spawned the development of TENS devices in the early 1970s as transcutaneous electrodes were used to evaluate patients as good candidates for a DCS. A significant number of patients obtained satisfactory pain control with TENS thus fostering its initial development.

TENS devices are now being manufactured by many companies. It is estimated that in the United States alone at least 30 manufacturers produce their own TENS units. International manufacturers exist in Canada, England, France, Sweden, Germany, Russia, China, Japan, and Israel. Similar portable electrical stimulators use invasive electrodes placed either around a peripheral nerve over the dorsal columns of the spinal cord or within various brain-stem sites. These stimulators thus differ from TENS units and are known as percutaneous (PCS), dorsal column (DCS), and deep brain (DBS) stimulators respectively.[8] The electrodes used with these electrical stimulators require surgical implantation thus taking them out of the realm of the physical therapist.

A TENS unit is small, portable, battery powered, and specifically designed for use by the patient at home. It thus becomes a modern alternative to drugs of both the narcotic and non-narcotic variety. In the United States, it is available only through physician prescription but in Japan it can be purchased over the counter.

TENS AND MEDICATION

TENS, like medicinal applications, may relieve part or all of a patient's pain for varying periods of time. However, the use of TENS is not governed by specific time intervals like medication in which dosages may for example be taken only once every 4 hours. There is no limit to the number of stimulation periods in a given day in which TENS can be used. TENS can thus provide sustained pain relief whereas medication will wax and wane in benefit as its effect wears off and a period of time must elapse before another dose can be taken.

Many side effects can occur from the use of drugs, especially the use of narcotics. Apart from the possibilities of addiction, narcotics may cause such effects as pruritis, cutaneous vasodilation, constipation, respiratory depression, lethargy, and a loss of mental acuity. Utilization of TENS will not cause any of these side effects but a small percentage of patients (less than 2 percent) may develop an allergic reaction to the electrode, its transmission medium, or tape patch.[9] Improper use of TENS can cause skin irritation in the form of erythema, actual burns of the pinpoint variety, blistering, or tissue damage. This usually occurs from improper placement of the electrodes or sparse application of transmission gel or pregelled electrodes that dry out. High frequency pulse rates are more likely to produce skin irritation than low frequency pulse rates. TENS, unlike medication, is difficult to use with a senile or aphasic patient and those with visual or hand dysfunction may have difficulty operating the device.

The positive effects of narcotics, besides pain relief, are sedation and mood enhancement. In comparison, TENS can provide sustained pain control along with continuous mental acuity that can allow for active patient participation in home or hospital therapeutic sessions. The use of TENS postoperatively, highlights the value of patient participation.

INDICATIONS, CONTRAINDICATIONS, AND PRECAUTIONS

TENS can be used adjunctively as a symptomatic means of pain control in a wide variety of acute, chronic, and postsurgical conditions. Whenever a physician prescribes medication for pain relief there are only a few reasons why TENS cannot be used instead. The only absolute contraindication to the use of TENS is the presence of a demand-type cardiac pacemaker: the electrical impulse produced by TENS may interfere with the action of a pacemaker.[10,11] TENS may also interfere with encephalographic and cardiac monitors; however, filtering devices are easily manufactured and can interface between the TENS device and the above mentioned monitors.[12,13]

There are specific precautions when using TENS which relate primarily to the area of electrode placement. Electrodes should not be placed directly on the eye. However, transcutaneous and subcutaneous electrodes have been successfully positioned on the supra- and infraorbital regions for pain control after eye surgery without any negative effects.[14] The following precautions should be considered when the use of TENS is contemplated:

1. Stimulation in the area of the carotid sinus nerves may produce laryngeal and/or pharyngeal spasm effecting blood pressure and respiration.

2. Stimulation over superficial aspects of bone such as the forehead and tibial shaft may not be tolerated well. The periosteum is highly innervated and is thus very sensitive to even mild stimulation.

3. Care must be taken when TENS is employed near or over the heart in patients with myocardial disease. The electrical energy produced by a TENS

unit, however, is not enough to cause cardiac fibrillation.[10] When used in the presence of cardiac disease, it is recommended that only a mild stimulation mode, known as conventional, be used and muscle contractions should not occur.

4. Caution is suggested when TENS is used on the head or neck in patients with epilepsy, or in those who have had transient ischemic attacks (TIAS) or a cerebrovascular accident (CVA). It is possible, although not documented, that TENS may trigger an epileptic seizure when stimulation is provided in this area. Certain stimulation parameters or programmed modes can produce significant vasodilation and may trigger detrimental vascular effects in patients with a history of TIAS or CVA.

5. The use of TENS during pregnancy is also considered to be precautionary. The effect on the unborn fetus is relatively unknown. However, TENS has been used successfully for pain control during labor and delivery.[15,16] Electrode placement in this instance is at T10-L1 and S2–S4 via paraspinally placed rectangular electrodes for control of stage one and stage two labor pain respectively. Bundsen and co-workers recommend placement of a pair of electrodes over the groin and lower abdominal region for the second stage of labor in addition to the S2–S4 placement. There have not been any harmful effects noted to the fetus or the newborn.[15,16] During pregnancy TENS can be placed in areas other than the abdomen as long as only the mild conventional stimulation mode is used. Muscle contractions must be avoided. In this form TENS is equivalent to that of a superficial massage in terms of intensity and depth of penetration. I have successfully used TENS for control of cervical and lumbar spine pain, after an auto accident involving two women who were in the third trimester of pregnancy. Electrodes were placed paraspinally via separate channels at the cervical and lumbar regions. TENS was used at home in lieu of medication and both women had normal deliveries and healthy babies.

THE ADJUNCTIVE ROLE OF TENS IN PAIN MANAGEMENT

TENS must be considered as an adjunctive modality within the framework of a comprehensive rehabilitation program for the patient with acute or chronic pain. A comprehensive program is one which consists of a thorough patient evaluation, specific treatment geared to correction of the dysfunctional structure or removal of irritation, pain control, and prophylaxis to prevent recurrence. TENS can only assist in one phase of such a program, namely that concerned with pain control.[17] TENS should therefore not be considered a sole treatment modality. It does not treat anything but merely serves as a means of symptomatic relief and/or control of discomfort. Unfortunately to the detriment of the medical profession, the modality itself, and also the patient, TENS has been severely abused. It is quite common to hear of situations in which the sole treatment for various types of pain, regardless of the cause, has been TENS. Furthermore, such treatment is frequently provided solely in the clinic on a periodic basis without any use of the device at home by the patient. The utilization of TENS in this manner is in no way comprehensive and treatment is only symptomatic in nature.

Treatment that consists entirely of TENS on a three times per week basis in the clinic should be equated with having a patient report to the clinic at the same frequency for two aspirins and a glass of water after which he may lie down on a plinth for 30 minutes! TENS must not replace definitive therapy that treats, restores function, and relieves irritation as opposed to just controlling discomfort. Optimal effectiveness with TENS occurs when it is used by the patient at home while specific treatment is provided in the clinic setting.

There is a distinct role for the use of TENS in the clinic when it is needed to relieve and/or control pain prior to, during, or after the performance of specific therapeutic procedures.[17-20] Techniques such as joint mobilization, contract relax stretching, transverse friction massage, and skin debridement are commonly painful to the patient. TENS can be used to allow for the performance by the therapist of the aforementioned procedures providing specific safety guidelines are followed. They are presented later on in this chapter.

There are also instances in which TENS may be the only viable modality that can be administered to the patient. Patients with pain syndromes such as trigeminal neuralgia, herpes zoster (shingles), and discomfort from severe functional changes due to rheumatoid or osteoarthritis may obtain satisfactory pain relief from TENS when nothing else is helpful.

The initial indication for TENS in the early 1970s was as a last resort modality for the patient with chronic pain. After all forms of medical intervention such as medication, physical therapy, psychotherapy, and surgery had failed TENS was prescribed. Only 25 to 50 percent of such chronic pain patients obtained satisfactory pain relief with TENS. If TENS is able to provide pain relief that is satisfactory to the patient and equal to or better than that obtained with medication, I consider the result to be positive. Clinical results now confirm that the greatest degree of efficacy with TENS is achieved when it is instituted early in the acute stage of pain. Satisfactory results with TENS as a means of pain control in acute pain patients is better than 80 percent. It is a rare occurance when I am unable to obtain satisfactory pain control with patients who have sustained acute cervical or lumbar strains, tendinitis, and other musculoskeletal injuries. The use of TENS in the acute stage is of course dependent upon early referral by the physician. Comprehensive rehabilitation programs which include the use of TENS at home can significantly decrease the development of chronicity.

THE TENS SYSTEM

A TENS device is about the size of a pack of cigarettes and thus easily worn by the patient via a belt clip. The unit consists of electrical circuitry powered by one or more batteries that produce and transmits electrical impulses to the skin via lead wire cables and surface electrodes. Batteries may be either of the alkaline, lithium, or nickel-cadmium rechargeable variety.

TENS units generate electrical impulses in specific waveforms which must be balanced so that a net positive or negative direct current (DC) potential does not occur. A galvanic effect from an unbalanced waveform can produce skin irritations and discomfort thus negating the repetitive usage that is required by many pain patients. The most common waveform is therefore termed *biphasic* which may also be called faradic or alternating current (AC). The positive and negative components need not be identical in shape as viewed on an oscilloscope. Asymmetrical biphasic waveforms can also be balanced and equal in energy. The amount of energy per pulse is a product of the amplitude (intensity) plus the pulse width (duration). Increasing or decreasing either parameter will alter the strength of the pulse.

The critical determinant of effective stimulation is not the shape of the waveform but the electrical parameters that the unit can generate. In order to be effective, a TENS unit must be capable of generating electrical energy sufficient to cause depolarization of the appropriate peripheral nerve. Subthreshold stimulation, although helpful in patients with neuropathies or areas where there is hyperesthesia, is not considered to be significantly better than relief obtained by placebo administration.[21-23] Standards for labeling, safety, and performance requirements for TENS devices have been developed by the Association for the Advancement of Medical Instrumentation (AAMI).[24]

The adjustable stimulation parameters are amplitude, measured in milliamps (mA), pulse duration measured in microseconds (μs), and pulse frequency or rate measured in cycles or pulses per second and expressed in terms of hertz (Hz). TENS units are available in single or dual channel formats. Dual channel units are much more common today and offer greater versatility in the management of two areas of pain or pain that is distributed through an extensive area. Single channel units may merely have an adjustable amplitude control or offer adjustment of two or all three parameters. Dual channel units with minimal manual adjustments offer independent amplitude controls per channel and at least a common pulse rate and pulse duration control. Common pulse rate and duration controls affect both channels simultaneously. Dual channel units are also available which offer independent pulse width and/or pulse controls per channel.

Stimulation Parameters

Stimulation parameters, if adjustable, commonly fall within the following range for the majority of manufacturers: amplitude 0 to 80 mA, pulse rate 1 to 150 Hz, and pulse duration 30 to 250 μs. The clinician can program a variety of stimulation modes with different adjustments of these parameters. Newer models offered by many manufacturers also provide for controls that may interrupt or burst the programmed parameters (burst or pulse-train stimulation) or modulate (fluctuate) one or more parameters. Devices that offer the clinician all of the aforementioned features are the most sophisticated units available.

Electrode Cables (Lead Wires)

Electrode cables (lead wires) allow for the transmission of the electrical impulses from the stimulator to the electrodes. They are available in various lengths and are usually color coded to denote channel separation and/or polarity. Each channel may have a common receptable for a dual lead wire cable or offer two receptables for single lead wires one of which is positive and the other negative. Cable bifurcators commonly known as "Y" adaptors allow for the use of more than two electrodes per channel. Electrode cables terminate in either a pin or snap connector for attachment to the electrodes. Adaptors are also available to convert pin leads to snap leads for added versatility.

Electrodes

The most common material used to manufacture transcutaneous electrodes is carbon silicone. These electrodes are available in various sizes and shapes, most frequently square, rectangular, or circular. A transmission medium is required as an interface between the electrode and the skin. Various conductive gels are available for this purpose and require hand application to thoroughly coat the surface of the electrode that lies against the skin. Pregelled electrodes are self adherent and also available in different sizes. They may be used for approximately 1 to 5 days without being removed.

Natural and synthetic polymer materials that are both conductive and adhesive are also available as an electrode interface. Karaya is a natural polysaccharide that is used in the manufacture of many types of self adhering electrodes.* Karaya is available in different degrees of thickness and thus varying amounts of impedence (resistance to electrical transmission). Aquapore is a new interface material that is 95 percent water with a very low impedence.†

NEUROPHYSIOLOGIC BASIS TO THE DEVELOPMENT OF STIMULATION MODES

A knowledge of the sensory changes and physiologic effects associated with manipulation of each stimulation parameter is essential for the clinician to explain to the patient the sensation to expect with TENS. Amplitude and pulse duration settings determine the total energy per pulse. As the total amount of energy progresses, a greater number of nerve fibers are recruited, the sensation

---

* Lec-tec Corp., 10701 Red Circle Drive, Minnetonka, MN 55343.
† TENS, Inc., 10215 County Line Road, P.O. Box 5030, Spring Hill, FL 33526.

becomes stronger, and the depth of stimulus penetration increases. The amount of energy per pulse further determines whether or not muscle contractions will occur. The pulse rate setting below 10 to 15 Hz allows for the sensation of individual pulses or muscle contractions but if the rate exceeds 15 to 20 Hz, electrical paresthesia or a tingling sensation occurs.

The normal human nervous system is easily able to perceive the sensation of each individual pulse as long as the frequency remains below 10 to 15 Hz. When the frequency exceeds 20 Hz, the nervous system has greater difficulty separating the sensation of each pulse and as a result, a merging of pulses occurs producing a constant electrical paresthesia. Various combinations of stimulation parameters can result in the production of an infinite amount of minor or major sensory changes.

A combination of low frequency (1 to 10 Hz) and low pulse energy (1 to 15 mA, 30 to 50 μs) may be below the perception threshold or produce a sensation of mild rhythmic pulsing without muscle contraction or fasciculation. Low frequency (1 to 10 Hz) and high pulse energy (30 to 60 mA, 150 to 200 μs) will cause strong rhythmic muscle contractions. Parameter settings of 50 to 100 Hz with a mild to moderate amount of pulse energy (15 to 30 mA, 50 to 150 μs) results in a continuous and comfortable electrical paresthesia. If the pulse energy is further increased upwards to 60 mA and 200 μs strong electrical paresthesia and muscle tetany will occur. Nonrhythmic muscle fasciculation may also occur if full tetany is not obtained or fatigue sets in. A complete description of the sensations and physiologic effects that occur with changes solely of one stimulation parameter while the other two are fixed is available from other publications.[25,26]

The aforementioned examples of parameter combinations and their resultant sensory effects may be minimized or maximized by other factors such as the interelectrode distance, electrode size, impedence, and electrode placement sites. As the distance between two electrodes of one channel decreases, less pulse energy is required to produce the desired sensation or effect. An increase in the interelectrode distance proportionately increases the amount of pulse energy necessary for the desired results. Lead wire bifurcators used to increase the number of electrodes per channel also results in the need for a greater degree of pulse energy.

The smaller the electrode, the greater the current density beneath it. Smaller electrodes therefore require less pulse energy to produce the sensory and motor effects obtained with larger electrodes. The higher the impedance of the electrode and its interface as well as the underlying skin, the greater the amount of pulse energy needed to produce the desired effect. Dry, scaly skin has a great deal of resistance to electricity and electrode placement at these areas is not recommended. Electrode placement sites at areas where there are acupuncture, motor, or trigger points as well as superficial peripheral nerve branches offers greater electrical conductance and lower impedance than areas which are not so densely innervated.[27-29] The greater the depth of the peripheral nerve from the skin surface and stimulating electrode, the greater the impedance between the two. The excitability characteristics of nerve fibers further provides scientific basis for the different stimulation modes. Basic neurophysiologic tenets state that myelineated nerve fibers conduct an electrical impulse at a faster velocity than nonmyelinated fibers.[30] In addition, the larger the diameter of the fiber, the more rapid is its conduction velocity. Larger diameter fibers also contain a greater volume of axoplasm, which is easily excitable. Therefore, the largest myelineated afferent nerve fibers (A-alpha and beta) are the most rapid conducting (40 to 120 m/sec) and also the easiest to excite or depolarize.

The direct opposite in conduction and excitability characteristics are the nonmyelineated C fibers. These fibers are very thin, lack a myelin sheath and thus conduct very slowly at a speed that does not exeed 2 to 3 m/sec.[30] C fibers have a smaller volume of axoplasm and require a greater amount of pulse energy for excitation or depolarization.

A-alpha and beta fibers mediate afferent information pertaining to touch, proprioception, and kinesthesis.[30] A-gamma fibers convey information relative to changes in muscle length. A-delta fibers, the smallest of the myelineated A fibers, mediate nociceptive information primarily related to superficial, sharp, easy to localize pain. C fibers mediate nociceptive information more indicative of deep, achy, hard to localize pain of the chronic variety.

A knowledge of these neurophysiologic factors and mechanisms relative to a variety of pain syndromes is necessary in order to understand the programming and administration of TENS. Based on the gate control theory of pain,[4] input from large proprioceptive fibers provide a balancing effect to small nociceptive fiber input at the dorsal horn of the spinal cord.[4,5,30–32] This is easily understood when one considers the effects which occur following a simple ankle sprain. If the individual who sustains an ankle sprain assumes a nonweightbearing position and does nothing to soothe the discomfort or distract his attention from the injured area, input from small nociceptive fibers predominates. This nociceptive input resulting from tissue damage and edema disrupts the normal dorsal horn input. Since there is no active or passive ankle movement, touch, temperature changes (heat or cold application), or mental stimulation in the form of music, television, or conversation; stimuli conducive to proprioceptive input is nonexistent and pain predominates. However, if the injured area is gently massaged, mobilized, or treated with cryotherapy or mental distraction is provided, pain perception will be decreased. These forms of stimuli provide large afferent fiber input.

THE STIMULATION MODES

A significant amount of the material presented in this section is adapted from a previous publication by myself specifically comparing the characteristics and role of the different stimulation modes.[33] Pain syndromes differ via their neurophysiologic mechanisms and the resultant quality, depth, intensity, and distribution of discomfort. The quality of pain that a patient perceives may also be indicative of involvement of more than one tissue structure. Pain arising from an arthritic joint is an excellent example. The quality of pain which stems from the synovial joint can thus be representative of each distinct structure which acts upon the joint. Furthermore, various tissue structures have different types and degrees of afferent innervation producing variations in pain quality and distribution. TENS units should therefore be capable of generating different stimulation modes to excite either a selective type or the full range of nerve fibers for the widest possible efficacy.

Recent clinical and technologic advances have led to the development of four distinctly different stimulation modes; conventional, strong low rate (acupuncturelike), pulse train (burst), and brief-intense. Alterations of these modes by forms of parameter modulation allow for programming of an infinite variety of sensory and motor stimuli.

Conventional

The stimulation modes differ significantly by many factors such as parameter settings, depth of tissue penetration, electrode placement techniques, speed of action, duration of pain relief, and physiologic effects. When TENS units first became commercially available in the early 1970s, manufacturer recommendations were for stimulation parameter settings to deliver only a mild, low intensity, and high frequency sensation which has come to be known as the conventional mode of TENS.

The conventional mode which has a wide range of clinical application is not universally effective for all pain syndromes or each patient in a group with a similar pain syndrome. The clinician who becomes familiar with and evaluates the efficacy of other stimulation modes will be able to enhance the effectiveness of TENS. Although two or more stimulation modes may be beneficial for a specific patient or pain syndrome one mode will usually provide greater pain relief that may also be longer lasting.[20,25]

The use of TENS solely as a last resort modality or by evaluation of only one stimulation mode or electrode array severely hinders its chances of success. TENS efficacy also decreases in proportion to the number of other intervention techniques that have preceeded its use.[32]

Stimulation parameters incorporating a high pulse rate (50 to 100 Hz), narrow pulse width (30 to 75 μs), and low amplitude (10 to 30 mA) produce a comfortable tingling sensation or electrical paresthesia without muscle contraction that is consistant with that of conventional TENS. This combination of parameters should selectively activate only large afferent fibers (A-alpha and beta).[34,35] Muscle contraction is to be avoided, although dependent upon the electrode array, mild muscle fasciculation is at times hard to eliminate.

On the basis of conventional TENS parameters, one should speculate that this mode would be best suited for the control of acute and superficial pain syndromes. Clinical experience, however, has shown that conventional TENS is also frequently beneficial in deep, achy, chronic pain syndromes and therefore remains the most widely used and clinically effective method of TENS.

A decrease in pain perception usually occurs quite rapidly with conventional TENS (1 to 20 minutes is the most common) and upon termination of treatment the duration of relief should at least equal the length of the stimulation period.[34-37] It is quite common in my clinical experience to see pain relief persist with this mode for 1 to 3 hours and occasionally longer. The most important factors that govern the degree and duration of pain relief with any stimulation mode are proper instruction in posture, body mechanics, and activities of daily living (ADL).

Strong Low Rate

A complete reversal of the stimulation parameters which give rise to the conventional mode programs the TENS unit to deliver the strong low rate or acupuncturelike mode. Stimulation parameters are consistent with those of invasive electroacupuncture, but surface electrodes are used in place of subcutaneous needle electrodes.[38,39]

The strong, low rate mode promotes intense, rhythmic muscle contractions without the sensation of electrical paresthesia. Depth of stimulus penetration is greater as parameter settings are sufficient to excite high threshold, smaller diameter, slow conducting afferent nerve fibers such as nonmyelineated C fibers. Efferent (motor) fibers which require a longer pulse duration for excitation are also activated. Proper programming for this mode requires a low rate (1 to 4 Hz), wide pulse width (150 to 250 μs), and amplitude to the highest comfortably tolerable level.[36-43]

Clinical experience has shown that the strong low rate mode is best suited for deep, achy, chronic pain syndromes. Onset of relief usually does not occur until at least 20 to 30 minutes of stimulation has elapsed and at times up to 1 hour is needed for an adequate evaluation. The duration of poststimulation analgesia may persist for 2 to 6 hours or longer.[36-43]

Pulse-Train

A combination of the parameters inherent in both the conventional and acupuncturelike modes produce what has been termed pulse-train or burst stimulation. High and low pulse rates are utilized simultaneously to deliver a sensation of slow rhythmic pulsing or muscle contractions (dependent upon the total energy per pulse) as well as a background electrical paresthesia. The burst frequency is usually fixed at 2 Hz and high frequency (70 to 100 Hz) pulses occur with each burst or train.[26,41,43-45]

The pulse-train or burst mode can also be delivered at high or low intensity. Low intensity (without muscle contraction) usage is merely a form of modulating the conventional stimulation mode. Switching from conventional TENS to burst produces a 2 Hz interruption in the steady paresthesia. Patients who dislike the sensation of a constant electrical tingling may prefer to have it interrupted twice each second. The perceived sensation is thus one of electrical paresthesia (from the high frequency pulses per burst) and a rhythmic pulsing twice each second. Clinically low intensity pulse train (burst) TENS seems to be most effective, as conventional TENS, in acute and/or superficial pain syndromes.

When delivered at high energy levels consistent with that of the strong low rate mode, this form of TENS is known as high intensity pulse-train (burst) stimulation. Stimulation parameters now consist of the same pulse rate but the pulse width and amplitude are increased to a level which produces strong but comfortable muscle contractions (two per second) plus a strong degree of electrical paresthesia. The mixture of both high and low frequency at an energy level sufficient to cause muscle contraction results in an increased recruitment of muscle fibers at less pulse energy than that needed with the strong low rate mode.[43,44]

High intensity pulse-train (burst) TENS seems to be more effective in deep, achy, chronic pain syndromes as does the strong low rate mode. The stimulation time required prior to an onset of pain relief and the duration of poststimulation analgesia with pulse-train (burst) TENS is dependent upon the energy level used and therefore corresponds well to the previously mentioned characteristics of both conventional and strong low rate TENS.

Brief-Intense

Brief-intense is the strongest and least tolerable mode, and thus not used as frequently as the other forms. Parameter adjustment for delivery of this mode requires a high rate (100 to 150 Hz), wide pulse width (150 to 250 μs), and amplitude to the highest tolerable level that is reasonably comfortable. The resultant sensation is one of a strong and continuous electrical paresthesia that will produce either muscle tetany or nonrythmic fasciculation depending upon electrode placement. Depth of penetration and stimulus strength is sufficient to excite and recruit the full range of motor and sensory nerve fibers.

Brief-intense TENS gives rise to a rapid onset of analgesia (1 to 15 minutes) yet the duration of poststimulation pain relief is quite short. Discomfort usually returns quickly after cessation of stimulation if nociceptive stimuli persist. This is very important to consider when use of this mode is contemplated. It is advisable not to use this mode for periods exceeding 15 minutes as significant ischemia can occur. When pain persists after the use of brief-intense stimulation, a decrease in the total energy per pulse can change the stimulation mode to that of conventional if ongoing pain control is necessary.

The brief-intense mode is primarily employed to obtain quick and profound analgesia which is sufficient to allow for the performance of specific therapeutic procedures such as skin debridement, suture removal, minor dental, and podiatric surgical procedures, joint mobilization, transverse friction massage, and contract-relax stretching when pain is a hindering factor.[17-20] When TENS is used in this manner, it is recommended that the clinician adhere to the following guidelines:

1. TENS should be initiated 5 to 15 minutes prior to the onset of the procedure. This should allow for the production of a degree of analgesia sufficient to promote patient tolerance to the therapeutic technique.

2. Stimulation should remain in progress while the technique is being performed.

3. When joint mobilization followed by contract-relax stretching are the desired procedures, active and passive range of motion (ROM) must be assessed before TENS is activated.

4. ROM should not exceed 20 degrees beyond the pretested range in any single treatment session.

These guidelines should eliminate any chance of soft tissue damage. It is important to state at this juncture that TENS allows breakthrough pain to occur. Since the patient is awake (not anesthetized), the clinician should be told if the pain becomes too unbearable. Brief-intense TENS obviously does not eliminate all the discomfort of the therapeutic procedure. However, if TENS can provide at least a 25 percent decrease in discomfort, then the patient should be able to tolerate some treatment. I have used brief-intense TENS quite successfully in this manner to rehabilitate patients with functional deficits from adhesive capsulitis.[18–20] Electrode placement techniques with the brief intense mode differ in regard to specific therapeutic procedures and is discussed in the electrode placement section.

Brief-intense TENS has also been used to initially break through deep persistent pain in patients with pancreatitis after which management could be achieved by the conventional mode.[46]

Modulation

Modulation of one or more stimulus parameters is the most recent addition to the methods by which TENS can be delivered. Oscillation of pulse rate and/or pulse energy parameters are the most common forms of modulation presently available in newer models manufactured by various companies. The degree of parameter modulation is usually within a range of 40 to 100 percent, plus or minus, from the preset level. A continuous oscillation occurs within a time factor of 0.5 to 1.5 seconds (dependent upon the manufacturer). Therefore, the number of pulses per second and/or the strength of each pulse shifts back and forth between the preset parameter level and the percentage of modulation. A review of the literature relative to the different stimulation modes and a complete listing of their specific characteristics is available.[20]

Modulation thus provides for variations in the depth of penetration and recruitment of high and low threshold nerve fibers. The value of modulation is threefold:

1. To increase comfort to irritating but effective stimulation.

2. To increase tolerance to the stronger stimulation modes. (strong, low rate and brief-intense).

3.   To decrease accommodation to mild continuous stimuli (conventional mode).

Many patients equate the sensation produced by modulation to that of a massage. Factors such as stimulation time prior to the onset of pain relief and its poststimulation duration are dependent upon the primary mode that is being modulated.

Clinical experience has shown that it is not possible to distinctly categorize each stimulation mode with a list of pain syndromes for which it is best suited. There is no single stimulation mode that is equally effective for all pain syndromes. The mode with the widest range of effectiveness, however, is conventional and thus it should be the first one to be evaluated with any patient or pain syndrome. Table 8-1 lists the adjustment guidelines in a step by step fashion that should be followed to easily program the different stimulation modes. The suggested settings are to be considered as intitial adjustments only. Readjustment and adaptation to individual patients and pain syndromes is necessary. Pulse width and amplitude settings can be increased or decreased from the

Table 8-1. The Stimulation Modes: Adjustment Guidelines

Mode	Step I: Pulse Rate	Step II: Pulse Width	Step III: Amplitude	Step IV: Readjustment
Conventional	Preset within 50–100 Hz	Preset within 40–75 μs	Slowly activate one channel at a time and increase until a smooth comfortable electrical paresthesia is obtained.	Electrical paresthesia should be perceived throughout the distribution of the pain. Increasing the pulse width can result in a spread of paresthesia, comfort can be increased and accommodation minimized by modulation or burst features.
Strong low rate (acupuncture-like)	Preset 1–4 Hz	Preset 150–200 μs	Slowly activate one channel at a time and increase to highest tolerable level producing rhythmic muscle contractions.	Comfort can be increased by use of modulation.
Pulse train (burst)	Preset within 70–100 Hz	Preset within 40–75 μs (low intensity) 150–200 μs (high intensity)	Slowly activate one channel at a time and increase to desired level. Paresthesia with rhythmic pulsing (low intensity). Paresthesia with rhythmic muscle contractions (high intensity) should occur.	Increasing pulse width can result in a spread of paresthesia if not perceived throughout distributions of pain.
Brief intense	Preset within 100–150 Hz	Preset within 150–200 μs	Slowly activate one channel at a time to highest tolerable level of paresthesia. Nonrhythmic muscle fasciculations or tetany should occur in conjunction with paresthesia.	Increase amplitude and/or pulse width if sensation decreases. Activation of modulation can increase comfort and tolerance.

given levels as they are dependent upon the depth and distribution of pain, interelectrode distance, number of electrodes per channel, size of the electrodes, and skin resistance. A short interelectrode distance between two electrodes of one channel will not require a large amount of pulse energy to obtain the desired result.

PRINCIPLES OF ELECTRODE PLACEMENT

A thorough discussion of electrode placement techniques must include information pertaining to optimal stimulation sites and the methods by which the electrode channels are arranged. Electrode placement sites and channel arrangements will also depend upon the specific stimulation mode that is to be used.

In order for TENS to be effective, the stimulus must be transmitted into the central nervous system (CNS). The dense innervation of the skin should permit an adequate stimulus to produce sensory input to the CNS. The strength of the stimulus and its efficacy can, however, be enhanced by electrode placement on optimal stimulation sites (OSS). These sites include the spinal column (specifically paraspinally overlying the posterior primary rami), superficial aspects of peripheral nerves, and acupuncture, motor, and trigger points. Greater specificity can be obtained by choosing sites at which two or more of the aforementioned entities exist simultaneously.

I have previously published articles and charts which have discussed in detail the anatomic relationship of acupuncture, motor, and trigger points to one another as well as to superficial aspects of peripheral nerves.[27-29] These specific points and superficial aspects of peripheral nerves represent anatomic areas that can be distinctly located by a knowledge of musculoskeletal and peripheral neuroanatomy. Furthermore, at least one or more specific points are always found to be located overlying superficial aspects of peripheral nerves, therefore, simulation sites used for motor and sensory conduction velocity testing are excellent areas for electrode placement. OSS become tender to palpation in the presence of a segmentally related pathology, are frequently located at indurated areas (bordered by bone), may give rise to referred pain upon pressure, and manifest a high electrical conductance with a decreased skin resistance in comparison to the surrounding or adjacent skin.[27-29] The characteristics of OSS allow them to be easily located by finger palpation. Once the pain distribution has been determined the therapist should palpate for sites of greatest tenderness within this area concentrating at superficial aspects of peripheral nerves coursing through or innervating the involved region. Palpation should also include muscle bellies, musculotendinous junctions, and paraspinally between the transverse processes of segmentally related spinal cord segments. Paraspinal tenderness is manifested at erector spinae motor/trigger points which correspond with bladder meridian acupuncture points as well as posterior primary rami.[27-29] The location of OSS can also be performed by scanning the painful region with probes that measure skin resistance.[28-29]

When OSS have been determined, the clinician must decide how to arrange the electrodes per channel. Channel arrangements and electrode placement sites may differ according to the stimulation mode. When using the conventional mode, electrode placement and channel arrangements must ensure that the sensation of electrical paresthesia is perceived by the patient throughout the entire distribution of pain. This requires at the very least one electrode each at the proximal and distal aspects of the pain distribution. An extensive longitudinal area of pain will necessitate two channels with electrodes arranged in a linear or overlapping pattern. A diffuse area of pain at the posterior aspect of the spine may require a criss cross technique. Electrodes of unequal size per channel may be needed to balance the distribution of electrical paresthesia by adjustments in current density at different skin impedence sites. Electrode placement overlying superficial aspects of related peripheral nerves is recommended.

A prime objective of the strong low rate mode is the production of rhythmic muscle contractions. Electrode placement on motor points of the desired muscle or superficial aspects of the mixed peripheral nerve innervating the specific muscles or myotome will allow for muscle contraction with the least amount of pulse energy. Muscle contractions within the area of pain, especially in the presence of muscle guarding, may not be tolerated by the patient. Effectiveness can still be obtained by electrode placement on motor points of segmentally related myotomes or superficial aspects of innervating peripheral nerves remote from the area of pain. The effectiveness of the strong low rate mode is enhanced by excitation of larger muscle groups.[20]

In the presence of severe low back pain with significant muscle guarding, conventional TENS at the painful region may not be effective. Such a patient will not be able to tolerate the strong low rate mode on the already contracted paraspinal musculature. However, the strong low rate mode may still be effective if electrodes are placed on the legs to produce rhythmic muscle contractions of the gastroc-soleus group. Channel arrangements for this technique would be termed dual channel-bilateral. Electrode placement would be just below the popliteal space and between the medial malleolus and heelcord unilaterally. This array would ensure stimulation of the tibial nerves. These muscles, although remote from the area of pain, are segmentally related via branches of the sciatic nerve which innervate them. Afferent input to the appropriate spinal segments will still occur and may provide activation of pain relief mechanisms. Strong literature support exists for the utilization of segmentally related myotomes.[20,29,43,47,48]

Electrode placement sites and arrangements with the pulse-train (burst) mode depends upon whether or not high or low intensity is utilized. When high intensity pulse-train stimulation is used, electrode placement sites and channel arrangements will be equivalent to that of the strong low rate mode. The recommendations outlined for the conventional mode holds true when stimulating with low intensity pulse-train TENS.

Brief-intense TENS, when applied at superficial aspects of mixed peripheral nerves innervating the area of pain, will produce muscle tetany. This is desired for therapeutic procedures such as skin debridement or suture removal when movement of the involved area is not wanted. When joint mobilization and/or contract-relax stretching is the treatment of choice, electrode placement should not produce muscle tetany as this will hinder joint movement. Electrode arrays for these procedures should produce nonrhythmic muscle fasciculation, and therefore are optimally arranged in a surround or criss-cross fashion at the area of pain and not specifically on superficial peripheral nerve sites. For optimal effectiveness, with the least amount of stimulus strength, electrode placement with the brief-intense mode should be as close to the area of pain as possible.

Although this chapter does not engage in a complete discourse relative to electrode placement techniques and stimulation sites, several anatomic relationships and physiologic processes are mentioned.

Head and Face

Electrical stimulation is not tolerated well on the head or face yet may be required to obtain adequate pain control in the presence of headaches, trigeminal neuralgia, temporomandibular joint syndrome (TMJ), and dental pain. The initial application of TENS in this area should begin at the suboccipital fossa where stimulation of the occipital nerves as well as the spinal tract of the trigeminal nerve can be accomplished without facial stimulation. Regardless of the specific pain syndromes involving the face or head, a single channel of two electrodes placed in the depression between the cranial attachment of the sternocleidomastoid and upper trapezius muscles should represent the first choice. Bilateral stimulation is recommended even in the presence of unilateral pain.[20,27–29]

The spinal tract of the trigeminal nerve has synaptic connections with the upper cervical spinal cord at the C2 to C4 level.[49–52] Therefore, suboccipital stimulation may be able to produce pain relief at any facial or cranial region. Electrode placement at the dorsal web space of the hand can also be an effective remote stimulation site to use for control of facial and head pain. Segmental innervation of the dorsal web space is C5–T1 and thus is not considered to be related to the spinal tract of the trigeminal nerve which may extend only as low as the C4 segment. However, upon examination of Penfields' somatomotor and somatosensory cortices one can see an interesting relationship.

Cortical cells which receive input from the thumb and index finger lie adjacent to those of the head and face. The cortical inhibitory surround theory or "busy cortex" provides a possible explanation for the effectiveness of remote unrelated stimulation sites.[53–55] Significant excitation of a specific cortical region may result in inhibition and decreased sensitivity of an adjacent or surrounding cortical region. Thus dorsal web space stimulation may cause an increase in the excitation threshold of the cortical cells representative of the face and head. Well known acupuncture points exist at the suboccipital fossa (GB20) and dorsal web space (L14).[28]

Electrode placement techniques incorporating both the suboccipital fossa and dorsal web space can also be evaluated prior to stimulation on the head and face.[20,29] Suboccipital stimulation should not produce muscle guarding nor promote reflex vasodilation. Thus the conventional mode is recommended. Dorsal web space stimulation can be accomplished with any mode other than brief-intense as long as the patient does not suffer from migraine headaches. Kaada has shown that the pulse-train mode when applied at the dorsal web space in patients with Raynauds disease produced a 7 to 10° C increase in skin temperature and concomitant pain relief, but also resulted in migraine type headaches in three of four patients.[56]

When stimulation at sites other than the face and head fails to produce satisfactory relief, electrode placement on the head or face may be necessary. This should first be tried with only one electrode at the appropriate area of pain and the other either at the suboccipital fossa or dorsal web space. A small facial electrode and larger suboccipital or dorsal web space electrode will minimize overflow of stimulation to other facial sites.[20–29] Low intensity stimulation is necessary in this area and use of a device called the *pain suppressor* which does not exceed 4 mA in amplitude, but mediates a pulse rate of approximately 15,000 Hz with a 15 Hz burst, is recommended as an initial application.[29] Transcranial stimulation is suggested by the manufacturer.[57–59]

Although there is literature support for the efficacy of TENS in trigeminal neuralgia, TMJ, and dental pain, reports relating to the use of TENS for headaches are sparse and purely anecdotal.[29,41,59–62] The use of TENS in the management of headaches should be purely adjunctive to a comprehensive approach which first determines the specific type of headache and initiates treatment that may consist of biofeedback, relaxation training, postural correction, and instruction in proper body mechanics as well as manual techniques for joint and soft tissue dysfunction. Many times such definitive treatment can eliminate the causative factor and dependency upon symptomatic modalities can be negated.[29–31]

Postoperative TENS

The use of TENS postoperatively falls into the category of acute pain management. Hymes and co-workers initiated the work in the use of TENS after surgery and established its efficacy in a wide variety of thoracic surgical procedures.[63,64] Postoperative pain control with TENS has also shown a concomitant decrease in the incidence of ileus and atelectasis.

Postoperative TENS is easy to perform once a program has been initiated. The operative site is usually known and electrode placement arrangements are commonly medial and lateral to the incision site. When a second surgical site is present, as in the case of bone taken from a donor site, a dual channel unit will be needed. A dual channel arrangement is also necessary when one pair of electrodes is placed overlying the ascending and descending colon to prevent the development of ileus and the other pair used for pain control at the operative site. Recommended stimulation parameters for postoperative pain control consist of a pulse rate between 50 and 100 Hz, pulse width of at least 100 to 200 μs and amplitude to a comfortable level of electrical paresthesia. When an extensive distribution of pain exists, pulse width, and amplitude may need to be increased. Parameter modulation can increase tolerance to higher levels of stimulation.

The effectiveness of postoperative TENS has been established for many types of surgery.[14,63–68] However, its efficacy is significantly diminished when used with drug-experienced as opposed to drug-naive patients.[69] Guidelines for the development and management of a postoperative TENS program are available.[70]

MODE OF ACTION

There is no singular explanation for the physiologic effects produced by TENS. Each specific stimulation mode may have different sites of action and thus can be explained by more than one theory. The gate control theory has already been mentioned as a plausible explanation for the physiologic effects of conventional TENS.[4,5] The cortical inhibitory surround theory may be one hypothesis for the action of high frequency TENS thus explaining some effects of the conventional, pulse-train, and brief-intense modes.[53–55]

Another explanation for the effects of high frequency stimulation is simply counterirritation. Gammon and Starr determined that counterirritation was most effective when applied at the locus of pain with a pulse rate of 50 to 60 Hz.[71]

The stimulation modes that produce strong rhythmic contractions have been shown to promote a release of neurohumeral substances known as enkephalins and endorphins.[23,42,43,72–75] Stimulation requirements, other than strong muscle contractions, (high pulse width and amplitude) to produce neurohumeral liberation include a low pulse rate (1 to 4Hz) and long induction period of at least 20 to 30 minutes. Naloxone reversiblity (a return of pain after relief from electrical stimulation upon naloxone administration) has been the criteria used to determine if an endorphin release took place.

Conventional TENS parameters have not shown reversibility via naloxone administration.[73–75] Naloxone is a morphine antagonist available in different strengths and formulations which may affect only selective brain stem sites.[75–77] There have not been enough definitive studies to strongly support the view that a neurohumeral liberation occurs from strong low rate and high intensity pulse-train TENS. The cerebrospinal fluid (CSF) endorphin level has, however, been elevated by strong low rate TENS.[78]

The best explanation for production of quick analgesia with brief-intense TENS is a conduction block.[79,80] The conduction block may be anodal, chemical, or ischemic.[81] All modes obviously have some effect at the segmental level related to the afferent input that they produce. The stronger modes also have a proposed supraspinal action that does not occur immediately, but possibly produces a summation mechanism. This summation mechanism involves various brain stem structures as well as the pituitary gland and may result in the initiation of neurohumeral liberation which can inhibit the release of substance P, a neurotransmitter needed to promote propagation of afferent nociceptive stimuli.[81] A complete discussion of theoretical possibilities relative to TENS including the complex relationship of serotonin and endogenous opioid peptides is available.[5,81]

EXAMPLES OF USES OF TENS

Cervical Spine

TENS is an excellent adjunctive modality in the comprehensive rehabilitation of patients with acute or chronic cervical spine dysfunction. Nordemar and Thorner found TENS to be very helpful in the management of patients with acute cervical strains.[83] In my clinical practice, many patients with whiplash injuries benefit from home use of TENS while out-patient treatment consisting of techniques to restore function, eliminate muscle guarding, remove irritation, and eliminate pain are performed.[29] Patients with chronic cervical problems and/or cervical radiculitis also can obtain pain relief with TENS.[29]

The conventional stimulation mode with a criss-cross electrode array is recommended for patients with bilateral cervical spine pain from the occipital to the cervical-thoracic junctions or below. When pain is referred from the neck to the upper extremity, a linear current flow with or without the overlapping of stimulation channels is the technique of choice.[20,29] Case study 1 discusses the adjunctive use of TENS for a patient with occipital neuralgia and headaches. Each case study that is presented in this chapter represents patients who were treated by me in my private practice. The evaluation, treatment goals, and plan are taken directly from the patients' charts.

Case Study 1

Evaluation. A 64-year-old female referred for treatment on September 13, 1983, with a diagnosis of cervical osteoarthritis. History dates to one day in July when she awoke with a "stiff neck". She saw her physician who recommended traction at home (18 lbs. for 30 minutes, four times per day). She obtained relief only when the traction was used, but this persisted for a short time after traction. Significant cervical hypomobility existed and she was subsequently hospitalized for 17 days in traction (3 lbs.) and received treatment solely of TENS and moist heat in the hospital physical therapy department. She was discharged with a Philadelphia collar which she was wearing almost 24 hours per day for the past 2 to 3 weeks.

The patient complained of periodic sharp pain that was subsequently replaced by an ache. Pain was primarily in the suboccipital region bilaterally and across the upper trapezius muscles. She also complained of right ear pain, occipital-vertex headaches and left ulnar paresthesia into the fourth and fifth fingers. Paresthesia was present only since the recent hospitalization. Pain was aggravated by combing her hair, coughing, emotional upsets, and active movement of the neck. Pain also occurred at night and she slept sidelying on a flat pillow.

Structurally, there was a significant forward head and round shoulder posture with a Dowager's hump. Active ROM of the cervical spine was severely limited in all directions as follows: forward bending by 50 percent, backward bending by 80 percent, bilateral rotation and sidebending by 75 percent and 85 percent respectively. There was soft tissue restriction, and pain occurred at end range in all directions. Passive ROM testing revealed similar limitations. Active ROM of the shoulders was within normal limits (WNL).

Strength of the C1 to T1 myotomes revealed weakness and some atrophy of the left abductor digiti quinti and first dorsal interosseous. Palpation revealed tenderness of the splenius capitus and upper trapezius muscles bilaterally (L>R). There was some visible muscle guarding at the left paraspinal region. Posterior-anterior (PA) glides and lateral oscillation of the cervical vertebrae could not be adequately tested as the patient could not assume a prone position. X-ray report stated the presence of neural foraminal encroachment at C3-C4 and C4-C5 plus narrowing at the C4-C5 level with degenerative arthritis.

Goals. Decrease pain, increase function, teach prophylaxis.

Treatment plan. High voltage galvanic stimulation followed by ultrasound, gentle joint mobilization, and soft tissue stretching techniques, manual and mechanical (intermittent) traction plus instruction in a home exercise program and proper cervical spine mechanics as well as gradual weaning from the cervical collar. Treatment to be given three times per week.

This patient had received a TENS unit while in the hospital for home use upon discharge. She, however, was not obtaining satisfactory pain relief with it as electrical paresthesia was not being perceived throughout the entire area of pain. She was using four electrodes at the appropriate stimulation sites (suboccipital and paraspinal at the cervical-thoracic junction) but channel arrangements were in a longitudinal fashion on each side of the spine.

Figure 8-1 illustrates the electrode placement sites and restructuring of the stimulation channels to that of a criss cross array. Current flow was thus across the cervical spine producing a greater perception of the electrical paresthesia at the locus of pain. The conventional stimulation mode was used and the patient instructed to place the electrodes on in the morning and use the unit on an as needed basis for periods of 20 to 30 minutes throughout the day.

Progress note. On October 3, 1983, the patient was able to go without the cervical collar for the major part of the day, but would develop discomfort if she performed housecleaning or activities requiring forward bending of the head. Pain had decreased in intensity by 50 percent and occurred periodically. The TENS unit provided at least 75 percent pain relief when needed and she stopped taking pain medications which had upset her stomach. Active ROM of the cervical spine demonstrated increases in all directions and was now limited by only 15 percent in forward bending and 50 percent in bilateral rotation and sidebending as well as backward bending. She was now able to comb her hair much more easily. Treatments were reduced to twice a week.

Progress note. On October 24, 1983, painful episodes continued to decrease in frequency and she was no longer in need of the TENS unit, which she was renting from a distributor. Active ROM of the cervical spine had, however, not

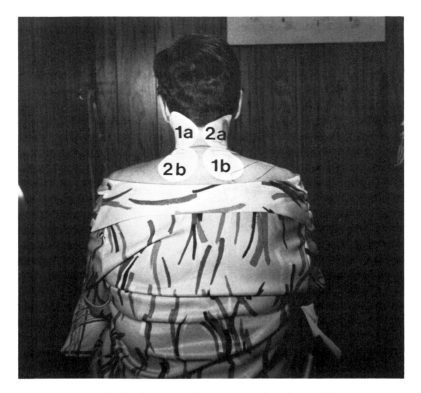

Fig. 8-1.   *Diagnosis:* Cervical osteoarthritis and occipital neuralgia.
    Electrode placement technique: criss-cross, dual channel.
    Electrode placement sites: 1a/2a suboccipital; 2a/2b, paraspinal at cervicothoracic junction.
    TENS mode: Conventional.
    Electrodes: Carbon-silicone.
    TENS unit: Dynex.
    Rationale: Provides for electrical paresthesia throughout distribution of pain.

increased beyond the ranges noted in the previous report. The left ulnar paresthesia remained unchanged and electromyographic studies were suggested. The TENS unit was returned to the distributor and pain relief when needed was being obtained in the form of a home traction unit and ice packs.

Progress note. On November 14, 1983, painful episodes were very infrequent and the intensity of pain very low. She, however, complained of bilateral ankle and knee pain which was severe enough to hinder ambulation. The right medial malleolus and left lateral malleolus were red, warm, and edematous. These areas had now replaced the cervical spine pain as her prime concern. This was immediately brought to the attention of the referring physician who subsequently admitted her to the hospital for further evaluation. Treatments were discontinued at this time with increased cervical active ROM noted. Limitations had decreased to 5 percent in forward bending, 40 percent in backward bending and sidebending bilaterally, 25 percent in right rotation, and 35 percent in left rotation.

Upper Extremity Pain

TENS is an extremely valuable adjunctive pain control modality for intrinsic joint pain, peripheral nerve injuries, amputations, and reflex sympathetic dystrophy.[29,84–86] Adequate pain control can be obtained by the use of TENS at home to allow for exercise and ROM as well as in the clinic to allow for treatment to be performed. Case study 2 highlights the extensive use of TENS for a patient who sustained a traumatic amputation of the distal phalanx of the middle finger.

Case Study 2

Evaluation. The patient is a 50-year-old female referred on May 13, 1982 for rehabilitation to the right hand. She sustained a traumatic amputation of the distal phalanx of the right middle finger from a machine accident while at work on March 23, 1981. Surgical revision was performed on May 26, 1981. Postoperatively, she suffered from headaches, right upper extremity (RUE) pain, paresthesia, and hyperesthesia of the hand (primarily of the distal end of the amputated finger) which was colder than the adjacent fingers and had a distal sensory deficit. Hand dynamometer readings of 40 lbs on the left and 20 lbs on the right for grip were attained.

The finger was hypersensitive to gentle touch and she was unable to tolerate whirlpool due to vibrating irritation. She complained of periodic edema and drawing of the amputated finger along with phantom pain. She returned to work in September of 1981 but could not continue due to increased RUE discomfort. The patient had become depressed and was under care of a psychiatrist.

Active ROM of the right shoulder, elbow, and wrist was WNL. Active ROM of the third metacarpophalangeal joint (MCP) was WNL but the proximal interphalangeal joint (PIP) was limited to 60 degrees, 75 degrees passively. Active ROM of the cervical spine was limited by 25 percent in rotation and sidebending bilaterally as well as backward bending.

Goals. Decrease pain and hyperesthesia, increase function.

Treatment plan. Evaluation with TENS for pain control, whirlpool with high voltage galvanic stimulation followed by ultrasound, joint mobilization, and therapeutic exercise as well as instruction in a home exercise program.

The results of the TENS evaluation revealed that five electrodes were needed to obtain adequate pain control (Fig. 8-2). The conventional stimulation mode was used. The patient was only able to perform the home exercise program adequately with simultaneous use of the TENS unit. Without use of TENS she states that "the finger feels stiff making it difficult to bend, and pain in the RUE occurs." TENS also controlled the finger hyperesthesia which allowed for the performance of joint mobilization and manual resistive exercises. The patient obtained a TENS unit for home use on rental from a distributor.

Progress note. On July 29, 1982, the patient was using the TENS unit daily turning it on about four times per day for 20 minute periods during which she would exercise.

Progress note. On September 22, 1982, the patient was able to make a complete fist, and active PIP flexion was measured to 80 degrees. RUE, cervical spine,

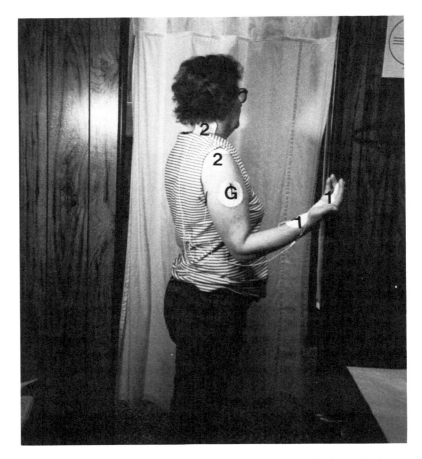

Fig. 8-2. *Diagnosis:* Reflex sympathetic dystrophy, hyperesthesia, and phantom pain following traumatic amputation of distal phalanx of middle finger.

Electrode placement technique: linear pathway.

Electrode placement sites: G, common positive at deltoid insertion. Negative electrodes of channel two at right cervical spine and musculotendinous junction of supraspinatus. Negative electrodes of channel one at volar surface of wrist and wrapped around finger proximal to end of stump.

TENS mode: Conventional.

Electrodes: Carbon-silicone.

TENS unit: Biostim System 10.

Rationale: Electrical paresthesia from the positive electrode to the shoulder and neck and to the forearm and hand to provide pain control throughout whole distribution of pain.

phantom finger pain, and hyperesthesia continued. Purchase of the TENS unit was recommended and agreed upon by the referring physician.

Progress note. On November 11, 1982, pain control still was only possible with TENS. Attempts at various desensitization techniques showed no progress and on November 7, 1982, she underwent a second surgical procedure for removal of neuroma formation at the distal end of the amputated finger. She now reported much less pain but had total sensory loss on the volar surface from the PIP crease to the end of the stump. Sensation, however, was intact at the medial, lateral, and dorsal surfaces. She reported a vibratory sensation and burning on the dorsum of the finger as well as the palmar surface of the hand whenever she reached for something.

Active ROM had decreased to 50 degrees at the PIP joint and grip strength to 10 lbs. Between December 15, 1982, and February 2, 1983, ROM and strength gradually increased, but discomfort at the volar surface of the amputated finger increased. The patient reported pain intensification upon movement which was controlled by TENS. Pain referral to the shoulder and cervical spine increased and active ROM began to decrease. She underwent another surgical revision on February 23, 1983, after which she complained of increased pain in the entire RUE and right cervical spine with evidence of causalgia and an apparent reflex sympathetic dystrophy. Treatment in the form of gentle mobilization techniques to the right shoulder and cervical spine was initiated along with intermittent mechanical cervical traction. The patient also obtained a home traction unit as this gave her good relief of cervical discomfort.

The increased discomfort necessitated evaluation of electrode placement techniques specifically to obtain pain control at the shoulder and cervical spine depicted in Figures 8-3 and 8-4 respectively.

The patient continued to regress and on September 22, 1983, she reported that she needed to sleep with the TENS unit on. Relaxation training was initiated. She has since burned the distal volar surface of the amputated finger two times due to sensory loss and a protective splint was fabricated. The patient continued to be very depressed, remained under psychiatric care, and continued physical therapy to regain function of the RUE and cervical spine. The TENS unit continued to provide pain relief of at least 75 percent.

Sensory Deprivation Pain Syndromes

Neuralgia/causalgia and phantom limb pain syndromes fall into the sensory deprivation category. As their names denote, these pain syndromes result in damage to either large or small afferent nerve fibers thus depriving the CNS of a balanced neural input. Perhaps the pain syndrome most representative of this category is shingles or herpes zoster (postherpetic neuralgia).

The herpes zoster virus has an affinity for the myelin sheath and thus selectively attacks the large A-fibers dampening the natural CNS proprioceptive input. Normal CNS balance is thus disrupted resulting in a decrease of the excitation threshold of the small diameter nociceptive fibers.[31,78-89]

Case study 3 discusses the role of TENS in the pain management of a patient with a severe case of shingles. The efficacy of TENS in various types of sensory deprivation pain syndromes (SDPS) supports its use in these painful conditions.[29,32,90-95] Further characterization of SDPS includes cutaneous hyperesthesia induced by non-noxious stimuli, severe intractable burning pain, and involvement of the autonomic nervous system.[89] Cutaneous hyperesthesia may negate the placement of electrodes at the involved area. When effective

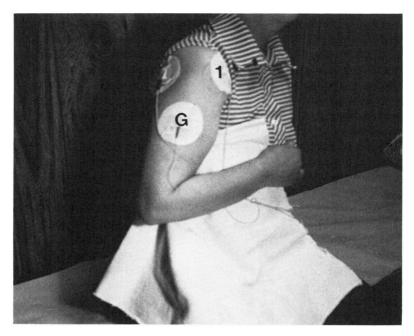

Fig. 8-3. *Diagnosis:* Reflex sympathetic dystrophy, hyperesthesia, and phantom pain following traumatic amputation of distal phalanx of middle finger.

Electrode placement technique: "V" shape pathway.

Electrode placement sites: G, common positive electrode at deltoid insertion. Negative electrode of channel one in depression below acromion anterially. Negative electrode of channel two in depression below acromion posterially.

TENS mode: Conventional.

Electrodes: Carbon-silicone.

TENS unit: Biostim System 10.

Rationale: Common positive electrode in series with negative electrodes to produce electrical paresthesia across shoulder.

Note: With a dual (isolated) channel unit a fourth electrode would be placed at the musculotendinous junction.

sites cannot be obtained on the side of the lesion, contralateral stimulation of the same dermatomes or peripheral nerve is recommended.[29,96]

Conventional TENS is the stimulation mode of choice with SDPS as it can produce large A-fiber input to the dorsal horn of the cord and hopefully provide a balancing effect. Care must be taken to avoid electrode placement over skin lesions where conduction is likely to be impaired.

Case Study 3

Evaluation. A 76-year-old man was referred on December 13, 1983, for evaluation with TENS as a means of pain control for postherpetic neuralgia. The onset

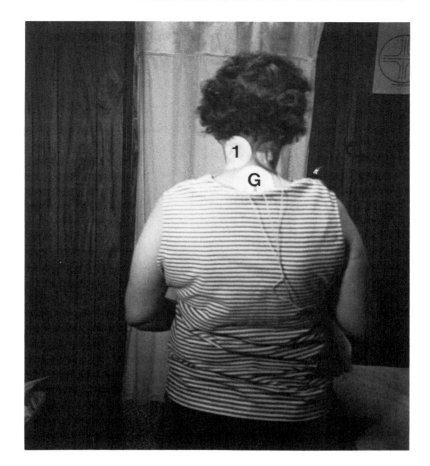

Fig. 8-4. *Diagnosis:* Reflex sympathetic dystrophy, hyperesthesia and phantom pain following traumatic amputation of distal phalanx of middle finger.

    Electrode placement technique: "V" shape pathway.

    Electrode placement sites: G, common positive electrode at cervico thoracic junction midline. Negative electrodes of channel 1 and 2 in suboccipital fossa.

    TENS mode: Conventional.

    Electrodes: Carbon-silicone.

    TENS unit: Biostim System 10.

    Rationale: Arrangement provides for sensation of electrical paresthesia throughout area of pain.

of pain was about 7 weeks before and skin lesions began within the first week. When seen, scab formation had fallen off but the skin rash remained. The patient also developed nausea, an enlarged abdominal area ipsilateral to the lesion, and muscle spasms of the abdominal region which occurred every 30 seconds for 2 hour periods.

    Pain was described as a burning and stabbing type with the feeling of a "hot needle" in his back. Pain was constant during the day and night and the area of involvement extended from the T10-L1 right paraspinal level laterally and anterior to the umbilicus. Pain was aggravated by sitting, lying on his back or stomach, and clothing rubbing against the involved skin area. He was unable to sit upright with his back against a chair. Cold applications and Tylenol helped him sleep and he took diazapam (Valium) and Percodan daily when pain became severe.

Goals. Establish pain control with TENS.

Treatment plan. The patient arrived with a TENS unit which he had been using at home for the past few weeks. He apparently had not been properly instructed in use of the unit nor evaluated for optimal electrode placement arrangements. He was only using one channel of two small electrodes placed proximal and distal to the skin lesions paraspinally. This arrangement only provided for minimal pain relief at the stimulated area and not the extensive distribution of the pain.

Instruction in operation of the stimulator consisted of turning it on until the electrical sensation appeared and then letting accommodation occur without any further parameter adjustment. He thus was using the unit 24 hours per day but at an intensity that did not provide for the sensation of electrical paresthesia. He stated that he had not been obtaining any significant pain relief.

Due to the extensive area of involvement, large rectangular postoperative electrodes were used in an attempt to block a large area of pain. Karaya electrodes were used so that tape would not be required. The initial electrode sites and dual channel array is illustrated in Figure 8-5. This consisted of one electrode pair placed at the right paraspinal region and just to the left of the midline beyond the anterior extent of the lesions. The second pair was placed above and below the lesions at the lateral rib cage. When the unit was activated after resetting pulse rate and width parameters for the conventional stimulation mode, the patient reported an immediate perception of electrical paresthesia with pain relief throughout the complete distribution of pain beyond that achieved from previous use.

The criss-cross arrangement depicted in Figure 8-6 was chosen as it was assumed that the most intense area of discomfort was the lateral rib cage. The second technique changed the direction of stimulation to a more distinct "X" fashion but did not significantly increase benefit.

Upon further questioning, the patient revealed that his most intensive areas of discomfort were at the back and abdomen which thus prompted a rearrangement of the electrodes to two distinctly separate areas as shown in Figure 8-7. This array immediately provided the best pain relief since the interelectrode distance was shortened and independent adjustment of amplitude could be performed as a criss-cross energy flow was not occurring.

Contralateral electrode placement (on the noninvolved side) was contemplated. However, this was not attempted as the patient stated that left sidelying was his only comfortable position in which to sleep or rest and he did not want to lie on the electrodes. Instruction was given to keep the electrodes in place 24 hours per day, but to try and turn the stimulation off every hour for at least 5 to 10 minutes or longer if possible. The skin beneath the electrodes was to be checked every 6 hours. He was told to maintain perception of the electrical paresthesia by periodic adjustment of amplitude and/or pulse width at a comfortable level which did not produce muscle contraction.

Followup by telephone was performed within a few days as the patient lived a considerable distance away. On December 20, 1983, he reported that use of TENS remained continuous with periods of no stimulation not exceeding 30 minutes. He had not had any pain medication since he left the office on December 13, 1983.

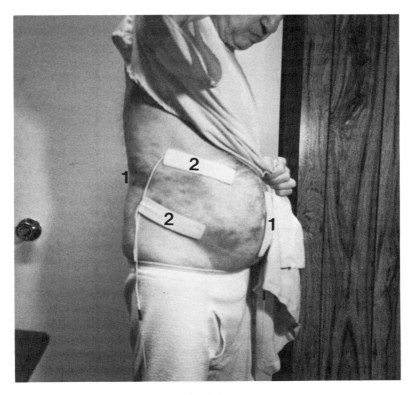

Fig. 8-5. *Diagnosis:* Herpes zoster (shingles).

Electrode placement technique: Dual channel criss-cross technique. Channel one electrodes at right paraspinal region (hidden) and to left of midline (anterior) beyond extent of lesions. Channel two electrodes placed superior and inferior to lesions at lateral rib cage.

TENS mode: Conventional.

Electrodes: Postoperative, karaya by Lec-tec.

TENS unit: 3M Tenzcare.

Rationale: To obtain electrical paresthesia throughout area of pain.

Stimulation was controlling the onset of abdominal muscle spasms which was very helpful to him. Although he continued to experience relatively constant discomfort, the use of TENS was "now taking the painful edge off" and providing greater relief than anything else (medication or cold applications) that was tried. The percentage of relief was estimated to be about 50 percent by the patient.

The role of TENS as a means of noninvasive and nonmedicinal pain control is perhaps best illustrated in the presence of SDPS. Patients with pain of this intensity and duration which occurs with SDPS can obtain ongoing pain control which usually is not apparent by the use of medication. Furthermore, TENS can accomplish pain control without the side effects inherent with the

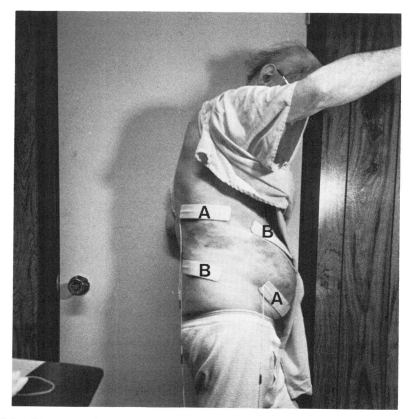

Fig. 8-6. *Diagnosis:* Herpes Zoster (shingles).
    Electrode placement technique: Dual channel criss-cross technique. Channel A electrodes at superior posterolateral rib cage and inferior anteromedial rib cage. Channel B electrodes at superior anteromedial region to inferior posterolateral rib cage.
    TENS mode: Conventional.
    Electrodes: Postoperative karaya by Lec-tec.
    TENS unit: 3M Tenzcare.
    Rationale: An attempt to improve energy flow (electrical paresthesia) across the lateral rib cage.

use of medication. Proper efficacy, however, can only be obtained in pain syndromes of this type by spending time evaluating the best electrode arrangements. Electrode placement above the level of the lesion is recommended for use with peripheral nerve injuries.

Back and Peripheral Joint Pain

TENS when used properly as an adjunctive technique is also very effective in the control of pain due to arthritic and mechanical dysfunction of the low back and peripheral joints.[29,45,90,96–99] In fact, patients with low back pain con-

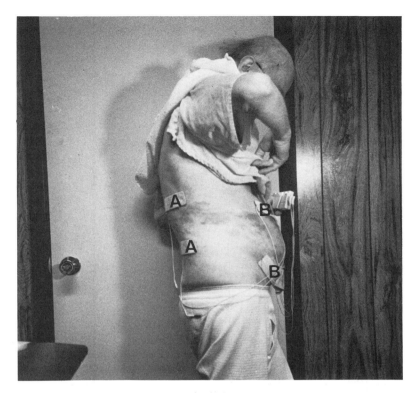

Fig. 8-7. *Diagnosis:* Herpes zoster (shingles).

 Electrode placement technique: Dual channel (isolated) Channel A, superior and inferior to lesions at posterior rib cage and spine. Channel B, superior and inferior to abdominal lesions.

 TENS mode: Conventional.

 Electrodes: Postoperative karaya by Lec-tec.

 TENS unit: 3M Tenzcare.

 Rationale: Isolate energy at the two most severe regions.

stitute the largest pain category in which benefit is obtained from TENS.[100–103] It is necessary to reiterate at this point that TENS is not a treatment for low back pain but should merely be used adjunctively for pain control at home while specific therapy to eliminate the cause of pain, correct the dysfunction if possible, and prevent recurrence is provided.[17,20,25,31] Case study 4 highlights the use of TENS for a patient with osteoarthritis of the lumbar spine and left knee.

Case Study 4

 Evaluation. A 66-year-old female was referred for evaluation with TENS on November 7, 1983. The patient had diagnoses of degenerative osteoarthritis of the lumbar spine and left knee, compression fractures of L1 and L2, as well as degen-

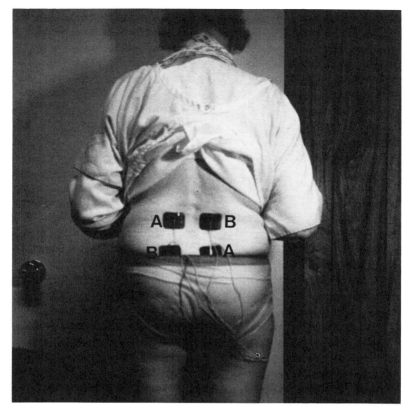

Fig. 8-8.   *Diagnosis:* Degenerative osteoarthritis of lumbar spine and left knee, compression fractures of L1 and L2.

Electrode placement technique: Dual channel criss-cross. Channel A at left superior paraspinal area and right inferior paraspinal area. Channel B at right superior paraspinal area and left inferior paraspinal area.

TENS mode: Conventional with modulation.

Electrodes: Bioform by Biostim.

TENS unit: Biostim Biomod.

Rationale: Criss-cross electrode array to concentrate energy at center of spine.

erative disc disease. Low back pain had become a constant ache and was increasing since July. Left knee pain was periodic and not as severe as the low back pain.

Back pain was aggravated by ambulation or standing and eased by sitting upright. Night pain was not a factor, only occurring slightly when turning. Discomfort was most severe in the morning even though she slept on a firm mattress. Previous treatment in the form of chiropractic kinesiology and the use of medication (Motrin and Ascriptin) did not provide sufficient pain relief.

The patient ambulated normally. Structurally there was a significant loss of the lumbar lordosis, rotation of the thoracic spine partially to the right, a forward

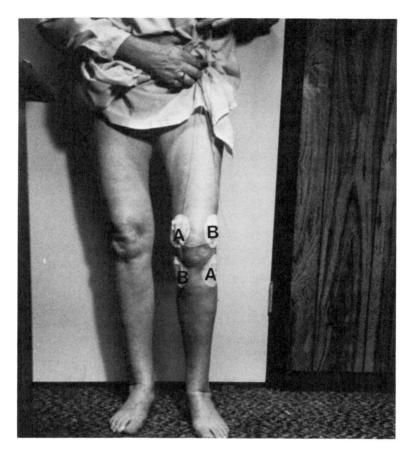

Fig. 8-9. *Diagnosis:* Degenerative osteoarthritis of lumbar spine and left knee compression fractures of L1 and L2.

    Electrode placement technique: Criss-cross, dual channel. Channel A at right superior to the patella and left by the fibular head. Channel B at left superior to the patella and right inferior with patella.

    TENS mode: Conventional.

    Electrodes: Bioform by Biostim.

    TENS unit: Biostim Biomod.

    Rationale: Provides a criss-cross current flow across the whole knee.

head and Dowager's hump. Active ROM of the lumbar spine was limited by 75 percent in backward bending and 50 percent in sidebending bilaterally with pain at end range. Straight leg raising (SLR) was not limited and did not produce pain. Strength of the L1 to S2 myotomes was WNL as was active ROM of the knees.

    Posterior-anterior glides and lateral oscillations revealed hypomobility throughout the lumbar spine. Palpation gave rise to local and referred tenderness at the left sciatic notch, popliteal space, and superficial aspects of the sural nerve. However, without provocation, sciatic pain was not present.

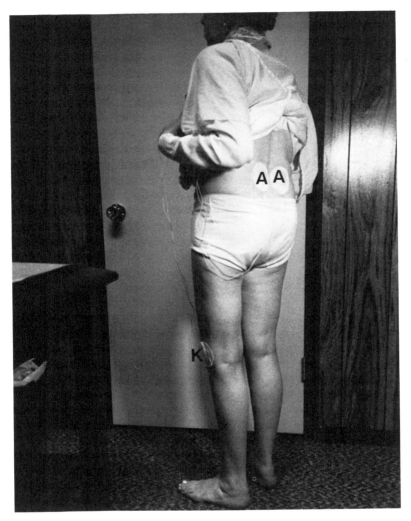

Fig. 8-10.   *Diagnosis:* Degenerative osteoarthritis of lumbar spine and left knee, compression fractures of L1 and L2.

Electrode placement technique: Dual channel isolated areas. Channel A, bilateral paraspinal; channel K, bilateral peripheral joint.

TENS mode: Conventional.

Electrodes: Biostim Bioform.

TENS unit: Biostim Biomod.

Rationale: Isolated channels to obtain pain controls at two separate areas.

Goals.   Obtain pain control with TENS and teach prophylaxis.

Treatment plan.   Evaluation with TENS determined that satisfactory pain relief was obtained with a dual channel criss-cross technique (Fig. 8-8). The conventional stimulation mode with and without the use of pulse rate and width modulation was preferred for the low back pain. A criss-cross technique about the left knee also provided satisfactory pain relief (Fig. 8-9).

The patient obtained a TENS unit on rental from a dealer on November 18, 1983, and was fully instructed in its use. In addition, at this time she was shown how to use one channel at the low back and the other at the left knee to obtain simultaneous pain control at both areas (Fig. 8-10). She was instructed in proper cervical and lumbar spinal mechanics to minimize the degree of pain.

Followup telephone conversation on November 26, 1983, revealed that the patient was obtaining 75 percent pain relief which persisted for 2 or 3 hours after a 30 minute stimulation period. On the clinic visit of November 14, 1983, 1 month after obtaining the unit for home use, the patient decided to purchase it. She was extremely pleased with the benefit obtained and was now getting 90 percent relief persisting for 2 to 4 hour periods after a 30 minute stimulation session. She had been able to eliminate the use of medication and increase her ADL within established guidelines. She was using the unit two or three times per day. The patient was thus discharged and further followup was done by mail questionnaire.

THE TENS EVALUATION

The successful evaluation of patients with TENS requires their presence in the clinic at a time of day when pain is most intense and when they are not under the influence of medication.[20] The evaluation should be performed in the position which produces pain providing that it is consistent with proper body mechanics. If patients are unable to assume a proper position due to dysfunction, then the evaluation should proceed in that position and as definitive therapy begins, proper posture should be emphasized.

The conventional stimulation mode should be used for the initial assessment of efficacy. This mode is mild without producing muscle contractions and should provide fast feedback of efficacy. The initial goal is to arrange the electrodes so that perception of the electrical paresthesia is perceived by the patient throughout the complete distribution of pain. Once this has been achieved the stimulation session should persist for at least 20 minutes. If satisfactory relief is not evident within 20 minutes, the electrodes should be rearranged and tried again. If all possible arrangements using the conventional mode with or without modulation are unsuccessful, further evaluation with another mode should be performed.

My second choice would be the strong low rate or high intensity pulse-train (burst) mode. A proper assessment of the effectiveness of these modes would now require 20 to 30 minutes at the minimum and possibly up to 1 hour. Failure to achieve success with any of the aforementioned modes would prompt me to try 5 to 15 minutes of brief-intense TENS after which pulse width and amplitude parameters would be decreased to the conventional TENS range. Parameter modulation could be used to promote tolerance to brief-intense stimulation.

The prime purpose of the TENS evaluation is to determine the stimulation mode and electrode placement sites and arrangement that provide the patient with the most significant degree of relief that persists the longest with the shortest possible stimulation period. I do not encourage any patient to rent a unit from a dealer unless satisfactory effectiveness is obtained in the clinic. Once this has been determined, the therapist should decide on the specific model and accessories that seem best suited for the patient. Consideration should be given to ease of operation, battery life, lead wire length, electrode size and shape, transmission medium, and form of adherence to the skin. The total package (unit and accessories) should then be ordered from the dealer (a prescription for rental of the device must be obtained) and the patient scheduled for another visit at the time of delivery. As a clinician I do not rent or sell TENS units. This is the domain of the dealer. The dealer should equally respect the domain of the clinician and not perform TENS evaluations.

When patients are to receive the TENS unit, I first have them read the manufacturer's manual in my waiting room and then review the total operation of the device, including electrode maintenance, battery replacement, and electrode placement. A complete TENS home instruction form is given to the patient that includes instructions in proper programming of the unit, the desired sensation, and length of the treatment period. Electrode placement sites and channel arrangements are drawn on the appropriate page of the instruction form, specific reminders highlighted, and the means by which long term effectiveness will be determined is explained. A complete TENS home instruction form has been developed for patient and clinical use.[104] If the patient is not being seen for specific treatments, a followup appointment is made. If everything is going well, the appointment can be cancelled, but if a problem develops I should be informed. At the very least, I will see the patient one more time just prior to the end of the initial month rental period. A followup questionnaire will then be given to the patient to complete.[104] A determination now needs to be made regarding purchase, continued rental, or return of the unit if pain has resolved or effectiveness is not satisfactory.

There are numerous factors, separate from proper utilization of the TENS unit, that can interfere with success, enhance it when it is minimal, and restore it when it ceases to be effective.[81] Perhaps the most important hindering factor is poor body mechanics. Patients with musculoskeletal pain of mechanical origin frequently do not obtain benefit from TENS because they are using the device to obtain pain control while performing improper ADL. The patient with low back pain who leaves the clinic feeling relieved while the TENS unit is functioning and immediately sits in a flexed position in his car will obtain a quick return of pain. Proper instruction by the therapist in the principles of proper body mechanics and postural exercises is of utmost importance to obtain satisfactory relief for a prolonged duration.

The use of specific types of medications or dietary supplements may either hinder, enhance, or restore benefit. Valium (diazepam), narcotics, and corticosteroids may hinder success while tricyclics and tryptophan may enhance and/or restore efficacy.[81,105-107]

If the effectiveness of TENS begins to wear off after long term use, reevaluation of the patient should be performed to determine if the original quality and distribution of pain has changed. A change in the characteristics of pain may require use of a different stimulation mode and/or electrode arrangement to regain effectiveness.

CONCLUSION

The intent of the chapter has been to provide a complete overview of TENS with emphasis on clinical application. Sections dealing with the stimulation modes, therapeutic applications, and the specific adjunctive role of TENS were covered in greater detail than others. TENS is a modality that seems specifically suited for physical therapists as it requires evaluation, hands on application, and time to achieve good results. Physical therapists see and treat their patients more frequently than the physician and also have education and training in electrophysiology and electrotherapeutics.

REFERENCES

1. Hymes A: A review of the historical area of electricity. p. 1. In Mannheimer JS, Lampe GN (eds): Clinical Transcutaneous Electrical Nerve Stimulation. FA Davis, Philadelphia, 1984
2. Taub A, Kane K: A history of local analgesia. Pain 1:125, 1975
3. Barcalow DR: Electreat relieves pain. Electreat Mfg Co, Peoria, 1919
4. Melzack R, Wall PW: Pain mechanisms: a new theory. Science 150:971, 1965
5. Wolf SL: Neurophysiologic mechanisms in pain modulation: relevance to TENS p. 41. In Mannheimer JS, Lampe GN (eds): Clinical Transcutaneous Electrical Nerve Stimulation. FA Davis, Philadelphia, 1984
6. Shealy CN, Mortimer JT, Reswick JB: Electrical inhibition of pain by stimulation of the dorsal column: preliminary clinical reports. Anesth Analg (Cleve) 45:489, 1967
7. Shealy CN, Mortimer JT: Dorsal column electroanalgesia. J Neurosurg 32:560, 1970
8. Ray CD: New electrical stimulation methods for therapy and rehabilitation. Ortho Review 4:29, 1977
9. Fisher AA: Dermatitis associated with transcutaneous electrical nerve stimulation. Current Contact News 21:24, 1978
10. Shealy CN, Maurer D: Transcutaneous nerve stimulation for control of pain. Surg Neurol 2:45, 1974
11. Eriksson MBE, Schuller H, Sjolund BH: Letter: Hazard from transcutaneous nerve stimulators in patients with pacemakers. Lancet 1:1319, 1978
12. Peper A, Grimbergen CA: EEG measurement during electrical stimulation. IEEE Trans Biomed Eng BME 30:231, 1983
13. Furno GS, Tompkins WJ: A learning filter for removing noise interference. IEEE Trans Biomed Eng BME 30:234, 1983
14. Ticho U, Olshwang D. Magora F: Relief of pain by subcutaneous electrical stimulation after ocular surgery. Am J Opth 89:803, 1980
15. Augustinsson LE, Bohlin P, Bundsen P, et al: Pain relief during delivery by transcutaneous electrical nerve stimulation. Pain 4:59, 1977

16. Bundsen P, Ericson K: Pain relief in labor by transcutaneous electrical nerve stimulation: safety aspects. Acta Obstet Gynecol Scand 61:1, 1982

17. Mannheimer JS, Lampe GN: Pain and TENS in pain management. p. 7. In Mannheimer JS, Lampe GN (eds): Clinical Transcutaneous Electrical Nerve Stimulation. FA Davis, Philadelphia, 1984.

18. Mannheimer JS: Transcutaneous electrical nerve stimulation for pain modulation during specific therapeutic techniques. Program Abstacts, second general meeting of the American Pain Society 56, 1980

19. Mannheimer JS: TENS as an adjunctive technique in hand rehabilitation. APTA Hand Section newsletter, 1983.

20. Mannheimer JS, Lampe GN: Electrode placement techniques. p. 331. In Mannheimer JS, Lampe GN (eds): Clinical Transcutaneous Electrical Nerve Stimulation. FA Davis, Philadelphia, 1984.

21. Thorsteinsson G, Stonnington HH, Stillwell GK, et al: The placebo effect of transcutaneous electrical nerve stimulation. Pain 5:31, 1978

22. Long DM, Campbell JN, Gucer G: Transcutaneous electrical stimulation for relief of chronic pain. Adv Pain Ther 3:593, 1979

23. Andersson SA: Pain control by sensory stimulation. p. 569. In Bonica JJ (ed): Advances in Pain Research and Therapy. Vol. 3. Raven Press, New York, 1979

24. AAMI Neurosurgery Committee: Proposed Standard for Transcutaneous Electrical Nerve Stimulators. Association for the Advancement of Medical Instrumentation. Arlington, 1981

25. Mannheimer JS, Lampe GN: Clinical Transcutaneous Electrical Nerve Stimulation. FA Davis, Philadelphia, 1984

26. Biostim Inc: Informative Series. Princeton, 1983

27. Mannheimer JS: Electrode placement for transcutaneous electrical nerve stimulation. Physical Therapy 58:1455, 1978

28. Mannheimer JS: Optimal Stimulation Sites for TENS Electrodes. Hibbert Co, Trenton, 1980

29. Mannheimer JS, Lampe GN: Electrode placement sites and their relationships. p. 249. In Mannheimer JS, Lampe GN (eds): Clinical Transcutaneous Electrical Nerve Stimulation. FA Davis, Philadelphia, 1984

30. Sinclair D: Mechanisms of Cutaneous Sensation. Oxford University Press, Oxford, 1981

31. Mannheimer JS, Lampe GN: Differential evaluation for the determination of TENS effectiveness in specific pain syndromes p. 63. In Mannheimer JS, Lampe GN: Clinical Transcutaneous Electrical Nerve Stimulation. FA Davis, Phildelphia, 1984

32. Wolf SL, Gersh MR, Rao VR: Examination of electrode placement and stimulation parameters in treating chronic pain with conventional electrical nerve stimulation (TENS). Pain 11:37, 1981

33. Mannheimer JS: TENS Update: the stimulation modes. Stimulus: Clinical Electrophysiology Section of APTA 8:10, 1983

34. Linzer M, Long DM: Transcutaneous neural stimulation for relief of pain. IEEE Trans Biomed Eng 23:341, 1974

35. Burton C, Maurer DD: Pain suppression by transcutaneous electrical stimulation. IEEE Trans Biomed Eng 21:81, 1974

36. Andersson SA, Holmgren E, Ross A: Analgesic effects of peripheral conditioning stimulation II. Importance of certain stimulation parameters. Acupunc Electrother Res 2:237, 1977

37. Andersson SA, Holmgren E: Analgesic effects of peripheral conditioning stimulation III. Effect of high frequency stimulation: segmental mechanisms interacting with pain. Acupunc Electrother Res 3:23, 1978
38. Holmgren E: Increase of pain threshold as a function of conditioning electrical stimulation: an experimental study with application to electroacupuncture for pain suppression. Am J Chin Med 3:133, 1975
39. Andersson SA, Holmgren E: Pain threshold effects of peripheral conditioning stimulation. p. 761. In Bonica JJ, Albe-Fessard D (eds): Advances in Pain Research and Therapy. Vol. 6. Raven Press, New York, 1976
40. Chapman CR, Wilson ME, Gehrig JD: Comparative effects of acupuncture on dental pain: evaluation of threshold estimation and sensory decision theory. Pain 3:2131, 1977
41. Chapman CR, Chen AC, Bonica JJ: Effects of intrasegmental electrical acupuncture on dental pain: evaluation of threshold estimation and sensory decision theory. Pain 3:2131, 1977
42. Eriksson MBE, Sjolund BH: Acupuncturelike electroanalgesia in TNS resistant chronic pain p. 575. In Zotterman Y (ed): Sensory Functions of the Skin. Pergamon Press, Oxford, 1976
43. Eriksson MBE, Sjolund BH, Neilzen S: Long term results of peripheral conditioning stimulation as analgesic measure in chronic pain. Pain 6:335, 1979
44. Fox EJ, Melzack R: Transcutaneous electrical stimulation and acupuncture: comparison of treatment of low back pain. Pain 2:141, 1976
45. Mannheimer C, Carlsson CA: The analgesic effect of transcutaneous electrical nerve stimulation (TNS) in patients with rheumatoid arthritis: a comparative study of different pulse patterns. Pain 6:329, 1979
46. Roberts HJ: Transcutaneous electrical nerve stimulation in the management of pancreatitis pain. South Med J 71:396, 1978
47. Handwerker HB, Iggo A, Zimmerman M: Segmental and supraspinal actions on dorsal horn neurons responding to noxious and nonnoxious skin stimuli. Pain 1:147, 1975
48. Gunn CC: Transcutaneous neural stimulation: acupuncture and the current of injury. Am J Acupunct 6:191, 1978
49. Elvidge AR, Li CL: Central protrusion of cervical intervertebral disc involving descending trigeminal tract. Archives Neurol Psychiat 63:455, 1950
50. Kerr FWL: Mechanisms, diagnosis, and management of some cranial and facial pain syndromes. Surg Clin North Am 43:951, 1963
51. Gobel S: Principles of organization in the substantia gelatinosa layer of the spinal trigeminal nucleus. p. 165. In Bonica JJ, Albe-Fessard D (eds): Advances in Pain Research and Therapy. Raven Press, New York, 1976
52. Edmeads J: Headaches and head pains associated with disease of the cervical spine. Med Clin North Am 62:533, 1978
53. Bresler DE, Froening RJ: Three essential factors in effective acupuncture therapy. Am J Chin Med 4:81, 1976
54. Liao SJ: Recent advances in the understanding of acupuncture. Yale J Biol Med 51:55, 1978
55. Bull GM: Acupuncture anesthesia. Lancet 2:417, 1973
56. Kaada B: Vasodilation induced by transcutaneous nerve stimulation in peripheral ischemia (Raynaud's) phenomenon and diabetic polyneuropathy. Eur Heart J 3:303, 1982
57. Shealy CN, Kwako JL, Hughes S: Effects of transcranial neurostimulation upon mood and serotonin production: a preliminary report. IL Dolore 1:13, 1979

58. Pain Suppression Labs Inc, Elmwood Park, NJ,

59. Markovich SE: Pain in the head: a neurological appraisal. p. 125. In Gelb H (ed): Clinical Management of Head, Neck and TMJ Pain and Dysfunction. WB Saunders, Philadelphia, 1977

60. Mumford JM: Relief of orofacial pain by transcutaneous neural stimulation. J Br Endo Soc 9:71, 1976

61. Appenzeller O, Atkinson R: Transcutaneous nerve stimulation in the treatment of hemicrania and other forms of headache. Minerva Med 67:2023, 1976

62. Hag KM: Control of head pain in migraine using transcutaneous electrical nerve stimulation. Practitioner 226:771, 1982

63. Hymes A: The therapeutic value of postoperative TENS. p. 497. In Mannheimer JS, Lampe GN (eds): Clinical Transcutaneous Electrical Nerve Stimulation. FA Davis, Philadelphia, 1984

64. Hymes AC, Yonehiro EG, Raab DE, et al: Electrical surface stimulation for treatment and prevention of ileus and atelectasis. Surg Forum 26:222, 1975

65. Stabile ML, Malloy TH: The management of postoperative pain in total joint replacement. Ortho Review 7:121, 1978

66. Alm WA, Gold ML, Weil LS: Evaluation of transcutaneous electrical nerve stimulation (TENS) in podiatric surgery. J Am Podiatric Assoc 69:537, 1979

67. Schuster G. Infante M: Pain relief after low back surgery: the efficacy of transcutaneous electrical nerve stimulation. Pain 8:299–302, 1980

68. Harvie KW: A major advance in the control of postoperative knee pain. Orthopedics 2:25, 1979

69. Solomon RA, Viernstein MC, Long DM: Reduction of postoperative pain and narcotic use by transcutaneous electrical nerve stimulation. Surgery 87:142, 1980

70. Lampe GN, Mannheimer JS: Postoperative TENS analgesia: protocol, methods, results, and benefit. p. 511. In Mannheimer JS, Lampe GN (eds): Clinical Transcutaneous Electrical Nerve Stimulation. FA Davis, Philadelphia, 1984

71. Gammon GD, Starr I: Studies on the relief of pain by counterirritation. J Clin Invest 2:13, 1941

72. Sjolund BH, Terenius L, Ericksson MBE: Increased cerebrospinal fluid levels of endorphin after electro-acupuncture. Acta Physiol Scand 100:382, 1977

73. Sjolund BH, Eriksson MBE: The influence of naloxone on analgesia produced by peripheral conditioning stimulation. Brain Res 173:295, 1979

74. Sjolund BH, Ericksson MBE: Electro-acupuncture and endogenous morphine. Lancet 2:1035, 1976

75. Abram SE, Reynolds AC, Cusick JF: Failure of naloxone to reverse analgesia from transcutaneous electrical stimulation in patients with chronic pain. Anesth Analg (Cleve) 60:81, 1981

76. Bausbaum AI, Fields HL: Endogenous pain control mechanisms: review and hypothesis. Ann Neurol 4:451, 1978

77. Buchsbaum MS, Davis GC, Bunney WE Jr: Naloxone alters pain perception and somatosensory evoked potentials in normal subjects. Nature 270:620, 1977

78. Sjolund BH, Terenius L, Eriksson MBE: Increased cerebrospinal fluid levels of endorphin after electro-acupuncture. Acta Physiol Scand 100:382, 1977

79. Ignelzi RJ, Nyquist JK: Direct effect of electrical stimulation on peripheral nerve evoked activity: implications for pain relief. J Neurosurg 45:159, 1976

80. Ignelzi RJ, Nyquist JK: Excitability changes in peripheral nerve fibers after repetitive electrical stimulation: implications in pain modulation. J Neurosurg 51:824, 1979

81. Mannheimer JS, Lampe GN: Factors that hinder, enhance and restore the effectiveness of TENS: physiologic and theoretical considerations. p. 529. In Mannheimer JS, Lampe GN (eds): Clinical Transcutaneous Electrical Nerve Stimulation. FA Davis, Philadelphia, 1984.

82. Mudge AW, Leeman FE, Fishbach GD: Enkephalin inhibits release of substance P from sensory neurons in culture and decreases action potential duration. Proc Natl Acad Sci USA 76:526, 1979

83. Nordemar R, Thorner C: Treatment of acute cervical pain: a comparative study group. Pain 10:93, 1981

84. Cauthen JC, Renner EJ: Transcutaneous and peripheral nerve stimulation for chronic pain states. Surg Neurol 4:102, 1975

85. Stilz RJ, Carron H. Sanders DB: Case history number 96: reflex sympathetic dystrophy in a 6 year old. Successful treatment by transcutaneous nerve stimulation. Anesth Analg 56:438, 1977

86. Parry CBW: Rehabilitation of the Hand. 4th Ed. Butterworths, London, 1981

87. Korr IM: Sustained sympathicotonia. p. 229. In Korr IM (ed): The Neurobiologic Mechanisms in Manipulative Therapy. Plenum Press, New York, 1978

88. Melzack R, Loeser JD: Phantom body pain in paraplegics: evidence for a central "pattern generating mechanism" for pain. Pain 4:195, 1978

89. Loeser JS, Black RG, Christman A: Relief of pain by transcutaneous stimulation. J Neurosurg 42:308, 1975

90. Meyer GA, Fields HC: Causalgia treated by selective large fiber stimulation of the peripheral nerve. Brain 95:163, 1972

91. Nathan PW, Wall PD: Treatment of postherpetic neuralgia by prolonged electrical stimulation. Br Med J 3:645, 1974

92. Bates JAV, Nathan PW: Transcutaneous electrical nerve stimulation for chronic pain. Anesthesia 35:817, 1980

93. Long DM, Hagfors N: Electrical stimulation of the nervous system: the current status of electrical stimulation of the nervous system for relief of pain. Pain 1:109, 1975

94. Law JD, Swett J, Krisch WM: Retrospective analysis of 22 patients with chronic pain treated by peripheral nerve stimulation. J Neurosurg 52:482, 1980

95. Laitinen L: Placement of electrodes in transcutaneous stimulation for chronic pain. Neuro Chirurgie 22:517, 1976

96. Mannheimer C, Lund S, Carlsson CA: The effect of transcutaneous electrical nerve stimulation (TNS) on joint pain in patients with rheumatoid arthritis. Scand J Rheumatology 7:13, 1978

97. Taylor P, Hallet M, Flaherty L: Treatment of osteoarthritis of the knee with transcutaneous electrical stimulation. Pain 11:233, 1981

98. Kumar UN, Redford JB: Transcutaneous nerve stimulation in rheumatoid arthritis. Arch Phys Med Rehab 63:595, 1982

99. Abelson K, Langley AB: Transcutaneous electrical nerve stimulation in rheumatoid arthritis. N Zealand Med J 96:156, 1983

100. Walmsley RP, Flexman NE: Trancutaneous nerve stimulation for chronic low back pain: a pilot study. Physiotherapy Canada 31:245, 1979

101. Paxton SL: Clinical use of TENS: a survey of physical therapists. Phys Ther 60:38, 1980

102. Gunn CC, Milbrandt WE: Review of 100 patients with low back sprain treated by surface electrode stimulation of acupuncture points. Am J Acupuncture 3:244, 1975

103. Seres JL, Newman RI: Results of treatment of chronic low back pain at the Portland Pain Center. J Neurosurg 45:32, 1976

104. Lampe GN, Mannheimer JS: The patient and TENS. p. 219. In Mannheimer JS, Lampe GN (eds): Clinical Transcutaneous Electrical Nerve Stimulation. FA Davis, Philadelphia, 1984

105. Inversen LL: The chemistry of the brain. Sci Am 241:134, 1979

106. Hosobuchi Y, Lamb S, Bascom D: Trypthophan loading may reverse tolerance to opiate analgesics in humans: a preliminary report. Pain 9:161, 1980

107. Ward NG, Bloom VL, Friedel RO: The effectiveness of tricyclic antidepressants in the treatment of coexisting pain and depression. Pain 7:331, 1979

9 | Biofeedback and Behavior Modification for Chronic Pain

Ian Wickramasekera

ACUTE AND CHRONIC PAIN

The adequacy of conventional medical methods of dealing with chronic benign pain has become increasingly doubtful.[1-3] Typical surgical procedures and analgesic drugs appear to either exacerbate the patient's pain problem or create new problems of drug tolerance and abuse, which may in fact increase pain. It is the chronicity of these problems that makes analgesic drug management an unsatisfactory long term solution. In fact, the response to most neurosurgical procedures is unreliable and the pain returns in 6 to 18 months.[3,4] Another major factor contributing to the search for new and promising methods of controlling pain has been the growing recognition that the parameters of acute and chronic pain vary widely and that conventional methods that work well for acute pain may in fact intensify and complicate chronic pain problems by creating "illness behavior."[5]

Acute pain is easy to localize and recognize, and may in fact be mediated through different pathways from chronic pain. These pathways include the (1) dorsal column postsynaptic system (DCPS), (2) spinocervical tract (SCT), and (3) neospinothalamic tract (NSTT), which are all rapidly conducting systems suited to convey phasic information.[6] Acute pain is marked by an increase in mytonia, heart rate, blood pressure, skin conductance, and peripheral vasoconstriction together with other indicators of sympathetic activation. From a psychological or behavioral viewpoint we are seeing the same signs that indicate fear or anxiety.

Chronic pain has been defined as any pain that has persisted for over 6 months and not responded to standard medical management such as drugs, physical therapy, and surgery.[7] Chronic headache and chronic low back pain account for over 50 percent of all chronic pain patients but chronic pain syndromes also include phantom limb pain, neuralgias, and causalgia. In chronic pain, most of the signs of sympathetic activation have adapted and the primary signs of chronic pain are insomnia, loss of appetite and libido, irritability, constriction of range of interests, inhibition of activity, and feelings of helplessness and hopelessness. From a psychological viewpoint these are the symptoms of depression. Hence, any approach to the chronic pain patient has to confront the patient's depressive affect, which can potentiate pain. Chronic pain appears to be mediated through slow conductive fibers in the paleospinothalamic tract (PSTT) and the spinoreticular tract (SRT) and are poorly discriminated and poorly localized pain systems.[6]

Most of the problems with conventional medical management of pain, particularly chronic pain, are due to two factors: (1) the failure to distinguish between acute and chronic pain, and to recognize that the parameters of these two types of pain are very different, and (2) the failure to recognize the large psychological and behavioral components in both acute and chronic pain, particularly the onset of the illness behavior syndrome in chronic pain patients.

ILLNESS BEHAVIOR SYNDROME AND CHRONIC PAIN

In chronic pain patients, a distinct behavioral and psychophysiologic syndrome develops that becomes superimposed upon and interwoven into any organic pathophysiology and that can persist long after the pathophysiology has cleared up. This illness behavior syndrome[5,7-9] has been variously described by several authors. Essentially, it consists of the patient assuming a social role that is in fact reinforced by a health care system that responds to chronic pain as if it were an acute medical problem. The five components of this role are (1) dramatization of complaints, (2) progressive dysfunction, (3) drug misuse, (4) progressive dependency and, (5) income disability. The patient's dramatization of diffuse and "metastasizing" pain complaints often produces unnecessary and unproductive medical interventions (e.g., surgery, drugs, and invasive tests) that further complicate the pain problem. Progressive dysfunction is often a consequence of low levels of physical activity and postural habits that cause contractures, myofibrositis, osteoporosis, overweight, and circulatory and respiratory disorders.[5]

A third feature of the illness syndrome is the misuse of drugs including narcotics and psychotropics which are prescribed for acute pain and anxiety conditions. Another feature is a tendency for the patient to abdicate self-reliance and to permit the complaints and environment to control his or her life. These patients float miserably and angrily from one physician to another with episodic visits to attorneys and insurance companies. The fifth feature of the syndrome is a growing dependency on income that continues to flow only if the patient continues to have pain and disability complaints.

Biofeedback

Biofeedback can be defined as the use of instruments to provide a person with immediate and continuing information feedback of typically unconscious changes in a biologic response such as in muscle tension, heart rate, blood pressure, or electroencephalogram (EEG). The rationale for use of biofeedback involves certain types of pains (e.g., muscle tension headache) such as those pains based on sustained contraction of muscles on the scalp and/or neck.[10] Electromyogram (EMG) feedback reduces the muscle tension that partly accounts for the pain reports.[11-14] High and sustained levels of muscular bracing may occur in response to the pain of tissue damage. This sustained muscle contraction may, if chronically maintained, limit mobility and can potentiate the pain due to tissue damage. EMG biofeedback reduces the muscle spasm that is potentiating the pain of organic origin.

Behavior Modification

Behavior Modification can be defined as the use of the principles of operant and respondent conditioning to alter either the perception of pain or pain behaviors. The general goals of behavior modification are to (1) reduce the probability of pain behaviors by withdrawing any and all reinforcers for pain behavior and to (2) increase the probability of well behaviors by re-engaging, through selective reinforcement, the patient to life roles that compose the well behavior repertoire. The well behavior repertoire is composed of those normal behaviors (e.g., work and play) that make productive, coping functional citizens. The basic assumption underlying the operant conditioning approach is that chronic pain behaviors (moaning, posturing, "down-time") are controlled by factors (reinforcers) other than nociception (aversive sensations) alone. Respondent or Pavlovian conditioning can occur when the pain of tissue damage (unconditioned response, UCR) has been paired or associated with neutral situations, sensations, or cognitions, so that these situations, sensations, or cognitions can operate like conditioned stimuli (CS) to elicit a conditioned pain response.[15-17]

Imaginal or in vivo desensitization procedures (using relaxation or other counter-conditioning stimuli) should reduce any respondently conditioned pain (conditioned response CR) or anxiety responses (CR) to situations, sensations, movements, or cognitions (CS) that were previously paired with the pain of tissue damage (UCR). Anxiety, of course, can potentiate even minimal sensory pain by triggering muscle spasm and fearful affect. Also, the neutral aspect of stimuli (CS), such as pills and injections reliably associated with the relief of pain through active ingredients (e.g., morphine and aspirin), may in highly conditionable subjects reduce pain through placebo mechanisms.[15,16]

Rationales for the Use of Psychological and Behavioral Procedures with Pain

There are several other general empirically established rationales for the use of psychological and behavioral procedures with acute and chronic pain problems. First, the most influential current theory of pain, the gate control theory,[18] assigns a major role to descending inhibitory pathways from the brain through which psychological variables, such as attention, reinforcement, distraction, anxiety, placebo effects, depression, and hypnosis, can profoundly influence the opening or closing of the gating mechanism in pain perception. The gate control theory postulates a presynaptic mechanism modulating peripheral nociceptive input in the region of the dorsal horn of the spinal cord. All of the above six psychological variables have been empirically shown to influence pain perception.[19,20]

Second, it has been known for many years that though the pain threshold is fairly fixed and universal in man, the threshold of pain tolerance is profoundly influenced by a variety of cultural, personality, learning, and situational factors.[21] Pain experssion seems to be determined by two factors. The first factor is based on cultural learning and ethnic membership. For example, Zborowski[22] showed that Old Americans and Irish Americans inhibit pain expression but that Italian and Jewish Americans encourage pain expression. The second major determinant of pain expression is individual personality. It has been found that the perception of pain is related to the degree of neuroticism[23,24] but that the expression of pain is related to the degree of extroversion.[25] Hence, neurotic introverts may suffer silently but neurotic extroverts freely express their pain.

It has been shown[8] that chronic pain behaviors are controlled by reinforcing consequences. Pain behaviors can be reinforced by attention, monetary rewards, feedback, sympathy, and escape from unpleasant activities or situations. For example, Beecher[26] found that the amount of pain medication prescribed for tissue damage was more closely related not to the amount of tissue damage but to the situation where the damage occurred. A given injury in civilian life requires more morphine than the same injury in the combat zone. An injury in the combat zone may be perceived as a relief, since it assures that the person will be removed from the battlefield and perhaps his life will be saved. For example, Beecher[26] also showed that comparable amounts of tissue damage generate quantatively variable requests for analgesics, depending on the location of the trauma. Review of over 1,000 postsurgical pain patients have shown that a placebo, an inert substance, can under double blind conditions reduce by 50 percent postsurgical pain in 36 percent of patients.

Fourth, it has been shown that attention and distraction can significantly modify the perception of pain due to tissue damage.[21] An example is the football player who may seriously lacerate himself during a game but discovers the injury only later in the locker room and then perceives pain.

Fifth, the reduction of depressive affect by drugs and psychotherapy can significantly increase pain tolerance.[20] It appears that the depletion of central serotonin may account for increases in both depression and chronic pain.[27] Anxiety can significantly amplify both acute and chronic pain.[20]

Sixth, there is now good evidence that people of high hypnotic ability can significantly reduce experimentally induced pain[28] and there is less complete evidence that they can also reduce clinical pain.[28,29] Nearly 70 percent of people of high hypnotic ability can reduce cold pressor pain significantly whereas only 13 percent of people of low hypnotic ability can do so. Hypnotic ability has been shown[30] to be a measurable, stable, and partly genetically determined individual variable that has clear consequences for both the reduction and possibly also for the amplification of pain perception.[31-33] It is likely that high hypnotic ability subjects have a lower pain tolerance or threshold level than people of low or moderate hypnotic ability if their cognitive ability to block pain is not mobilized.[31,33]

Biofeedback and Pain

Biofeedback includes several techniques that use bioelectric instrumentation to provide a patient with information about changes in biologic responses to which the person is typically unaware. First, the biologic response (e.g., EMG) to be controlled is identified and assessed to secure a baseline or moment to moment changes. This information is quantified and translated into information that is immediately fed back to the patient in a visual or auditory display. Biofeedback appears to fit an operant learning model in some respects, and by trial and error the subject learns to recognize the subjective sensations and subtle internal changes that are associated with changes in specific biologic responses.

Biofeedback has been used in the therapy of several types of pain, but the best established use is in the area of severe chronic muscular and vascular headache. In a pioneering study, Budzynski and Stoyva[34] were able to confirm Sainsbury and Gibson's[35] observation of a correlation between tension in scalp and neck muscles and frontalis EMG activity. This observation became the basis for a set of clinical procedures (training in reducing frontal EMG and home practice of relaxation) that have been shown to reliably reduce both the intensity and frequency of muscle contraction headache both during therapy and with long term follow up.[11,12,14,36,37] Subsequent large scale clinical applications and other replication studies have routinely confirmed the clinical efficacy (75 to 80 percent) of the EMG biofeedback procedure for tension headache but it is still not clear what the active ingredients are in the procedure and if the procedure is always superior to simple progressive muscle relaxation therapy.[38] There is evidence to suggest EMG biofeedback may be unnecessary for people of high hypnotic ability to learn frontal EMG reduction[39] and may in fact retard their rate of acquisition of the relaxation skill. But this group (high hypnotic ability) is less than 10 percent of the general population. For people of high hypnotic ability, who have skeptical attitudes towards verbal-instructional procedures (e.g., hypnotic inductions, autogenic training, and muscular exercises) EMG feedback may be at least initially the treatment of choice, because of the high credibility set and placebo effects generated by the medical-electronic instruments.[15]

The use of peripheral skin temperature feedback training and autogenic phrases was reported to be effective in reducing the frequency and intensity of migraine headache by Sargent et al[40] and these results were confirmed by Wickramasekera.[13] Since then several other types of biofeedback investigations[41-43] have confirmed the efficacy of the temperature or pulse amplitude feedback procedures for the therapy of vascular headache. As with EMG biofeedback, the active ingredients and mechanisms have not been isolated nor has the size of the placebo component been identified. But repeated clinical trials have confirmed that the standard procedures are effective with over 75 percent of patients with severe chronic vascular headache as determined by a 2-year follow up. It now appears that either EMG or temperature feedback will help vascular headache and the earlier claim of specificity[13] has not been supported.

It is less certain that biofeedback procedures alone will be effective with other nonheadache type pain syndromes.[44-51] But in combination with procedures such as cognitive behavior modification, operant behavior modification, verbal relaxation instructions, psychotherapy, and hypnosis, biofeedback may significantly contribute to pain relief through cognitive mechanisms (increased self-esteem, perceived environmental mastery). These positive results which are incompletely understood today, persist even on a 6-month follow up. The other types of pain syndromes treated with biofeedback include chronic rheumatoid arthritic pain,[45] chronic low back pain, peripheral nerve injury, cancer pain, phantom limb, stump pain, and post-traumatic pain.

Several clinical rationales for the use of biofeedback as a primary or secondary procedure in the management of chronic pain have been proposed. Pain can have both psychological and biologic components. The psychological components of pain perception include anxiety, reinforcement, attention, depression, and suggestion.[20,21,28] Anxiety and fear can induce reflex muscle spasm, vasomotor changes, and local ischemia, all of which can amplify pain syndromes that involve muscles, tendons, and joints.[52] Suggestion and hypnosis can dramatically influence pain perception[28] in superior hypnotic subjects. It seems that extended clinical biofeedback training increases the hypnotic ability of people with low or moderate hypnotic ability (90 percent of the population). Both logically and empirically, there is reason to believe that extended biofeedback training in combination with positive expectations can even temporarily increase hypnotic ability.[53] Logically, the biofeedback training situation is similar to the sensory restriction situation and there is evidence that sensory restriction can temporarily increase suggestibility.[54-57] In the biofeedback training situation, the person sits for extended periods quietly limiting internal and external sensory input to a single auditory stimulus. Empirically, several studies have shown that EMG and EEG feedback can temporarily increase hypnotic ability.[13,54,58–60] This is not to imply that the informational feedback variable is unimportant in reducing pain perception but that it is inevitably confounded with increasing suggestibility in effective clinical biofeedback training. Effective clinical biofeedback training implicitly and explicitly positively manages the patient's expectancies both before and during low arousal training in ways that may even modestly increase the hypnotic ability of 90 percent of the population.

Biofeedback devices can be useful in helping the patient who is unaware of being physiologically activated. Objective credible evidence from an EMG or temperature monitor can motivate a patient to work at reducing an EMG signal or to attempt to warm his or her hands. The therapist may need to sample multiple physiologic response systems (e.g., EMG, temperature, skin conductance, and heart rate) to determine which patient response system is most reactive to psychosocial stressors and which functions as the patient's "window of vulnerability." The window of vulnerability is that physiologic system that is most reactive to stress, and is hence most likely to develop pathophysiology. On the other hand, the failure of a symptom to respond to low arousal physiologic feedback training from several response systems may indicate that the symptom is under the control of a more cognitive or social variable and requires psychotherapy or behavior modification.

BEHAVIOR MODIFICATION FOR PAIN

Cognitive behavior modification is an effort to self-regulate events (e.g., thoughts, anticipations, fantasies, and images) occurring inside the "black box," or the head. This approach is based on the assumption that a patient's perceived pain response to an aversive stimulus (trauma) is very largely a function of the type of cognitive self-statement images evoked before, during, and after aversive sensory stimulation. Laboratory studies have shown that the best predictor of patient response to an aversive stimulus of procedure is the patient's general cognitive attitude towards the event. Patients who "catastrophize" are very likely to experience high levels of pain. Catastrophizers make self-statements like "How I hate injections; I can't stand them; here we go again; that great big needle hurts awfully; I can't stand this suffering; and I am going bananas." Confident use of cognitive strategies for coping with pain are the next best predictor of pain tolerance. One study[61] found that 85 percent of catastrophizers and only 39 percent on noncatastrophizers reported a decrease in pain tolerance during a cold pressor pain test.

There are several types of cognitive strategies that seek to alter the appraisal of the pain situation and/or to divert attention away from the pain. There are at least six common cognitive strategies that have been variously classified by Scott and Barber[62] and Turk et al:[63]

1. *Imaginative inattention* involves ignoring the painful stimulus by engaging in a vivid mental image incompatible with pain such as attending a fun party or making love during aversive stimulation.

2. *Imaginative transformation* of pain involves interpreting the present sensations as something other than pain or minimizing those sensations as trivial or unreal. A patient can imagine the pain affected limb as numbed by Novacaine or having mechanical limbs, such as those of the Six Million Dollar Man.

3. *Imaginative transformation of the context* involves changing the context of the painful situation. For example, "I am James Bond and have been shot in a limb while driving my car."

4. *Focusing attention on the physical features* of the environment such as getting absorbed in watching TV or counting the holes in the ceiling during pain induction.

5. *Mental distractions* involve focusing attention on various thoughts without producing vivid images. For example, doing mental arithmetic or singing battle songs during painful stimulation.

6. *Intellectualization* involves focusing attention on that part of the body that has been hurt, but doing so in an objective, detached abstract way; by analyzing pain sensations in a quantitative, scientific way and avoiding subjective involvement in the event.

Implementing a Behavioral Pain Therapy Program

There are several steps that are critical to implementing an effective behavioral pain therapy program.

Identifying and Defusing Patient Resistance

Identifying and defusing patient resistance begins long before the initial patient contact and starts with educating referral sources to the nature of the procedures used, their rationales, limitations of the procedures, and data on their efficacy. It is also important to provide the referring sources with prompt feedback on the referral. It is important to be alert and aware of how the individual patient construes for himself why he or she is in your waiting room and what he or she expects to find out and hear. The approach to the patient's intrapersonal private monologues during the initial visit can open or close the door to a therapeutic alliance.

Translating Pain

It is critical up front to help the patient start translating pain from a simple conventional acute tissue damage model to a three channel (verbal-behavioral-physiologic) psychophysiologic model in which different variables may control different channels. For example, the pain may reside mainly in the motor (behavioral) channel, and its increase or decrease may be simply a function of activity. Alternatively, the pain may, in rare instances, be exclusively in the verbal, subjective or psychogenic channel, that is mainly delusional in character but is associated with inhibition of motor activity. Of course 95 percent of chronic pain is psychophysiologic and involves complex interactions between cognitive anticipations, social and financial incentives and disincentives, residual tissue damage, and perhaps muscle spasm and peripheral vasoconstriction as a reaction to the tissue damage. The reactive muscle spasm, chronic myotonia, and peripheral vasoconstriction, plus the cognitive anxiety and uncertainty about the duration of the pain can further potentiate any sensory component of the pain. It is likely that the social and financial consequences of the tissue damage can reinforce the pain behaviors and the patient role can insulate the patient from the natural consequences of confronting fears of returning to work and being unable to cope with any changes on the job. These are all complexities of chronic pain into which patients need to be lead or educated.

Setting Realistic Limited Goals for Therapy

Therapy goals have to be individualized, modest, and include some short term goals such as reducing use of the narcotic pain medications and psychotropics, and increasing activities in relation to recreation or "fun time." Another specific goal is to reduce down time (time spent sitting or laying down). These goals may include spending more time playing with grandchildren, eating out, going to religious services, losing weight, learning to swim, or walking for an hour. Acquisition of coping skills may include learning to use EMG feedback to reduce muscle spasm in the back or learning to warm one's hands to dilate peripheral blood vessels. For those who have hypnotic ability, the acquisition of self-hypnotic skills may be important in coping with pain. The skills could include learning to identify topics, events, and persons who elicit a stress response in the patient, and learning how to avoid, deal with, or desensitize one's reactions to these persons or events. This may also include learning to extinguish catastrophizing cognition and learning to replace them with coping cognitive self statements and imagery. For example, learning to increase the frequency of self-statements such as "I can handle this present pain, I know it will reduce in intensity eventually, I can turn my attention to enjoyable memories until this passes."

Arranging Conditions for the Generalization and Maintenance of Progress

It is critical to ensure that coping skills and procedures learned in the clinic or consulting room transfer to the patient's natural habitat. An important part of this provision involves building short and long term follow up of all patients into the initial role induction of the new patient. It also involves training the patient to practice learned skills in the natural habitat (at the "scene of the crime") and learning to recognize and mobilize resources in the environment to support the acquired changes in coping with the pain. During periods of acute exacerbation it is very easy for these patients to relapse into their previous maladaptive methods of dealing with stress and pain.

ACKNOWLEDGEMENT

I would like to thank R. Giannetti, Ph.D., for editorial comments on this chapter.

REFERENCES

1. Bonica JJ: Importance of the problem. In Bonica JJ, Ventofriddo V (eds): Advances in Pain Research and Therapy. Vol. 2. Raven Press, New York, 1979
2. Pagni CA, Maspes PE: A Critical Appraisal of Pain Surgery and Suggestions for Improving Treatment: Recent Advances on Pain Pathophysiology and Clinical Aspects. Springfield, Ill., Charles C Thomas, 1974
3. White JC, Sweet WH: Pain and the Neurosurgeon: a forty-year experience. Springfield, IL, Charles C Thomas, 1969
4. Kerr FWL: The structural basis of pain: circuitry and pathways. In Ng KYL, Bonica JJ (eds): Pain, Discomfort, and Humanitarian Care. Elsevier, New York, 1980
5. Brena SF: The Mystery of Pain: Is Pain a Sensation? Management of Patients with Chronic Pain. Spectrum Publications Inc., Jamaica, New York, 1983
6. Melzack R, Dennis SG: Neurophysiological foundations of pain. In Sternbach RA (ed): The Psychology of Pain. Raven Press, New York, 1978
7. Sternbach RA: Pain Patients: traits and treatment. Academic Press, New York, 1974
8. Fordyce WE: Behavioral methods for chronic pain and illness. CV Mosby, St. Louis, 1976
9. Blackwell B: Biofeedback in a comprehensive behavioral medicine program. Biofeedback and Self Regul 6:445–472, 1981
10. Wolf HG: Headache and other head pain. 2d Ed. Oxford University Press, New York, 1963
11. Budzynski TH, Stoyva JM, Adler C: Feedback-induced muscle relaxation. In Barber T, DiCara L, Kamiya J, Miller N, Shapiro D, Stoyva JM(eds): Biofeedback and Self-Control. Aldine-Atherton, Chicago, 1970
12. Wickramasekera I: EMG feedback training and tension headache: preliminary observations. Am J Clin Hyp 15(2):83–85, 1972
13. Wickramasekera I: The application of verbal instructions and EMG Feedback training to the management of tension headache: preliminary observations. Headache 13(2):74–76, 1973
14. Cox DJ, Freundlich A, Meyer RG: Differential effectiveness of electromyograph feedback, verbal relaxation instructions, and medication placebo with tension headaches. J Consult Clin Psychol 43:892–898, 1975
15. Wickramasekera I: The Placebo Effect and Biofeedback for Headache Pain. Proc San Diego Biomed Symp. Academic Press, New York, 1977a
16. Wickramasekera, I: A conditioned response model of the placebo effect: predictions from the model. Biofeedback Self Regul 5:5–18, 1980

17. Wickramasekera I: A conditioned response model of the placebo effect: predictions and postdictions from the model. In White L, Tursky B, Schwartz G(eds): Placebo: Clinical Phenomena and New Insights. Guilford Press, 1984
18. Melzack R, Wall PD: Pain mechanisms: a new theory. Science 150:971–979, 1965
19. Sternbach RA: Pain: A Psychophysiological Analysis. Academic Press, New York, 1968
20. Sternbach RA: Treatment of the chronic pain patient. J Human Stress 4:11–15, 1978
21. Melzack R: The puzzle of pain. Basic Books, New York, 1973
22. Zborowski M: People in pain. Jossey-Bass, San Francisco, 1969
23. Bond MR: The relation of pain to the Eysenck Personality Inventory, Cornell Medical Index and Witley Index of Hypochondriasis. Brit Psychiatry 119:671–678, 1971
24. Bond MR: Personality studies in patients with pain secondary to organic disease. J of Psychosom Res 17:257–263, 1973
25. Lynn R, Eysenck HJ: Tolerance for pain, extraversion and neuroticism. Percep Mot Skills, 12:161–167, 1961
26. Beecher HK: Measurement of subjective responses: Quantitative effects of drugs. Oxford University Press, New York, 1959
27. Sternbach RA, Janowski DS, Huey LY, Segal DS: Effects of altering brain serotonin activity on human chronic pain. pp. 601–606. In Bonica JJ, Abbe-Feesard D (eds): Advances in Pain Research and Therapy. Vol. 1. Proc on the First World Congress on Pain. Raven Press, New York, 1976
28. Hilgard ER, Hilgard JR: Hypnosis in the Relief of Pain. Vol. 1. Kaufmann Inc., Los Altos, CA, 1975
29. Gottfredson DK: Hypnosis as an anesthetic in dentistry. Doctoral dissertation, Department of Psychology, Brigham Young University. Dissertion Abst Int 33(7–13):3303, 1973
30. Hilgard ER: Hypnotic Susceptibility. Harcourt and Brace, New York, 1965
31. Wickramasekera I: A model of the patient at high risk for chronic stress related disorders. Paper read at Annu Conv Biofeedback Soc Am. San Diego, CA, 1979
32. Wickramasekera I: Clinical Research in a behavioral medicine private practice. Behav Assess 3:265–271, 1981
33. Wickramasekera I: A model of people at high risk to develop chronic stress related symptoms. Paper presented and published in the Proc Int Stress and Tension Control Soc., England, 1983
34. Budzynski TH, Stoyva JM: An instrument for producing deep muscle relaxation by means of analog information feedback. J Appl Behav Anal 2:231–237, 1969
35. Sainsbury P, Gibson JG: Symptoms of anxiety and tension and the accompanying physiological changes in the muscular system. J Neurol Neurosurg Psychiatry 17:216–224, 1954
36. Budzynski TH, Stoyva JM, Adler CS, Mullaney DJ: EMG biofeedback and tension headache: A controlled outcome study. Semin Psychiatry 5:397–410, 1973
37. Hutching DF, Reinking RH: Tension Headaches: What form of therapy is most effective. J Biofeedback Self Regul 1:183–190, 1976
38. Wolpe J, Lazarus AA: Behavior therapy techniques. Pergamon Press, New York, 1966
39. Qualls PJ, Sheehan PW: Electromyograph biofeedback as a relaxation technique: A critical appraisal and reassessment. Psychol Bull 90:21–42, 1981
40. Sargent JD, Green EE, Walters ED: Autogenic feedback training in a pilot study of migraine and tension headaches. Unpublished manuscript, 1972
41. Friar LR, Beatty J: Migraine: Management by trained control of vasoconstriction. Consult Clin Psychol 44:46–53, 1976

42. Medina JL, Diamond S, Franklin MA: Biofeedback therapy for migraine. Headache 16:115–119, 1976

43. Andreychuck T, Skiver C: Hypnosis and biofeedback in the treatment of migraine headache. Int J Exp Clin Hypn 23:172–183, 1975

44. Coger R, Werback M: Attention, anxiety, and the effects of learned enhancement of EEG in chronic pain: A pilot study in biofeedback. In Crue BL Jr (ed): Pain: research and treatment. Academic Press, New York, 1975

45. Wickramasekera I, Truong XT, Busch M, Oer C: The Management of Rheumatoid Arthritic Pain: preliminary observation. In Wickramasekera I (ed): Biofeedback, Behavior Therapy and Hypnosis. Nelson-Hall, Chicago, 1976

46. Gentry WP, Bernal GA: Chronic pain. In Williams RB, Gentry WD (eds): Behavioral Approaches to Medical Treatment. Ballinger, Cambridge, 1977

47. Newman RI, Seres JL, Yospe LP, Garlington B: Multidisciplinary treatment of chronic pain: Long-term follow-up of low back pain patients. Pain 4:283–292, 1978

48. Seres JL, Newman RI: Results of treatment of chronic low back pain at the Portland Pain Center. J Neurosurg 45:32–36, 1976

49. Swanson DW, Swenson WM, Marita T, McPhee MC: Program for managing chronic pain: program description and characteristics of patients. Mayo Clin Proc 51:401–408, 1976

50. Hendler N, Derogatis L, Vaella J, Long D: EMG biofeedback in patient with chronic pain. Dis Nerv Sys 38:505–574, 1977

51. Melzack R, Perry C: Self-regulation of pain: use of alpha feedback and hypnotic training for control of chronic pain. Neurol 46:452–469, 1975

52. Bonica JJ: International symposium on pain. Adv Neurol. Vol. 4. Raven Press, New York, 1974

53. Wickramasekera I: On attempts to modify hypnotic susceptibility: some psychophysiological procedures and promising directions. Ann NY Acad Sci 796:143–153, 1977

54. Pena F: Perceptual Isolation and Hypnotic Susceptibility. Unpublished Ph.D. Thesis. Washington State University. Pullman, Washington, 1963

55. Sanders RS, Reyher J: Sensory deprivation and the enhancement of hypnotic susceptibility. Abnorm Psychol 74:375–318, 1969

56. Wickramasekera I: The effects of sensory restriction on hypnotic susceptibility. Int J Clin Exp Hypn 17:217–224, 1969

57. Wickramasekera I: The effects of sensory restriction on susceptibility to hypnosis: a hypothesis and more preliminary data. Abnorm Psychol 76:69–75, 1970

58. London P, Hart J, Lebovits M: EEG alpha rhythms and hypnotic susceptibility. Nature 219:71–72, 1968

59. Engstrom DR, London P, Hart JL: EEG alpha feedback training and hypnotic susceptibility. APA Proc 5:837–838, 1970

60. Wickramasekera I: Effects of EMG feedback training on susceptibility to hypnosis: preliminary observations. Proc 79, Annu Conv Am Psychol Assoc 6:785–787, 1971

61. Spanos NP, et al: The effects of hypnotic susceptibility suggestions for analgesia and the utilization of cognitive strategies on the reduction of pain. Abnorm Psychol 88:282–292, 1979

62. Scott DS, Barber TX: Cognitive control of pain: effects of multiple cognitive strategies. Psychol Rec 27:373–383, 1977

63. Turk DC, Meichenbaum D, Genest M: Pain and Behavioral Medicine—A Cognitive Behavioral Perspective. The Guilford Press, New York, 1983

10 | Pain and the Pediatric Patient: Psychological Aspects

John V. Lavigne   Michael J. Schulein
Julie A. Hannan   Yoon S. Hahn

While there has been a notable increase in the study of the psychological aspects of pain in the last two decades, most of the basic research and clinical studies have been conducted with adults. Though there may well be ethical, pragmatic, and economic reasons for this, pain in children remains a significant problem. Like adults, many children suffer unnecessarily from pain in the form of headache, abdominal pain, or pain related to trauma or chronic diseases. Economic consequences of pain may be greater among adults than children; still, the long term consequences of pain for the child cannot be overlooked. In particular, when pain interferes with a child's education or a rehabilitation program, the impact on the quality of the child's life can be significant.

This chapter begins with a brief discussion of important theoretical assumptions involved in the study and treatment of pediatric pain patients. This includes an approach to conceptualizing pain experiences and pain-related behaviors, developmental aspects of pain, and assessment approaches to pain in children. Following this, we highlight relevant areas of the literature on the psychological aspects of pain in children. Finally, we present an overview of clinical considerations useful in approaching pediatric patients with pain problems.

ASSUMPTIONS AND PRINCIPLES

Because so much of the research has been conducted with adults, the study of pain in children must draw upon the theoretical principles and clinical methods developed with that age group. This approach can be useful clinically, but it also has its limitations. The child is constantly developing; in particular, the child's manner of thinking changes radically as he or she matures. These changes are related to the child's understanding of illness[1] and there are some preliminary indications that this may also affect the child's experience of pain.[2] Although this area has not been well explicated, the child's developmental status may even render certain treatment procedures ineffective, while increasing the effectiveness of others. Our approach to understanding the psychological aspects of pain in children must involve a downward extension of principles and techniques used with adults as they interact with developmental considerations.

Pain as a Psychological Experience

Of critical importance to the study of pain in children is the belief that there is a psychological component to the experience of pain. This concept is prominent in two recent definitions of pain:

1. [Pain is] an unpleasant sensory and emotional experience associated with actual or potential tissue damage, or described in terms of such damage.[3]
2. [Pain is] a reaction related to actual or impending tissue damage on the basis of the stimuli that arouse it and on the basis of the responses measured to indicate evidence of its presence.[4]

As these definitions imply, pain is partly a sensory experience, but the emotional aspects of the experience of pain, in *anticipation or response* to the sensory aspect of pain are integral parts of the pain experience. In addition to the emotional aspects, there are cognitive, motivational, and behavioral components of the pain experience.

Theoretical Underpinnings

With our current state of knowledge, pain management in children involves an eclectic theoretical perspective and multimodal approaches to treatment. At different times nonmedical treatments of pain may rely upon concepts from theories of hypnosis, behavior modification, sensory control of pain through transcutaneous electrical nerve stimulation (TENS), and cognitive theories of development. However, most of the work involved in clinical applications of psychological knowledge of pain can be understood within the combined frameworks of the gate control theory of the psychophysiological nature of pain, and a cognitive-behavioral perspective on psychological processes and behavior.

The gate control theory of Melzack and Wall[5,6] provides a theoretical basis for the use of psychological techniques in pain management as well as both sensory, peripheral procedures such as TENS and physical therapy regimens. While this theory is open to criticism,[4] it does explicate ways in which psychological processes are primary elements in the actual experience of pain as well as the behavior of the individual. By integrating the role of psychological and sensory processes in pain experience, the gate control theory suggests that psychological approaches to pain management can influence the experience of pain itself and not simply serve to "cover up" pain. It further suggests that "hypnosis, anxiety reduction, desensitization, attention, distraction, and other behavioral approaches can be effective alternatives and supplements to pharmacology and surgery."[4]

Also of importance have been contemporary behavioral theories of human behavior. There are disputes within the field about how important cognitive processes are for understanding behavior. In relation to pain control, the broader cognitive approach seems to be the most important. A cognitive-behavioral approach can subsume views about how reinforcement and avoidance conditioning can influence pain behavior as well as the role of hypnosis in pain control.

Classification of Pain

Real versus Psychogenic: A False Dichotomy

The Diagnostic and Statistical Manual[7] of the American Psychiatric Association defines a condition of psychogenic pain as the "complaint of pain, in the absence of adequate physical findings and in association with evidence of the etiological role of psychological factors." This definition implies that such a condition can be clearly delineated in opposition to "real" pain.

Fordyce[8] has forcefully brought home some of the dangers of the tendency to falsely dichotomize pain into "real" versus "psychogenic" pain. As Lavigne and Burns[9] subsequently noted:

> In the minds of professionals and parents, a distinction is made between explainable, "real," organic pain versus unexplainable, imaginary, or "fake" psychogenic pain. This overly simplified, unproductive dichotomy is sustained by the notion that "real" pain is a simple, purely sensory, and well-understood phenomena. In fact, the experience of pain is much more complicated, involving sensory, cultural, and psychological influences.

The consequences of such a false dichotomy cannot be ignored. There is a natural tendency to respond empathically and sensitively to the child with real pain. In contrast, there is a tendency for the psychogenic pain patient to be viewed as malingering, as faking the pain and somehow "willfully" resisting efforts to be cured. This can elicit anger on the parent or the professional treating the child and eventually interfere with the child's treatment.

One problem with the dichotomous approach to pain classification is that the management of the psychological aspects of pain can be important for many patients who cannot be classified as psychogenic pain patients. For this reason, and since psychological processes are involved in the experience of pain for everyone, it is probably best to conceptualize the psychological aspects of pain as falling along a continuum. At one end of the continuum, psychological procedures are of minimal importance in affecting the intensity of frequency of the child's pain, and medical factors are of maximal importance. At the other end, psychological factors play a major role in determining the intensity and frequency of the patient's pain, and medical considerations are of minimal importance. Psychogenic pain conditions constitute the extreme point along this continuum. According to that conceptualization, the more the psychological component increases, the more important is the management of the psychological aspects of pain in the overall treatment plan.

Respondent versus Operant Pain Behavior

Recognizing this, there are certain basic distinctions that can be important in deciding how to evaluate and manage pediatric pain problems. In particular, it can be important to determine the degree to which a child's pain is respondent rather than operant and chronic rather than acute.

Respondents are behaviors emitted in response to a stimulus and occurring "automatically when the stimulus is adequate."[8] Operant behaviors are controlled by their consequences and "come to occur because they are being followed by positive or reinforcing consequences."[8] Respondent pain behavior occurs when the peripheral noxious stimuli (e.g., tissue damage resulting from a burn) are sufficiently intense to "open the gate" (a la Melzack and Wall[6]), allowing painful sensations to enter into consciousness and eliciting pain-related behaviors (e.g., moaning and guarding the injured area). When pain-related behaviors are systematically followed by reinforcing consequences such as social attention, or avoidance of aversive activities such as school attendance, then operant pain behavior may be established. If reinforced adequately, operant pain behavior may be elicited even in the absence of noxious peripheral stimulation.

Respondent and operant pain behaviors can either coexist or occur independently. When they coexist, they can be present in different proportions (i.e., the person may be showing predominantly respondent versus primarily operant pain).

The distinction between operant and respondent pain is important although, clinically, the distinction cannot always be made with absolute confidence, largely because the two types of pain behavior can coexist. Nonetheless, certain treatment techniques can be utilized if operant pain behavior is present that would not be helpful with primarily respondent pain problems. This is discussed more fully in the clinical section later.

Pain Behaviors

In the course of considering the nature of a child's pain experience while planning an intervention program, it is useful to analyze the complex set of events, thoughts, and behaviors, that constitute the child's pain. Fordyce[8] places emphasis upon examing observable pain behaviors which include:

1. Autonomic signs such as blanching and pulse rate changes.
2. Vocal but nonverbal signs of pain that include gasps, moans, and crying.
3. Visible, nonverbal manifestations of pain, such as compensatory posturing and careful movements.
4. Verbal pain reports, such as statements of being in pain and descriptions of pain.
5. Requests for help, medication, back rub, and being held.
6. Functional limitations or restricted movements, including an interruption of normal activity. One aspect of this involves a reduction in normal, healthy activity or the inability to engage in desirable, rehabilitative work.

Acute versus Chronic Pain States

Fordyce[8] makes a critical point:

> Each of these sets of behaviors meets different contingencies or consequences in the environment. As a result, verbal and nonverbal behaviors are not only somewhat free to vary from each other; they in fact do vary from each other far more than we often are ready to accept.

As the pain problem becomes more chronic, the likelihood increases that these behaviors will not occur together. Thus, the likelihood increases that verbal pain behavior will occur without the presence of autonomic signs; or avoidance behavior (e.g., resisting school and avoiding physical therapy exercises) without autonomic signs.

DEVELOPMENTAL ASPECTS OF PAIN

While it is commonplace to note that children develop in the complexity of their thinking and behavior, it is still somewhat surprising to realize that their experience of pain and their pain-related behavior show developmental changes as well.

Some physicians have contended that neonates do not experience pain during the first week, and sometimes the first month of life. This argument is based upon the belief that complete myelinization of nerve fibers is necessary for pain to be experienced. Swafford and Allen[10] have questioned that belief, noting that myelinization "proceeds rapidly when the (nerve) tracts are utilized in their physiological tasks" and that there are differences in the rate at which myelinization occurs across infants. Because of this, the claim that neonates do not experience pain is dubious, and certainly it contradicts the everyday experience of health care workers and parents alike.

What may change over time is the child's pain threshold, the child's pain-related behavior patterns, the child's ability to communicate about pain, and the nature of his or her cognitions about pain.

Pain Threshold

Haslam[11] conducted a study in which children between the ages of 5 and 18 years were subjected to different levels of pressure applied to the tibia. The children were asked to report the level at which it began to "hurt." There was a significant correlation between age and the pain threshold, with the pain threshold increasing with age. While useful, the implications of this study are limited in scope because pain thresholds vary with the type of pain the person experiences.[4] More importantly, responses to laboratory pain often are not the same as responses to pain in real-life situations, probably because the behavioral/emotional components of pain are minimized in the laboratory. Thus, the relationship of age to pain intensity may be different for diseases or injuries, as will be discussed in the section on cognitive aspects of pain perception.

Pain Behavior

Children's behavior in situations when they are about to experience pain or have experienced pain can vary with age. Katz and co-workers[12] have conducted an observational study of children of different ages who were about to receive a bone marrow aspiration (BMA) or were actually receiving a BMA. They had observers note the children's behavior on 13 different characteristics (verbal expressions of pain, crying, musuclar rigidity, requests for emotional support, screaming, needing to be restrained, being carried into or out of the room, flailing, refusal to be placed in appropriate position on the examining table, clinging, stalling, requesting termination of the procedure, and verbal expressions of fear). Because it is virtually impossible to always distinguish between anxiety and pain, they described this as a behavioral distress rating procedure. They rated the children in four phases of the procedure: (1) in the waiting room as they were called to the treatment room, (2) in the treatment room while they were being undressed, (3) from the time their skin was cleansed, a local anesthetic was administered, the BMA was performed, and the needle was removed, and (4) during the time that an adhesive bandage was placed on the child until he or she left the room.

The children in the study were divided into younger (under 6.4 years of age), middle (6.6 to 9.11 years of age), and older (10.0 to 17.9 years of age) groups. During the third rating period, in which the BMA was conducted and both sensory and distress aspects of pain were likely to be present, the two younger groups both showed more behavioral signs of distress than did the older group. When all the phases were combined, the younger children showed the widest range of distressed or anxious behaviors. The young children expressed pain and distress by crying, screaming, verbal expressions of pain and resisting so that they needed to be restrained. Physical restraint was not needed with the intermediate age group. Children in the intermediate age group were more likely to express pain verbally, and muscular rigidity in painful situations began to be prominent. For the oldest children only two ways of displaying distress were prominent: verbal expression of pain and muscular rigidity. The authors observed a developmental trend toward less diffuse vocal protest and skeletal activity along with increased muscle tension and verbal expression of pain.

The younger children also showed distress over more rating periods, and girls showed more behavioral signs of distress at all ages and in all phases of the procedure than did boys. Girls were more likely to cry, cling, and request emotional support, while boys were more likely to engage in stalling tactics.

Using a modification of the Katz, Kellerman, and Siegal rating scale, Jay et al[13] also rated children's distress during a BMA. Similar to the Katz et al study, age was a significant predictor of behavioral distress. Children in the 2- to 6-year-old group were more likely than older children, to exhibit crying, screaming, the need for restraint, and verbal resistance. There was also a tendency for the younger children to engage in flailing and requesting emotional support. Younger girls were more likely to exhibit verbal resistance than older girls or boys at any age. There were no age differences in nervous behavior, information seeking, muscular rigidity, verbal fear, and verbal pain behavior. Overall, the children in the 2- to 6-year-old age group exhibited more total distress than did children in the 7- to 12- or 13- to 20-year-old age brackets. With the one exception noted above, they did not find sex differences like Katz et al did.

Jay and co-workers also took pains to note that older children did not exhibit as much behavioral distress as young children, but that does not mean that they did not experience distress. As the older children gained in the ability to control the expression of pain, their distress may only have been observable through self-report.[13]

In addition, it should be noted that pain-related distress during a discrete, time-limited treatment procedure is not the same as pain-related distress due to an illness or trauma. In the latter situation, the pain may be more chronic or episodic, and the child may begin to associate pain with punishment, with a deterioration in his or her physical condition, or both. More prolonged distress may result. As the child responds to the pain, anxiety, and restrictions of activity that accompany the pain and illness, a variety of other behavioral changes may be noted. For example, the child experiencing prolonged pain may begin to eat poorly, exhibit sleep changes, and seem "out of sorts." These types of changes have not been carefully delineated, but case studies have reported a variety of behavioral responses and ways of perceiving pain that may occur at different developmental stages. These are described more fully in Table 10-1.

Developmental Changes in Pain Cognitions

There may also be developmental changes in the child's thinking about pain that may affect how intense the pain seems to be. Beales et al[2] have reported that adolescents with juvenile rheumatoid arthritis (JRA) are likely to find joint pain to be more severe and unpleasant than 6- to 11-year-old patients. The children's comments suggested that pain was more likely to remind the older children of the implications of their disease—including its limiting effects on their activities, and the possibility that the disease was getting worse—and this could increase the severity of their pain. Their method of analyzing the children's comments was faulty, however, since the ratings were not done in a reliable manner. Thus, the results of the study must be accepted with some reservations.

Exactly why such changes might come about is not yet known. Probably at

Table 10-1. Developmentally Related Pain Perception and Response Styles

Age (years)	Response	Perception
Infant (0–3)	Diffuse body movements Crying Reflexive withdrawal Feeding problems Sleep disturbance	
Preschooler (3–5)	Crying Clinging to parent Regression in verbal and/or motor skills Enuresis, encopresis Panic Nightmares Clenching lips Rocking Verbal report	Viewed as punishment Concrete, egocentric thinking with no ability to relate the pain to time or future events
School-aged	Verbal report Passivity Withdrawal Crying	Viewed as loss of control Heightens preexisting fears of bodily harm Some understanding of reasons for pain Some ability to see pain as time-limited and related to outcomes
Adolescence	Verbal report Crying Depressive behavior	Viewed as threat to peer identification and emancipation from parents Cognitive interpreting similar to adults

least three factors are relevant. First, it is known that children's concepts of illness follow stages of cognitive development first described by Piaget. Gradually children become more capable of understanding the systemic nature of disease processes in a more articulated fashion. While no studies have been done directly concerning the child's concept of pain,[14] it is likely that conceptions about pain follow a similar pattern. Second, as the child grows older, he or she has more direct experience with pain. Their experience can sometimes serve to sensitize the child to pain or, conversely, contribute to habituation to painful experiences.[12,13] Finally, children learn about pain by observing how others, including their parents, respond to it (modeling effects). There are some indications in both the medical and dental literature[15-17] that children exposed to pain will be more likely to develop pain conditions on their own or respond with increased anxiety in painful situations.

ASSESSMENT

These developmental changes in pain perception and pain behavior have obvious implications for the development of pain assessment instruments for children. An adult pain instrument, for example, might require more cognitive and verbal sophistication than a child is capable of and, thus, it might not be useful for most age groups. Similarly, when the norms for behavioral measures of pain are developed, the norms must be sensitive to behavioral changes across age groups.

The existing pain scales can be divided into two categories: self-report indices and behavioral observation.

Self-Report Scales

Both verbal self-report indices of pain and visual analogue scales have been used with children. The verbal scales for children are five- or ten-point rating scales. The child is asked to rate the intensity of pain on an imaginary scale, with 0 indicating no pain, and the highest number representing incapacitating pain. While usually a useful tool with adolescents and older grammar school-age children, younger school-age children may have trouble translating the intensity of their pain into a numerical score, and preschool children will almost always have difficulty doing so.

The visual analogue scales offer interesting possibilities for use in pediatric pain assessment. Jay et al[13] report the use of a pain thermometer on which children rate their pain on a drawing of a thermometer. Ratings range from 0 (low) to 100 (high). The pain thermometer represents a creative adaptation of a verbal rating scale utilizing a concrete representation familiar to and suitable for grade school children. The thermometer context, however, may lead some children to confound pain intensity with heat. Careful questioning may be important with younger children who display more concrete thinking to ensure that the child's rating represents an estimate of pain intensity rather than the sensation of heat. A simple alternative procedure[18] asks children to rate pain intensity along a 10 cm line without reference to a thermometer.

Hester[19] utilized poker chips to give children a concrete reference in measuring pain. The child is instructed to take up to four chips to determine the intensity of his or her pain. The chips are called "pieces of hurt" and the child is instructed to take as many chips as he or she is experiencing pain. The poker chip tool appears best suited for 4- to 8-year-olds who are very concrete in their thinking style. The procedure has only been validated on pain associated with injections and, therefore, needs validation with other pain-inducing events, and physical conditions.

Behavioral Observation Methods

The last category of measurement tools, behavioral observations, may also be the most promising. In the measurement of pediatric pain, behavioral observation systems could provide a valuable addition to traditional verbal scales or visual analogues. Systematic observation of a child's distress could provide clinically valuable data to compare with rating scale data. For example, if intense pain was reported on a verbal scale while few pain behaviors were systematically observed, the clinician might speculate that (1) the child was overly sensitive to somatic signals, perhaps due to excessive anxiety, (2) the child was trying to control behavioral expressions of pain/discomfort, or (3) verbal pain reports and other pain behaviors were not closely correlated because of differential reinforcement of these behaviors. These possibilities could be investigated and perhaps provide key information in guiding treatment.

Despite the apparent advantages to the use of behavioral observations in the assessment of pediatric pain, only two studies were found that utilized behavioral observations. In two papers discussed earlier, Katz et al[12] and Jay et al[13] both reported clinical studies utilizing highly reliable behavioral observation systems during BMA procedures.

Both techniques appear to measure pain (behavioral distress) that occurs during painful medical procedures. While these scales are still primarily research instruments, the authors' multidimensional approach to pain measurement is commendable. Unfortunately, as Katz et al[12] note, behavioral observation systems tend to be very situation-specific and it is currently unclear whether these coding systems could be adapted to the measurement of pain having a less clean-cut etiology and longer duration.

LITERATURE REVIEW

It is convenient to talk about three different categories of pain-related conditions. These include:

1.   Physical disorders of unknown etiology in which pain is the major presenting complaint. Recurrent abdominal pain is the primary example of this.

    2. Pain related to a physical disorder or trauma, either acute or chronic, in which a physical etiology is clearly present or some form of pathophysiology can be identified. This category includes pain associated with tension headaches, juvenile rheumatoid arthritis, and burns, among others.

    3. Pain related to a medical procedure, such as a BMA.

    As discussed earlier, there will be a psychological component to pain arising from all of these sources, and the different conditions may sometimes overlap. The clinical and research literature on pediatric pain includes studies of the psychological aspects of the determinants and correlates of pain in children, as well as studies of treatment procedures. The treatment procedures that have been used with pediatric pain patients include (1) individual and family therapy treatment procedures designed to alleviate family or personality problems and, ultimately, reduce or eliminate pain, (2) treatment approaches designed to modify physiologic or neurophysiologic processes, including relaxation training, biofeedback, and TENS, (3) operant treatment strategies involving reward and punishment procedures to alter pain-related behavior, and (4) cognitive/behavioral treatment procedures designed to modify cognitive processes related to pain. These techniques can include the use of distraction and teaching coping skills, as well as self-hypnosis.

    This section reviews the research on several representative types of pain and pain-related disorders in children. Each section considers the personality, family, and treatment studies that have been conducted with that painful condition. Both clinical and controlled treatment studies are considered. Pain related to treatment procedures is discussed along with the diseases with which that procedure is associated. The interested reader may wish to review Turner and Chapman[20,21] for a summary of the treatment outcome studies using relaxation training, biofeedback, operant procedures, and hypnosis and cognitive-behavioral treatments with adults.

Recurrent Abdominal Pain

    Of all the painful conditions that occur among children, recurrent abdominal pain (RAP) has been studied the most extensively, and it warrants review for that reason. While there is no standard definition, RAP generally involves chronic abdominal pain that persists for weeks and sometimes months. The pain can vary in intensity and frequency, with some children complaining that it is present almost all of the time, while others reporting pain-free periods. The pain can interfere with the child's activities, and often causes them to miss school and some recreational activities. Occasionally, the children may have difficulty falling asleep, but the pain seldom awakens them at night. In an extreme case we reported elsewhere[9] a boy with RAP that had no identifiable medical basis who missed over 100 days of school across 3 years. Gradually, he became unable to walk outside or play actively for more than 20 to 30 minutes without experiencing pain and having to rest.

    When RAP was defined as three or more episodes of abdominal pain in 3 months and at least one episode the previous year,[15] the disorder showed both age and sex differences in its rate of occurrence. Between 5 and 8 years of age, the rate was slightly higher for boys (10 to 12 percent) than girls (8 to 12 percent). Subsequently, there was a dramatic increase at age 9 and 10 years for girls (to 30 percent) while the rate for boys remained steady. The rate then declined to near zero for both sexes by age 15.[22]

For children who present with RAP, a medical disease basis can be identified in only 5 to 10 percent of the cases. For the 90 to 95 percent of the children for whom a medical basis for the abdominal pain cannot be identified, an attempt to identify psychological causes for the pain is often made. The clinical and research studies have attempted to identify personality problems or family interaction patterns associated with RAP. Based upon these studies the typical RAP patient has been described as sensitive, trying to please adults, insecure, and worried;[23] high strung, fussy, and excitable;[16,24] anxious, timid, and apprehensive;[16,24] exhibiting undue fears;[16,24] and impulsive and demanding, or superachievers.[25]

The children also tend to come from families that are "pain-prone;" that is, families in which a relative had pain or somatic complaints, particularly GI symptoms.[16] The occurrence of pain is sometimes noted to be stress related, with school and social events, excitement and punishment, and parental marital problems implicated as stressful events.[25,26]

While these studies certainly suggest that psychological problems may be implicated in RAP, the quality of the research supporting these findings is almost uniformly poor. The personality and family studies seldom include control groups or reliable ways of assessing the child's personality characteristics or sources of stress. The studies are suggestive but not conclusive.

Treatment Studies

Most of the treatment studies of RAP patients also have serious methodological shortcomings. Studies to date have examined the effectiveness of support and reassurance with the child and family, family therapy, and behavior modification (operant) procedures.

Three studies have examined the prognosis for abdominal pain when the children and families were treated with reassurance that the disease was not serious and would subside. When Liebman[25] treated 119 children with reassurance and suggestions for changing the environment to reduce stress, 88 percent showed significant improvement or complete remission of symptoms. In contrast, Christensen and Mortensen[27] reported that 50 percent of the RAP patients treated as children continued to have abdominal pain.

Neither of these studies had control groups of treated patients, but a study by Apley and Hale[28] of RAP patients included a control group. In the long term followup conducted 8 to 20 years after treatment, both groups had comparable numbers of children who had not improved (approximately one third). When the symptoms did abate, it did so more quickly for the treated patients than the untreated patients. None of these studies, however, used adequate methods of defining the nature of the treatment or how many sessions were devoted to counseling, support, or reassurance. Also, none adequately defined the outcome variables (i.e., specified clearly what significant improvement really meant). Thus, we do not know the answers to certain clinically relevant questions such as who does reassurance work with, how much reassurance is enough, and what constituted effectiveness reassurance and support?

Liebman et al[29] reported a family therapy treatment procedure in which emphasis was placed upon removing family interaction patterns that might encourage symptom maintenance, restructuring parental roles within the family into more appropriate channels, and improving family communication. These treatment strategies may be combined with operant behavioral procedures such as reward programs for regular school attendance. This package of treatment procedures produced success in 8 of 10 patients, with the other 2 reporting only minor relapses. In a second series[30] these authors reported success with all 19 of their patients, with RAP being reduced to levels that did not interfere with functioning. Eight of the patients, however, also required long term psychotherapy.

These results are somewhat promising but the methodology is still somewhat problematic. Rating of improvement was not precise and it is not clear whether the "active ingredient" in the treatment program was the reassurance, rearranging the family relationships, or the reward program.

Two reports of behavioral treatment strategies have also been reported. The first, a well controlled single-case study,[31] used time-out to reduce verbal reports of pain in a 10-year-old girl with a 1-year history of stomach pains. The time-out procedure involved removing the girl from activities and social attention when pain reports were made. Pain reports were reduced from one or two a day to one a month. In another study,[32] a boy with frequent stomach cramps was treated with "covert positive reinforcement" to reduce stomach cramps. In this procedure the child imagined that he was in a situation in which cramps usually occurred and that he was handling them so well that he was praised by important people in his life. Complaints of cramps were eliminated after a few sessions.

Both of these procedures show promise, but they were only used with single cases. As a result we do not know how widespread their effectiveness is.

Headache and Migraine

Like abdominal pain, headaches are a relatively common form of pain experienced by children. Bille's[33] survey of a large school population in Denmark indicated that almost 60 percent of the children had experienced headaches. There were 6.8 percent who had recurrent, nonmigrainous headaches, while 4 percent of the school children between the ages of 7 and 15 years had migraine headaches. These were defined as paroxysmal headaches separated by pain-free intervals along with one or more of the following symptoms:

nausea, scotoma or related phenomena, one-sided pain, and positive family history among the parents or siblings.

Compared to abdominal pain, there are relatively few studies of tension headache or migraine in children that investigate personality, stress, or family factors. Stresses are thought to be associated with migraine among children, but this is not well documented because the studies rely upon retrospective reports.[34,35] By definition, there is also an increased incidence of migraine among the first-degree relatives of the children.

In a single-group study, Krupp and Friedman[35] reported that migraine patients tended to be sensitive, exhibited strong needs for approval, and were serious and concerned about their responsibilities. One fourth of their patients were considered to be neurotic. Their conclusions are weakened by the use of rating measures of unknown reliability and lack of a control group included for comparison purposes.

Two other studies of migraine patients did include control groups. Based upon psychiatric ratings, Maratos and Wilkinson[36] found that the migraine patients were significantly more likely than controls to be seen as emotionally disturbed. Unfortunately, the children in the two groups were not evaluated by psychiatrists who were unaware of their group membership, so there is a possibility of bias in their ratings. Also, the children in the two groups were not matched on socioeconomic class membership of their families. This is an important variable to match the children on because it correlates with the frequency of problem behaviors in children. Thus their conclusions were again weakened by methodologic shortcomings.

A study by Bille[33] also lacked the necessary matches between control and migraine patients but used more reliable rating measures. In this study, girls with migraines were more likely to report that they were anxious than were control girls who did not have headaches. This pattern was not seen among the boys. Children with migraine were also rated by their parents as more sensitive, more tidy, and more anxious. They were described as less self-controlled when frustrated and showing less physical endurance than controls. By history, children with pronounced or frequent migraine exhibited more sleep disturbance, more night terrors, more headbanging, and more severe temper tantrums.

While the methodologic limitations in these studies are apparent, the personality characteristics identified in these studies show certain similarities. These children show tendencies toward anxiety, worries, sensitivity, and obsessive-compulsive traits reflected in a preference for orderliness and tidiness. These characteristics may contribute to the occurrence of headache and migraine in children patients.

Treatment Studies

While headache management has received a great deal of attention among adults, treatment studies of headache among children are scarce. Olness and MacDonald[37] reported success with skin temperature biofeedback and self-hypnosis in the treatment of migraine for a few uncontrolled single-case studies. In a better controlled series of three pediatric patients with migraine, Labbe and Williamson[38] also have reported success with skin temperature biofeedback and relaxation training. These preliminary reports are promising and need to be extended to larger numbers of children.

Cancer

Pain in children with cancer has received more attention than any other form of pain associated with an identifiable disease. Two careful research projects outlining observational techniques and developmental changes during a BMA have been discussed earlier.[12,13]

Published reports concerning the management of pain in pediatric cancer patients have been almost entirely anecdotal. Beales[39] has advocated the use of carefully planned distraction techniques during painful procedures and modifying the meaning that the pain has for the child as pain control techniques. He has not presented data to support the effectiveness of these procedures with pediatric cancer patients, however. Uncontrolled case studies have also indicated that hypnosis can be useful in relieving pain in pediatric cancer patients. Hypnotic techniques have been used to reduce pain during BMA[40–42] and spinal taps as well as the pain related to the disease itself. The methodology of these reports has not been sufficient to provide strong support for their effectiveness.

We have been able to locate only one study[43] in which data were collected on the child's subjective ratings of discomfort both pre- and post-training in hypnosis. In this study, pain ratings were obtained before, during, and after the child had a BMA performed. These ratings indicated that the self-reported level of pain decreased after hypnosis training was instituted. The authors also report that hypnosis reduced self-reported headache and backache pain. Careful inspection of the visually presented data suggests that the adolescents' pain ratings actually declined on the morning *before* the hypnosis training was instituted. Possibly these pains were subsiding naturally, rather than due to the hypnosis training.

Burns

Clinical investigations have yielded some important examples of how children cope with and respond to pain. Stoddard[44] has noted that children who have been burned may show signs of regression, withdrawal, anxiety, sleep problems, and acting out in response to pain. Savedra[45] observed that children cope with pain by asking the staff to be gentle, requesting a postponement of treatment, trying to distance themselves from the threat through such actions as avoiding treatment and running away, distracting themselves, sleeping more, and trying to avoid displays of pain by other children on a burn ward.

Beales's[46] interviews with pediatric burn patients suggested that a number of factors might increase the anxiety and pain that they experienced both before and during treatment procedures. Some of the children believed that any movement of the affected area during treatment procedures would interfere with the healing process and should be resisted. This belief seemed to be based upon their prior experiences with minor injuries. Being restrained during treatment procedures seemed to increase fear and heighten the sensation of pain. Exposure to instruments while the staff prepared for a procedure, exposure to the damaged area and watching the treatment procedure, and overhearing anxiety-arousing conversation between staff members during treatment also heightened distress.

Treatment

These clinical observations have led to suggestions about managing pain among pediatric burn patients. Stoddard[44] recommends that children be adequately prepared for painful treatment procedures, especially by using parents to provide emotional support. When actual physical holding cannot be done, psychological holding procedures such as telling a story to the child, reinforcing appropriate uses of denial, and employing hypnosis or other distraction techniques can be used.

Beales[46] argues that modifying any cognitions that heighten anxiety should reduce the burned child's pain. This involves adequate preparation, with the medical staff taking "every opportunity to explain and justify to the patient what is being done, and will be done, to him"[46] well in advance. Anxiety-arousing practices before and during a treatment must be reduced, and any incorrect beliefs that a child has about the injury or the procedures must be altered.

While neither Stoddard not Beales provides case studies or empirical support for these procedures, a series of case studies by Elliott and Olson[47] provided partial support for the use of distraction and relaxation techniques. These authors conducted a series of controlled case studies with four patients who had been burned. Their procedures were designed to help them relieve the pain the children experienced during debridement, hydrotherapy, and dressing changes. The treatment package included (1) teaching the children distraction techniques (e.g., doing mental arithmetic problems and looking for objects hidden about the room), (2) relaxing breathing exercises, and (3) emotive imagery designed to help the patients reinterpret the context of the pain by imagining themselves in a heroic situation (e.g., during hydrotherapy, imagining that they were swimming in an effort to save a friend) or a relaxing situation (e.g., swimming during hydrotherapy). Trained observers used an adaption of the Katz, Kellerman, and Siegel[12] behavioral distress scale for burned-related treatment procedures. The ratings were taken under three conditions: (1) during a baseline rating prior to the initiation of any psychological treatment, (2) during the procedure when a psychologist was present and acting as a coach, and (3) during a procedure after the treatment techniques had been reviewed by the psychologist and patient, but the psychologist was not in the room. In general, the treatment package led to reduced distress while the psychologist was present, but the reduction in distress was not observed when the psychologist was not present. Thus, the technique seemed useful but could not be generalized to a time when the child could not be coached directly.

Using an alternative behavioral approach, Varni and co-workers[48] described the operant behavioral treatment of a 3-year-old girl with chronic pain resulting from severe second- and third-degree burns. The child was required to wear a Jobst stocking and splints as part of the treatment. Verbal and nonverbal pain behaviors were observed and recorded in three settings—a clinic office, in her room, and during physical therapy. The child was systematically rewarded for engaging in healthy activities such as engaging in physical therapy and refraining from crying. Displays of pain were ignored. Using a multiple baseline design, it was demonstrated that the procedure reduced displays of pain and increased participation in therapy. As the authors note, the ability to increase healthy behavior was perhaps more important than the reduction of pain indicators.

Sickle Cell Anemia

Zeltzer et al[49] have reported two single-case studies of young men, aged 20 years, who were successfully treated for pain control with sickle cell disease via hypnosis. These authors reported that there are no other studies of hypnosis with sickle cell disease. The hypnotic procedure used progressive relaxation techniques and eye fixation to induce hypnosis, and the patients were instructed to increase sensations of bodily warmth and dilation of blood vessels. Thermal biofeedback equipment was used to monitor peripheral skin temperature. Both patients reduced the number of emergency room visits, the number of hospitalizations, and the total length of hospitalizations over an 8-month period after hypnosis training compared to the 12 months prior to treatment. It remains to be seen whether these procedures are generally successful with young adults and can be used by younger patients, who may have more difficulty than adults in applying their training outside the treatment session. Also of interest is the use of counseling with one of the patients in addition to the hypnosis training; it is not clear whether this counseling may have been an active ingredient in the treatment's success.

Juvenile Rheumatoid Arthritis

Studies of JRA have been concerned with measuring the level of pain that JRA patients experience and examining factors that influence the intensity of the child's pain. Scott et al[50] had children rate the severity of their pain on a visual analogue scale. Most patients, under the age of 17 years, were able to complete the scale. The patients tended to report relatively low levels of pain, and the authors concluded that pain ratings could not be used as indicators of the effectiveness of treatment in children because of this "floor" effect. Also, as discussed in the section on developmental changes, adolescent JRA patients are more likely to find the joint pain to be unpleasant and severe than are younger children, possibly because of their growing awareness of the implications of the pain for their disease course and their future.[2] Apart from these two basic studies we have not been able to locate any treatment studies using psychological procedures with JRA patients.

Hemophilia

Varni and co-workers[51] have recently published a report detailing the treatment of a 9-year-old with hemophilia who had developed an inhibitor to the Factor VIII in the antihemophilic concentrate. This made the control of bleeding difficult using conventional therapy. The pain resulting from the uncontrolled bleeding led the child to take analgesics that produced even more bleeding. Treatment involved using self-regulation therapy for pain control. This procedure included instruction in relaxation training, meditative breathing exercises, and guided imagery techniques. In the year after the self regulation training was initiated, the child's pain intensity and use of medication decreased, the child's range of motion and quadricep strength increased, and the child had fewer days of hospitalization and fewer days of school absence.

Reflex Sympathetic Dystrophy Syndrome

Reflex sympathetic dystrophy syndrome (RSDS), or causalgia, is an unusual pain condition among children. RSDS can include pain that often has a burning sensation, swelling and trophic skin changes in the affected area, vasomotor instability, and a reduction in motion of the extremity.[52] Onset of the condition can follow a variety of precipitants, including fractures, infections, and soft tissue trauma. While the condition has long been recognized in adults, only two case studies with children have been reported. One study reported success with electrical stimulation at acupuncture points,[53] while another reported success with transcutaneous electrical nerve stimulation (TENS).[54] Both are anecdotal, uncontrolled case reports, however. In addition, Lavigne et al[55] have treated three cases using a multimodal approach that included relaxation training, hypnosis, social reinforcement, physical therapy, and TENS. Elements of this procedure will be discussed in the clinical section below.

CLINICAL CONSIDERATIONS

Because pain is so complex, there are distinct advantages to evaluating and managing pain within the context of a multidisciplinary team. Expert evaluations concerning the child's medical, psychological, and physical therapy needs can then be rendered. As a logical consequence of working as a team, each member also begins to gain crossdisciplinary knowledge about pain assessment and management. Obviously, a team approach is not available for all clinicians. When it is not, the physical therapist still must have a general sense of the kinds of psychological information that might prove useful in managing the pediatric pain patient.

As the literature reviewed earlier attests, there is relatively little definitive information about the personality and family factors that affect pain in pediatric patients. A number of treatment approaches appear promising with a variety of conditions, but no treatment procedures have received extensive empirical support. As a result, the clinician cannot always design a treatment strategy that arises from a solid, clear-cut, empirical base. Nonetheless, diagnostic and treatment decisions must be made based upon the best information available. What follows is a description of certain psychological and physical therapy considerations that are important in evaluating and treating children in pain.

ASSESSMENT PROCEDURES

Parent Interviews

The clinician has several methods available for gathering the information necessary for managing the child's pain problem. Important sources of information include separate interviews of the child and parents. When seen alone, both the child and the parents are usually more spontaneous in describing the child's experience of pain, and the child often may have a slightly different perspective on the pain experience than the parents have. This would not be obvious if the child and parents were interviewed together and the child experienced unspoken pressure to agree with the parents. Information about parent-child interaction patterns can be gathered by observing the parents and child interact during a physical therapy session.

Certain elements of the parent interview are particularly important, both for assessing the nature of the child's pain and planning an intervention program.

Pain Behavior

Particularly for chronic pain states and pain associated with diseases, it is important to gather information about the onset of the child's pain, how long the pain has lasted, the pattern of occurrence, and situations in which pain occurs. It is useful to obtain information about how the child shows that he or she is in pain (e.g., whether the child signals that pain is occurring through verbal pain reports, requests for pain medication, pain behaviors such as grimacing or limping, reduced activity, avoidance of normal activities, or physiologic indices of pain). This information should be elicited from the parents and, to the extent possible, from the child. In the course of obtaining this information it is critical to learn how other people respond to the indications of pain in order to determine if any regular pain-consequence relationships have been established (e.g., pain behaviors elicit excessive attention).

Family Characteristics

Family stresses can influence the child's experience of pain and have a direct effect on the conduct of a treatment program. Stresses that should be inquired about include marital problems, problems in the child's relationship to either parent, and financial problems or major changes in family members' lives. By eliciting anxiety or causing depression in the child, these stressors might enhance the intensity or frequency of the pain that the child experiences.

The child's siblings, parents, and grandparents serve as models of pain and illness behavior for the child. Through direct observation and hearing about their medical problems indirectly, the relatives' physical problems may heighten the child's awareness of physical sensations, including painful sensations. Gradually, the child may become sensitized to even minor indications of pain or other physical symptoms. Eventually this could lead the child to experience pain more frequently or intensely than necessary. Occasionally the child may even unconsciously imitate the pain behavior being displayed by the relative.

It is important to examine the timing between the stressors and the child's pain. Family stressors that occurred long ago are less likely to influence the child's pain than recent stresses or illnesses.

Temperament, Development, and Behavior Problems

The parents are the primary source of information about the child's general behavior and psychological development. A description about the child's developmental history (for younger children) and academic performance (for school age children) might help the clinician develop an appreciation for the child's level of cognitive sophistication. In addition, the parents can also be important sources of information about any misconceptions that the child may have expressed about the pain he or she is experiencing, the nature of the child's disease, and the child's expectations about pending medical procedures and physical therapy.

Also important in treatment planning is the child's temperament.[56] These characteristics are concerned with the style of the child's behavior rather than what the child actually does. For example, two children may be engaged in an exercise that causes some pain; both may try to escape from the exercise, but they may vary considerably in the *intensity* with which they respond. Various temperamental characteristics and their assessment are described more thoroughly elsewhere.[56]

There appear to be three clusters of temperamental characteristics that are important to recognize. The *easy child* tends to exhibit very regular behavior patterns, shows a positive approach to new situations, generally exhibits a positive mood, is not too intense in responding to situations, and is highly adaptable to change. Even when in pain, this child generally can enter into a physical therapy program with little difficulty when provided with adequate care and support from the family and the therapist.

The *difficult child* tends to be more irregular in habits and negative in response to new situations, adapts slowly to change, is often negative in mood, and responds negatively and intensely to new situations. When such a child is experiencing pain during physical therapy, he or she can indeed be difficult to manage. Regularity in the use of the same therapist to treat the child will be more important with the difficult child than with the easy child. Also, reward programs for complying with treatment may be helpful with such children even when the operant component of their plan is small (see section on operant pain management below).

The *slow-to-warm-up child* tends to be mildly negative in response to new situations and very slow to adapt to anything new. His or her mood will be less negative than that of the difficult child, and the manner of reacting will be less intense. The slowness to adapt will be the major source of difficulty in physical therapy. The slow-to-warm-up child is likely to make the best progress when treated consistently by the same therapist and adequately prepared for any changes in treatment arrangements.

Finally, developing a sense of the behavior problems that the child exhibits can be critical. This can be done by interviewing the parents and using a screening checklist.[57] In particular, an anxious child might require more explanation about treatment and more support than most children. A noncompliant child who chronically resists adults' directives may require more structured management procedures (e.g., reward systems, and clear standards of performance to earn rewards) in treatment.

The Child Interview

The child interview is important in gathering information about the child's understanding of the disorder, any surgical procedures he or she may have had, and what the child expects from therapy. Pain elicited during therapy, for example, may make the child afraid that he or she is getting worse, and such misperceptions need to be corrected. This part of the assessment must be ongoing since the child's concerns may change during treatment.

Self-Reports of Pain

A third source of information involves obtaining a self-report of the child's pain experiences. The child might be asked to rate the pain on a 0 to 5 or 0 to 10 scale or by using a visual analogue, as described earlier in Chapter 2. It is often helpful to ask the child to rate how bad the pain was at the worse point during a physical therapy session and overall during the session. Similarly, the therapist can make his or her own rating for comparisons purposes (based upon behavioral observations, as described below). The child who is to do exercises at home can provide ratings on a daily basis also. When the therapist has been comparing his or her pain ratings with the child's ratings during physical therapy sessions, the therapist can develop a better sense of the level of pain the child is experiencing while at home and adjust treatment plans accordingly.

Behavioral Observations

The third source involves direct observation of the child to learn about the child's pain behavior. Records can be obtained of the child's verbal pain expressions (e.g., reports of hurting), vocal pain behaviors (e.g., crying and moaning), nonverbal pain behavior (e.g., limping and grimacing), physiologic pain indicators, requests for pain medication, and reduction or avoidance of healthy behavior (e.g., resisting physical therapy exercises and being bedridden). We have found it helpful to rate whether these behaviors are present or absent in physical therapy, at home, and on the inpatient floors. It also is helpful for the therapist, nurse, and sometimes (e.g., when most treatment is done on an outpatient basis) the parent to rate their estimates of the child's pain intensity globally.

The behavioral ratings can serve several purposes. For example, in the initial assessment phase, behavior ratings measure how the child expresses pain and how other individuals in the environment respond to the child's pain behavior. This information can be used in determining whether operant treatment methods can be used productively. Thus, it might be noted that the child's parents respond too solicitously to minor expressions of pain or that they ignore verbal expressions of pain but respond to minor behavioral expressions (e.g., limping). It can also become clear that the child's verbal expressions of pain and the child's behavioral expressions of pain are discrepant. Thus, the child might be expressing intense reports of pain verbally but few indications of other behavioral signs of pain. In this case, operant procedures might be useful to shape lower, and more appropriate, levels of verbal pain reports. Finally, it sometimes happens that children cannot give reliable verbal pain reports (e.g., always reporting pain levels at 10) and behavioral reports may have to be relied upon to monitor the child's level of pain.

Physical Therapy Considerations

The physical therapist's assessment should include appropriate assessments of range of motion (ROM), muscle tone, strength, sensation to touch, balance, coordination, proprioceptive and kinesthetic sensations, postural alignment, gait analysis, functional disabilities, and activities of daily living and normal/abnormal movement patterns.

Clinical Decisions

At the end of the initial assessment, the clinician or pain team has gathered observations about the child's current functioning, historical information, self-report data, behavioral observations of the child's pain behavior and information about the social and medical factors that elicit pain or are the consequences of the pain. At that point, a clinical decision must be made about the degree to which operant factors are involved in the pain picture. There are no absolute rules governing this. It is a judgmental matter; the stronger the evidence that environmental factors are supporting pain behavior, the more likely it is that operant pain behavior is present. There should be positive indications that operant pain behavior is present; the absence of medical findings to account for the pain is not sufficient. Among the guidelines that Fordyce[8] has articulated that we have found useful for determining if operant pain is present with pediatric patients are the following:

1. Operant pain is more likely to be present when there are indications that rewards for pain behavior, such as social attention, are occurring at a high rate.

2. Pain that occurs regularly (e.g., every day or several times per day) is more likely to have an operant component than pain that occurs at long intervals. When pain occurs on a regular basis, there is a greater likelihood that it can be maintained by rewards such as parental attention or avoidance of unpleasant activities at home or at school.

3. An operant component to the pain is likely to be present if the pain is diurnal and rarely occurs at night.

4. Operant pain is more likely to be present when the pain is elicited by unpleasant tasks (e.g., school attendance) than pleasant tasks (e.g., going to a ballgame).

5. The costs of pain to the individual must be assessed. The more that pain keeps the individual from pleasurable activities, the less likely it is that operant pain is present. It is really the ratio of costs versus the benefits that the clinician must examine to decide whether significant operant pain is present.

This is especially important to keep in mind with pediatric patients because there are almost always some positive consequences of pain in the form of increased parental attention and expressions of concern. Also, when pain has become firmly established on an habitual basis, it may also begin to incur some costs and still have an operant component. Thus, the child who has operant pain that has been maintained by parental attention and school avoidance may occasionally miss a birthday party and still have a strong operant component to the pain.

6. Pain that begins with a respondent basis (e.g., pain beginning with a clearly documented sickle cell crisis) can be prolonged by the operant factors described above.

7. The child's pain may sometimes serve to improve family relations or interactions or to produce an alliance in the family that the child may see as

desirable. When pain is maintained on a frequent, recurrent basis by such conditions, the pain can also have an operant component.

8.   Pain-related behavior may be exacerbated by anxiety or depression. When the pain serves to avoid the anxiety-arousing situation, it can be operant (e.g., when the child is afraid of school and pain behavior results in staying home, then the pain behavior is operant). At other times, the child's anxiety is aroused by the anticipation of pain (e.g., when the child is afraid of the pain that he or she might experience during physical therapy). This may sometimes occur when the child would actually not experience much pain, but the child lacks confidence that he or she can do the physical therapy exercises without undue pain. At such a time a combination of respondent (e.g., relaxation training) and operant techniques (e.g., rewards for doing exercises) can be used. The reward procedures may serve to reduce the anxiety directly by showing the child that he or she can, indeed, participate in the exercises and cope successfully.

To the degree that operant pain behavior seems to be present, then operant treatment procedures can be used. Conversely, when the conditions do not seem to be present to maintain the operant pain behavior, and the child's medical condition and anxiety seem to account for the occurrence of pain, then respondent treatment procedures must be tried. Of course, combinations of these procedures must sometimes be used when both operant and respondent pain conditions seem to be present.

TREATMENT PROCEDURES

Rationale for Treatment

It is important for the parents and the child to understand the rationale for treatment whenever nonmedical treatment procedures are to be used in pain control. It is critical for the parents and the child to understand that the staff believes the child is in pain and is *not* "faking it" or that it is "all in the child's head." The child is not thought to be emotionally disturbed; rather, the staff is proposing ways to help reduce the pain without using medication (or to supplement medication). When operant pain is present, the treatment procedures should reduce "habit pain" that is occurring automatically rather than deliberately. It is also helpful for the child and the parents to understand that the nonmedical procedures can actually stop the occurrence of unnecessary pain, and not simply cover up a pain problem. To do this, it can be helpful to provide a simplified, concrete explanation of the gate control theory of pain to both the child and the parents. As part of this, the family can be taught that the nonmedical treatments can serve to "close the gate" and directly reduce the pain sensations and unnecessary pain behavior. Physical therapy is part of this process because it promotes a return to healthy behavior; the more the child engages in healthy behavior through physical therapy, the more likely it is that the gate will be closed.

When explaining the details of the child's physical therapy program, it is usually beneficial to explain the treatment methods to the parents first and then allow them to explain the treatment to the child in suitable language. The information can later be reviewed with the child and any misunderstandings can be corrected.

Operant Procedures

Operant treatment procedures are designed to modify environmental factors that are encouraging pain behavior and discouraging normal, healthy behavior from occurring. Operant techniques are designed to (1) eliminate stimuli that elicit pain behavior whenever possible, (2) alter the consequences of the pain behaviors that encourage the behaviors to occur, and (3) gradually shape and increase healthy behavior with physical therapy, walking, playing, attending school, and other activities of daily living. In physical therapy, this process begins with goal setting. Treatment goals should be discussed with the parents and the child when the child is of an appropriate age. When reasonable, it is best to attempt to achieve the child's goals first because this will usually facilitate better cooperation when working toward other goals. All of the goals for treatment should be as specific and simple as possible.

In daily treatments, it may be helpful to develop goals for each session. The goals should be attainable and increases should be made in small increments. The child should not work to exhaustion, because this increases the likelihood that the session will end in pain and resistance to further treatment. Rather, the child should work toward a specified criterion. Natural rewards in the form of praise and attention should always occur when the child meets a goal. In addition, rewards in the form of privileges, activities, or material rewards are sometimes useful when natural rewards are insufficient. To maintain interest, the child might be given a choice between two treatment activities or the order in which activities occur. This can heighten the child's sense of having some control over the treatment.

When pain behavior, especially verbal pain behavior and crying, are occurring at a high rate, they can sometimes interfere with treatment. These pain behaviors can be usually reduced when the child is being praised for healthy behavior, rewards are being provided for meeting goals, and the inappropriate pain behaviors are no longer being rewarded by parental attention. While some crying can usually be expected, particularly among young children, low levels of crying can usually be tolerated when they do not interfere with treatment.

Similar processes of rewarding healthy behavior and ignoring inappropriate pain behaviors can be used with healthy behavior at home or on an inpatient floor. For example, the child might be rewarded for walking in the hospital and for returning to school for increasingly longer periods of time when at home.

Finally, it should be remembered that an infant or toddler usually does not remain in a static posture for a long period of time. Treatment procedures should be developed that incorporate as many different positions and activities as possible.

Case Example

AB was an 8-year-old girl with cerebral palsy who underwent adductor myotomies and iliopsoas release. She was seen subsequently as an inpatient for physical therapy. During an initial trial of physical therapy lasting several weeks, she made poor progress. She would complain of extensive pain during the therapy sessions and refuse to perform exercises. Crying and verbal complaints were prominent responses. Her mother was often present during treatment sessions. AB would look to her for help and support and would often want her mother to rescue her from engaging in the exercises. While the parents were not actively trying to interfere with treatment, the mother's attention during treatment sessions seemed to be interfering with the child's progress by increasing verbal pain reports, crying, and resisting treatment. In addition, the family was not providing much verbal praise or even eye contact when AB was showing some effort in physical therapy. The parents' presence was felt to be useful therapeutically if managed correctly so they were instructed to use differential attention during the sessions. They were to provide verbal praise and eye contact when AB met treatment goals even when pain behaviors (moaning, crying, etc.) were forthcoming. If AB failed to cooperate, they were to turn away or avoid eye contact and not provide verbal comments. The second aspect of treatment involved providing parental attention and food snacks immediately after a good therapy session (in which she met most treatment goals). The parents were simply to leave the room for a brief period if she had a poor session. Attention and low calorie snacks were also to be provided during the physical therapy sessions if she was making a good effort. Although more precise standards were desirable, deciding what was a good effort was left to the therapist's judgment because the exercises varied often and a set schedule of exercises could not be arranged. Using a shaping process, more difficult tasks were gradually expected of the child. Following this plan, AB's effort improved, pain behaviors decreased within a few days, and the child's ability to support weight and stand properly increased significantly.

Respondent Pain

Treatment techniques to be used with respondent pain problems include distraction, relaxation training, hypnosis, cognitive-behavioral modification, modifying cognitions that increase pain and teaching coping skills, biofeedback techniques including skin temperature biofeedback and electromyographic (EMG) biofeedback, and TENS. Relaxation training, for example, might alleviate pain by reducing muscle tensions in the painful area, serving as a distractor as the child does the exercises, modifying the child's expectations about the pain by teaching the child a coping skill, or inducing a hypnotic-like state. This technique simultaneously serves some of the purposes of distraction techniques, cognitive-behavioral techniques, hypnosis, and biofeedback.

In deciding which of these procedures to use, our preference is to choose the least elaborate, most natural technique possible because the simpler, more natural technique is the most likely to be applied outside of the training sessions. Other considerations being equal, a biofeedback procedure or TENS is more likely to be held in reserve than a technique that does not require any apparatus, such as distraction or relaxation training.

Distraction techniques can be useful for pain related to a medical procedure and with brief, episodic pain associated with a disease. Care must be taken to ensure that distraction begins before the treatment procedure. Natural distractors, such as watching TV, playing a game, and conversation are important during treatment. School attendance and visits from friends and relatives can serve the same purpose for the outpatient. Relaxation training and hypnosis, especially procedures using imagery and fantasy (e.g., taking fantasy trips and engaging in pleasant activities) may help relieve pain, through distraction and by providing the child with a better sense of self-control. Cognitive behavioral procedures such as teaching coping self-statements (e.g., teaching the child to instruct himself or herself to remain calm and that the pain won't last and he or she can handle it) or reinterpreting pain sensations (e.g., teaching them to label the sensations as discomfort rather than pain) may also be useful.

EMG biofeedback and temperature biofeedback are effective in certain circumstances. EMG biofeedback can be used in any situation in which relaxation training might be appropriate, and sometimes enhances the effectiveness of relaxation training. Skin temperature biofeedback may be helpful with headaches and possibly for pain related to sickle cell anemia. TENS can be used in situations in which there is localized pain, especially if it is prolonged. TENS seems to have the advantage of being a treatment that the patient can sustain when distractors and relaxation cannot be sustained.

Case Example

CZ was a 13-year-old girl with RSDS who presented with pain in her right groin and thigh. Pain was elicited whenever the leg was touched or attempts were made to move the leg. She also frequently experienced feelings of numbness, and the leg appeared partially swollen and discolored, and sometimes cold to the touch. Evaluation of her pain suggested that operant pain behaviors were minimal, but she had developed some anticipatory anxiety about moving her leg during physical therapy. Initial attempts to improve the ROM of her leg solely through exercises and the application of heat were ineffective. Based upon reports that TENS can be helpful with RSDS patients, TENS was then initiated. An increase in ROM was noted, but her pain reports did not diminish. Subsequently relaxation training was initiated, coupled with cognitive-behavioral procedure in which she was taught to tell herself to relax and to interpret the sensations in her legs as discomfort rather than true pain. ROM increased considerably after this. With continued physical therapy, and social reinforcement through praise for complying with exercises, her pain was eliminated and she regained normal functioning.

REFERENCES

1. Bibace R, Walsh ME (eds): Children's Conceptions of Health, Illness, and Bodily Functions. Jossey-Bass, San Francisco, 1981
2. Beales G, Keen JH, Holt PJL: The child's perception of the disease and the experience of pain in juvenile chronic arthritis. J Rheumatol 10:61, 1983
3. International Association for the Study of Pain Subcommittee on Taxonomy: Pain terms: a list with definitions and notes on usage. Pain 6:249, 1979
4. Weisenberg M: Pain and pain control. Psychol Bull 84:1008, 1977
5. Melzack R, Wall PD: Pain mechanisms: a new theory. Science 150:971, 1965
6. Melzack R, Wall PD: The Challenge of Pain. Basic Books, New York, 1983
7. American Psychiatric Association: Diagnostic and Statistical Manual of Mental Disorders. Washington DC, 1980
8. Fordyce WE: Behavioral Methods for Chronic Pain and Illness. CV Mosby, St Louis, 1976
9. Lavigne JV, Burns WJ: Pediatric Psychology: An Introduction for Pediatricians and Psychologists. Grune & Stratton, New York, 1981
10. Swafford LI, Allen D: Pain relief in the pediatric patient. Med Clin North Am 52:131, 1968
11. Haslam DR: Age and the perception of pain. Psychonomic Science 15:86, 1969
12. Katz SR, Kellerman J, Siegal SE: Behavioral distress in children with cancer undergoing medical procedures: developmental considerations. J Consult Clin Psychol 48:356, 1980
13. Jay SM, Ozolins M, Elliott CH, Caldwell S: Assessment of children's distress during painful medical procedures. Health Psychol 2(2):133, 1983
14. Willis DJ, Elliott, CH, Jay S: Psychological effects of physical illness and its concomitants. p. 28. In Tuma JM (ed): Handbook for the Practice of Pediatric Psychology. John Wiley & Sons, New York, 1982
15. Apley J: The Child with Abdominal Pains. Blackwell Sci Pub, London, 1975
16. Gordon DA, Terdal L, Sterling E: The use of modeling and desensitization in the treatment of a phobic child. J Dent Child 2:102, 1974
17. Forgione AG, Clark RE: Comments on an empirical study of the causes of dental fears. J Dent Res 53:496, 1974
18. Abu-Saad H: The assessment of pain in children. Issues in Comp Nurs 5:327, 1981
19. Hester NK: The preoperational child's reaction to immunization. Nurs Res 28:250, 1979
20. Turner JA, Chapman CR: Psychological interventions for chronic pain: a critical review. I. Relaxation training and biofeedback. Pain 12:1, 1982
21. Turner JA, Chapman CR: Psychological interventions for chronic pain: a critical review. II. Operant conditioning, hypnosis and cognitive-behavioral therapy. Pain 12:23, 1982
22. Bain HW: Chronic vague abdominal pain in children. Ped Clin North Am 21:991, 1974
23. Stone RT, Barbero GJ: Recurrent abdominal pain in childhood. Pediatrics 45:732, 1970
24. Apley J, Naish N: Recurrent abdominal pains: a field survey of 1,000 school children. Arch Dis Child 33:165, 1958
25. Liebman WM: Recurrent abdominal pain in children: a retrospective survey of 119 patients. Clin Pediatr 17:149, 1978

26. MacKeith R, O'Neill D: Recurrent abdominal pain in children. Lancet 2:278, 1951
27. Christensen MF, Mortensen O: Long-term prognosis in children with recurrent abdominal pain. Arch Dis Child 50:110, 1975
28. Apley J, Hale B: Children with recurrent abdominal pain: how do they grow up? Brit Med J 3(Jul):7, 1973
29. Liebman R, Honig P, Berger H: An integrated treatment program for psychogenic pain. Fam Process 15:397, 1976
30. Berger HG, Honig PJ, Liebman R: Recurrent abdominal pain: gaining control of the symptom. Am J Dis Child 131:1340, 1977
31. Miller AJ, Kratochwill RT: Reduction of frequent stomachache complaints by time out. Behav Ther 10:211, 1979
32. Wasserman TH: The elimination of complaints of stomach cramps in a 12-year-old child by covert positive reinforcement. Behav Therapist 1:13, 1978
33. Bille B: Migraine in school children. Acta Paediatr Scand (Suppl) 51:136, 1962
34. Burke EC, Peters GA: Migraine in childhood. Am J Dis Child 92:330, 1956
35. Krupp GR, Friedman AP: Migraine in children: a report of 50 children. Am J Dis Child 85:146, 1953
36. Maratos J, Wilkinson M: Migraine in children: a medical and psychiatric study. Cephalgia 2:179, 1982
37. Olness K, MacDonald J: Self-hypnosis and biofeedback in the management of juvenile migraine. J Dev Behav Ped 2:168, 1981
38. Labbe EE, Williamson DA: Temperature biofeedback in the treatment of children with migraine headaches. J Pedia Psychol 8:317, 1983
39. Beales JG: Pain in children with cancer. p. 59. In Bonica JJ, Ventafrida V (eds): Advances in Pain Research and Therapy. Vol 2. Raven Press, New York, 1979
40. LaBaw W, Holton C, Tewell K, Eccles D: The use of self-hypnosis by children with cancer. Am J Clin Hypn 17:233, 1975
41. Olness K: Imagery (self-hypnosis) as adjunct therapy in childhood cancer. Am J Pediatric Hematology/Oncology 3:313, 1981
42. Dash J: Hypnosis for symptom amelioration. p. 215. In J Kellerman (ed): Psychological Aspects of Childhood Cancer. Charles C Thomas, Springfield, IL, 1980
43. Ellenberg L, Kellerman J, Dash J, et al: Use of hypnosis for multiple symptoms in the adolescent girl with leukemia. J Adol Health Care 1:132, 1980
44. Stoddard FJ: Coping with pain: a developmental approach to treatment of burned children. Am J Psych 139:736, 1982
45. Savedra M: Coping with pain: strategies of severely burned children. Matern Child Nurs J 5:197, 1976
46. Beales JG: Factors influencing the expectation of pain among patients in a children's burn unit. Burns 9:187, 1982–1983
47. Elliott CH, Olson RA: The management of children's distress in response to painful medical treatment for burn injuries. Behav Res Ther 21:675, 1983
48. Varni JW, Bessman CA, Russo DC, Cataldo MF: Behavioral management of chronic pain in children: case study. Arch Phys Med Rehabil 61:375, 1980
49. Zeltzer L, Dash J, Holland JP: Hypnotically induced pain control in sickle cell anemia. Pediatrics 64:533, 1979
50. Scott PJ, Ansell BM, Huskisson EC: Measurement of pain in juvenile chronic polyarthritis. Ann Rheum Dis 36:186, 1977
51. Varni JW, Gilbert A, Dietrich SL: Behavioral medicine in pain and analgesia management for the hemophilic child with Factor VIII inhibitor. Pain 11:121, 1981
52. Kozin F, McCarty DJ, Sims J, Genant H: The reflex sympathetic dystrophy syn-

drome. I. Clinical and histologic studies: evidence for bilaterality, response to corticosteroids and articular involvement. J Med 60:321, 1976

53. Leo KC: Use of electrical stimulation at acupuncture points for the treatment of reflex sympathetic dystrophy in a child. Phys Ther 63:957, 1983

54. Stilz RJ, Carron H, Sanders DB: Reflex sympathetic dystrophy in a 6-year-old: successful treatment by transcutaneous nerve stimulation. Anesth Analg 56:438, 1977

55. Lavigne JV, Schulein M, Hahn YS, et al: Multimodal treatment of reflex sympathetic dystrophy syndrome in children. Presented at the Midwest Pain Society, Las Vegas, Nevada, 1986

56. Thomas A, Chess S: Temperament and Development. New York: Brunner/Mazel, 1977

57. Achenbach TM, Edelbrock CS: Manual for the child behavior checklist and child behavior profile. In Burlington VT (ed): Child Psychiatry. University of Vermont, 1982

Index

Page numbers followed by *f* represent figures; numbers followed by *t* represent tables.

297